VACCINE NATION

VACCINE NATION

HOW IMMUNIZATION SHAPED INDIA

AMEER SHAHUL

First published in 2025 by Macmillan
an imprint of Pan Macmillan Publishing India Private Limited
707 Kailash Building
26 K. G. Marg, New Delhi 110001
www.panmacmillan.co.in

Pan Macmillan, The Smithson, 6 Briset Street, Farringdon, London EC1M 5NR
Associated companies throughout the world
www.panmacmillan.com

ISBN 978-93-6113-306-0

1 3 5 7 9 8 6 4 2

Typeset in Adobe Jenson Pro by R. Ajith Kumar, New Delhi
Printed and bound in India by Thomson Press India Ltd.

FSC www.fsc.org
MIX
Paper | Supporting responsible forestry
FSC® C010615

To the millions of lives lost –
because a vaccine didn't arrive in time,
because they couldn't afford one,
because the country didn't have one,
or because no one had yet invented one.

This book is a tribute to their memory,
a reminder of what was lost

CONTENTS

PREFACE

IT WAS DURING THE DEVASTATING SECOND WAVE OF COVID-19 in 2021 that the seed for this book was planted. After leaving IBM's advocacy and public policy team, I was working with a healthcare policy advocacy group in India, driven by a deep curiosity about how global pharmaceutical lobbies shape public health policy and influence governments.

I had just completed my first book, *Heavy Metal: How a Global Corporation Poisoned Kodaikanal,* and the publisher was running it through legal review in both India and the UK. One evening, while working on a related project, I was searching for reliable information on the history of vaccine development in India. To my astonishment, I found no single comprehensive source that chronicled India's legacy of vaccine research and vaccine making.

What started as a personal inquiry soon branched out into an epic spanning colonial-era science, post-Independence ambition and global leadership. It became increasingly clear to me that India's complex and largely unsung vaccine story needed to be told. When a hastily put-together concept note was sent around, to my surprise, three top publishers expressed immediate interest.

But enthusiasm alone wasn't enough. The real work was piecing together a historical narrative that had never been fully documented. It took four more years of painstaking research – digging through dusty archives, tracking down old journals and newspapers, consulting out-of-print books, scouring through online resources and sitting with the vaccine legends who are still alive – to bring this story to life.

I came to realize during this journey that few innovations have influenced human survival and progress as profoundly as vaccines. From a world of 1 billion human beings at the beginning of nineteenth century to over 8 billion today, vaccines have played a defining role – saving lives, reducing child mortality and transforming public health through the generations.

By the time Edward Jenner died in January 1823, his pioneering smallpox vaccine had already saved thousands across Europe. And what's more – he had sparked a revolution. Jenner's work laid the scientific and moral foundations for a field that would become central to modern medicine: immunology. Building on that legacy, Louis Pasteur would later push the boundaries even further with his groundbreaking research on rabies and anthrax, cementing vaccination as a pillar of preventive healthcare.

But while these milestones were reshaping the Western world, what was happening in India?

For much of the nineteenth century, India remained on the margins of this scientific awakening, held back by colonial apathy, fractured health infrastructure and a civilizational gulf that kept Western science at arm's length. It wasn't until the 1890s, with the arrival of Russian-born British scientist Waldemar Haffkine, that the country saw its first organized attempt at vaccine research. I was confronted with many questions even at the starting point of India's vaccine story. How did Haffkine gain the trust of both his colonial masters and the Indian people to launch the world's first vaccines for cholera and plague – right here in colonial India? And how did he eventually lose the trust of both?

The British did establish vaccine institutes in the early twentieth century, but why were they nestled in hill stations, designed to serve colonial officers instead of India's masses? Why was public health treated as a convenience, not a commitment? Why did life-saving science flourish in Europe while the vaccine landscape in India remained a footnote? My enquiries led me to reflect on the stark dichotomy in healthcare that prevailed between the West and the rest; driven not just by skin colour, but also geography, poverty and access to education.

As I moved from the Haffkine era into the next chapter of India's public health journey, I realized it wasn't until the final years of colonial rule – amid rising nationalist fervour and the global upheaval of World War II – that the British began to take disease control more seriously. I'm sure my readers would be equally curious to find out what triggered this sudden urgency. Was it genuine concern for India and its people, or merely a last-ditch effort to salvage imperial credibility and soften Britain's legacy of plundering nations, leaving them impoverished and broken?

Some seeds had been sown by the time independence was attained – through health surveys, expert committees and early public health experiments – that hinted at a broader vision. But who would carry that vision forward? Could an independent India, emerging from centuries of subjugation and the trauma of Partition, muster the will and resources to do so? With a piecemeal health system and scarcely any indigenous production capacity, but guided by the ideals of self-reliance and equity, that's exactly what India set out to do.

The early targets were clear: tuberculosis and smallpox – two scourges that had devastated families and communities alike. India was among the first countries to join the global BCG vaccination programme against TB, launching pilot projects as early as 1948, with support from WHO and UNICEF.

By the late 1970s, the pieces were slowly falling into place. Institutional capacity, albeit still shaky, was beginning to take shape. And then came a turning point: India's launch of the Expanded Programme on Immunization (EPI) in 1978. But what did 'expanded' immunization really mean for a country where access to even basic health services was uneven at best? And how did the EPI enable India to realistically prevent six critical diseases – tuberculosis, diphtheria, pertussis, tetanus, polio and measles?

As India's vaccine strategy continued to evolve, homegrown institutions came into focus. Unlike most developing countries at the time, India wasn't wholly reliant on imports. State-run production hubs like the Pasteur Institute in Coonoor, the Haffkine Institute in Mumbai and the Central Research Institute in Kasauli quietly ramped up manufacturing. In the face of rising demand, early coverage was far from ideal. Still, the scaffolding was being built for something larger, more ambitious. The foundations laid during this phase would become the backbone of India's national immunization efforts.

Then came the 1980s – a decade of consolidation. Making vaccines work in the real world is not just about vials and syringes. It's about getting them to the right place, at the right time, in the right condition. India turned its focus to cold chain logistics, health worker training, vaccine awareness and disease surveillance. Even as the systems improved, a new challenge began surfacing – vaccine hesitancy. Driven by misinformation, cultural beliefs and occasional distrust in government-led programmes, this hesitation would emerge as a silent barrier to full immunization coverage.

In 1985, measles immunization was introduced, targeting one of India's deadliest childhood killers. Why did it take so long to reach this point? And what would it take to make sure no child slipped through the cracks? Polio emerged as the next great frontier. Endemic for generations, the disease demanded a bold, aggressive national response. Could India mobilize at the scale required to defeat it? Could it overcome the last-mile challenges in rural heartlands and urban slums alike?

By 1990, India's vaccination programme still had its limitations – coverage remained uneven and quality varied. But make no mistake – what had been built was monumental: a comprehensive national immunization programme stitched together through sheer effort, endurance and an ever-evolving vision. A programme that would soon scale up into one of the largest vaccine delivery systems on the planet.

As I traced this journey, I realized that strategy and systems alone don't drive transformation. People do. The immunization story I was writing wasn't just about institutions and infrastructure – it was also about individuals.

No story of India's vaccine journey is complete without its constellation of quiet heroes. Not the ones etched in bronze or splashed across magazine covers, but those who toiled behind the scenes, often unrecognized yet always relentless. They came from different corners of the country; from different faiths, disciplines and walks of life. Scientists, doctors, administrators, entrepreneurs – men and women who defied the odds not for fame, but for a larger purpose.

Each one brought along a missing piece of the puzzle. A molecule here, a breakthrough there; a bold policy change, a stubborn refusal to give up. And together, they built more than vaccines. They built the nation's self-reliance. They built systems that would ensure all Indians received the best of global technology. They built a quiet revolution – one that would, in time, place India not at the margins, but at the very core of global immunization.

The 1970 Patents Act, which replaced colonial-era patent laws, marked a watershed moment in India's pharmaceutical and vaccine journey. By abolishing product patents for food and medicines and allowing only process patents, the door was opened for Indian companies to legally reverse-engineer patented vaccines using alternative methods. This critical shift broke the stranglehold of multinational corporations and gave rise to a generation of homegrown firms that combined scientific ingenuity with public health purpose. The result was a thriving ecosystem of affordable vaccines tailored to the needs of India and the rest of the developing world.

For the next three decades, this legal framework fuelled an era of creative reengineering, making lifesaving vaccines and drugs accessible to millions. The most intriguing piece of the puzzle was how Indian firms continued to find inventive ways to navigate the system, sustaining their global competitiveness even after product patents were reintroduced.

This quiet revolution of science and sovereignty didn't unfold overnight. But by the time economic liberalization swept through India in 1991, the groundwork had already been laid. A generation of scientists had been trained. Public institutions had grown more capable. A clutch of daring biotech entrepreneurs had begun to emerge – restless, ambitious and unafraid to compete with the West on their own terms. This became one of the most compelling parts of the story as I delved behind the scenes of invention, entrepreneurship and the manoeuvres of transnational companies to protect their turf.

The old state-run model, sturdy but sluggish, began giving way to nimble private players that combined scientific rigour with business agility. I tried to capture this tectonic shift in its minute details. What followed was not just industrial growth, but the rise of a new kind of national confidence. Indian vaccines no longer needed validation; they were becoming the global standard.

As agencies like UNICEF and WHO took notice, Indian firms went from backroom suppliers to frontline partners in global health. And soon, they moved beyond that orbit, venturing directly into international markets, taking on multinationals and reshaping the economics of vaccines across continents.

With the dawn of the twenty-first century, India was no longer just participating in the global vaccine story – it was authoring an entirely new chapter. A chapter written not just in patents and production numbers, but in lives saved, diseases contained. The world had begun to look eastward – not for charity, but for solutions.

By the time India joined the global patent regime in 2005, the country was home to a thriving ecosystem of public and private institutions engaged in developing and producing cutting-edge vaccines and biotechnologies. Indian scientists and firms were now contributing not only to global vaccine access but also to the furthering of science, developing novel platforms and low-cost technologies suited to the realities of the Global South. Innovations such as the indigenous rotavirus vaccine and IIT Bombay's development of a

CAR-T cell immunotherapy for certain cancers at one-tenth the cost of similar therapies in the West furthered India's scientific confidence.

Its prowess was further reinforced during the Covid-19 pandemic. While much of the world struggled with supply shortages and vaccine nationalism, the country's premier medical research system, Indian Council of Medical Research, developed the indigenous COVAXIN using a time-tested inactivated virus platform. Simultaneously, it leveraged public–private partnerships to produce and deploy COVISHIELD at an unprecedented scale. In record time, India vaccinated its 1.4 billion citizens, not only safeguarding its own population but also supporting dozens of low- and middle-income countries (LMICs) with timely vaccine supplies through bilateral aid and the COVAX initiative. At a moment when global solidarity faltered, India's vaccine diplomacy offered a powerful counter-narrative.

In the following pages, you will come across a sea of little-known facts, anecdotes and personalities that have shaped the chronicle of vaccine science in India. From R&D to public policy, my effort has been to unearth hitherto unmined details, place known facts in perspective, unveil unsung heroes and celebrate them. I have tried to narrate this story with honesty and depth, acknowledging both the triumphs and the tensions that have defined India's unprecedented vaccine journey.

I am certain you will find these revelations as thrilling and enlightening as I did while uncovering them, and come away with a renewed pride in India's scientific spirit. As you read, you will find that this is not just a story about vaccines – it is the story of a nation discovering its voice, asserting its autonomy and quietly rewriting the rules of global health.

Wishing you a rewarding and thought-provoking read.

PART I

THE EARLY DAYS
(1875–1930)

1

SNAKEBITE TURNS SAVIOUR

DAYS AFTER INDIRA GANDHI TOOK OFFICE AS THE PRIME minister of India in 1966 in the national capital of New Delhi, a mare at a stud farm in Pune was bitten by a snake some 1,500 kilometres away. Neither the snake nor the mare could have known their encounter would soon find a significant place in the history of India and beyond. This seemingly minor incident would lead to the birth of an enterprise that would go on to immunize billions of children around the world and become one of the world's largest vaccine* makers.

This was no ordinary mare, though; the animal belonged to a horse breeder in Pune, 150 kilometres east of Bombay. The young Cyrus Poonawalla was running a stud farm set up by his dad Soli Poonawalla in 1946. Over the decades, the farm produced some of the best stallions† for racing in Bombay and other cities and won many trophies and laurels. It wasn't surprising then that the Poonawalla Stud Farms had gained renown as a dependable source of champion horses for racing, an entertainment sport brought to India by the British as a pastime for their officers and later embraced enthusiastically by Indians. Poonawalla Stud Farms, as it is known,

* A substance that helps the body build immunity against specific diseases by training the immune system to recognize and combat harmful germs.

† Male horses that are not castrated and are used for breeding.

was then run by Soli's children Cyrus and Zavary and has produced 287 winners of classic races to date.[1]

However, Soli had been faced with a daunting problem: what to do with the horses at the end of their racing careers? He soon devised a solution: all the worn-out horses would be sent to retire and die at the Haffkine Institute, a government-owned facility dedicated to making vaccines that was located in the suburbs of Bombay. Desperately looking for healthy horses to extract serum* for vaccine production, the institute had welcomed this arrangement. They needed them in considerable numbers.

Upon taking charge of the stud farm, Cyrus Poonawalla had continued using most of the systems put in place by his father, including the arrangement with the Haffkine Institute. But given his attachment to these golden-agers, Cyrus treated any injury to them as personal hurt. So when he was informed that one of his best mares had been bitten by a snake, he instantly contacted the Haffkine Institute for anti-venom serum†. After all, the institute had ample stock since it was involved in the production of anti-venom.[2]

There was one challenge. The use of anti-venom in those days was not authorized by the government. Without any blanket permission in place, the institute had to seek one-time clearance from both the local government in Bombay and the central government authorities in New Delhi.

With no health minister appointed by PM Gandhi as yet and the ministry still being in its formative stages, securing the approval to inject anti-venom took four to five days. By the time permission came through, the mare had already died.

Cyrus was horrified. Had bureaucracy killed his mare, or the lack of systems? If he had been running a vaccine production centre, his

* The clear part of blood that contains antibodies and is used in vaccines or treatments to fight diseases. Plural: sera.

† A treatment made from antibodies that can neutralize snake venom and save the lives of people or animals bitten by venomous snakes.

horse could have been saved. Instead, he had been donating valuable horse serum to the institute by gifting them his horses.

From this tragedy emerged an opportunity – a new business idea began to take shape in his mind. Over the next few days, he decided not to gift any more mares and stallions to the Haffkine Institute. Rather, he set up a brand-new serum-making company. This venture, which would soon become the Serum Institute of India, would start its operations rough and ready from a shed on the stud farm.

The decision also marked the end of a long relationship between the Poonawallas and the Haffkine Institute – a pioneering biopharmaceutical research centre, which had been set up by a Soviet-born researcher who had laid the foundation for India's vaccine journey almost a century earlier.

2

HAFFKINE'S INDIAN EXPERIMENT

THE GANGETIC DELTA WAS HISTORICALLY KNOWN AS A BREEDING ground for *vibrio cholerae,* the comma-shaped bacteria responsible for Asiatic cholera.*[1] For decades, it was widely believed that the disease originated in the river itself. It was only by 1854 that an epidemiological study† by British scientist John Snow disproved this notion, demonstrating that the true source was contaminated drinking water. This discovery marked a significant shift in the understanding of cholera's transmission.

Stagnant water, often associated with poor living conditions, has long been the nursery for the multiplication of bacteria. Asiatic cholera had its origins in the Indian subcontinent, with one of the earliest recorded mentions appearing in Dutch physician Jakob de Bondt's *De Medicina Indorum* in the seventeenth century. By the turn of the twentieth century, at least six major pandemics‡ had hit the Indian subcontinent.

The first known cholera pandemic broke out in the current-day city of Jashore in Bangladesh. After multiplying rapidly through the

---

* A historical term for a deadly form of cholera that originated in Asia, especially the Indian subcontinent.

† A scientific investigation that looks at how diseases spread and what causes them in populations.

‡ A disease outbreak that spreads across multiple countries or continents, affecting many people.

Hindu religious congregation of Kumbh Mela, it reached Calcutta in 1817. Soon after, the disease made it to Burma (Myanmar), South India and Ceylon (Sri Lanka), through the moving British military battalions. In less than three years, it arrived on the shores of Siam (Thailand), killing over 100,000 people just on the island of Java in Indonesia. The very next year, some 18,000 people perished of the disease in Iraq and through Turkey, the pandemic entered Europe. Thereafter, it disappeared from most regions in the next few years, except for the Gangetic delta of Bengal.

The next outbreak was in 1826, lasting almost a decade, then ravaging through North America and Europe. The third outbreak was by 1846, mostly in South America, including Brazil, and parts of Africa and had lasted for almost fifteen years or so. The next was mostly in Spain, starting in 1863 and lasting over twelve years. The fifth outbreak was in India in 1881 and spread to the rest of Asia, Europe and extended all the way up to South America.

Therefore, when Soviet-born British researcher Haffkine set out for India, he had great hopes of carrying out a large-scale field study of cholera vaccinations in the Indian region. More so because it was coming soon after his requests for field trials were turned down by the Russian and Siamese (Thailand) governments.

Upsetting his field trial plans, when he landed in Calcutta in March 1893, cholera had not been a serious concern as the outbreak had somewhat ended in the Indian region and had moved over to other parts of the world.

In addition, Haffkine faced multiple problems in convincing people to participate in field studies, what are known today as clinical trials.* At the time, vaccination was carried out over a course of two injections set apart by a few weeks, and people weren't even sure how an illness in the intestine could be prevented by administering an injection under the skin of an arm. Help arrived serendipitously through the support of the military and medical cops attached to the British Army.

* Tests done on people to check if a new medicine or vaccine is safe and effective.

On his first voyage to India in March 1893, one of his fellow travellers happened to be the Surgeon Captain of the British Indian Army, C. C. Manifold. After exchanging pleasantries, Haffkine moved on to discuss his proposed cholera vaccinations with the surgeon captain. Impressed by what he had heard, Manifold offered the Army's full support to the scientist and agreed to get vaccinated himself. He was administered the attenuated vaccine* above the twelfth rib† on his left side while he was onboard the ship to India.

For the next four days, Manifold waited for 'possible adverse reaction'‡, documenting what he was feeling on an hourly basis. He published a report on his experience in the *Indian Medical Gazette*, where he concluded that the discomfort and the pain caused by the inoculation§ were so trivial that its fear should not deter anyone from getting vaccinated.[2]

Once in the saddle in Bengal, Haffkine began vaccinating soldiers of the Indian Army in Calcutta. The initiative soon extended to regiments stationed in the northwest provinces, Oudh (current-day Uttar Pradesh) and Punjab, spanning regions in present-day India and Pakistan. By the end of 1893, nearly 10,000 British and Indian soldiers and officers had been vaccinated, with at least 65 per cent also receiving the second dose.

As the army vouched for the vaccine's safety, the campaign moved to rural areas with sizeable populations. Haffkine travelled extensively, reaching the farming communities of Bengal, the tea estates of Assam, the hinterlands of the United Province and as far away as Kashmir and North West Province. The real challenge, however, was in finding people for the crucial second dose, though there was no shortage of volunteers for the first.

---

* A vaccine made from a weakened form of the disease-causing germ that doesn't make people sick but trains the immune system.

† The lowest rib in the human ribcage, often used as a reference point for injections.

‡ An unwanted or harmful effect that sometimes happens after taking a medicine or vaccine.

§ Another word for vaccination – giving a shot to protect against a disease.

Haffkine seized this opportunity to assess the vaccine's efficacy* against the Asiatic cholera, demonstrating its safety during trials. Initiating a broader vaccination campaign, he sought to study cholera cycles in endemic† villages. However, British authorities mandated that the vaccinations be voluntary, limiting the controlled trials he had envisioned.

Over time, Haffkine refined his approach, abandoning the primary attenuated vaccine in favour of the second, more effective version. Despite meticulous record-keeping, he found the trials yielded inconsistent results, underscoring their limitations. While it showed promise in some cases, issues with standardizing dosages and assessing efficacy persisted.

By the end of his first year, running up to March 1894, a total of 22,703 people had been vaccinated. By the second year, another 19,473 persons had received the attenuated vaccine, bringing the total to 42,176 in just two years. Considering the population of the British Indian territories at the time exceeded 200 million, this was a significant start. Despite the challenges of travel, vaccine supply and limited government cooperation, Haffkine managed to inoculate diverse populations – over 70,000 people by 1896.

As he himself noted, the choice of localities and participants was largely determined by the willingness of the individuals; but at the same time, in every location, efforts were made to focus operations on populations living under similar conditions.[3]

For much of the first year, vaccinations were carried out in non-cholera-infected areas, as the endemic had temporarily subsided in Calcutta. This left the challenge of conducting clinical trials in active outbreak zones.

In March 1894, however, cholera broke out in the Kattal Bagan *bustee*. Dr William John Ritchie Simpson, the city's Health Officer, scrambled together a team to find solutions to contain the outbreak.

---

* How well a treatment or vaccine works to prevent or cure a disease.

† A disease that is regularly found in a particular area or among a specific group of people.

He had heard about the arrival of vaccination and of Haffkine's work. He shot off a letter to Haffkine, requesting help in identifying cholera bacilli* in the affected area. For Haffkine, this was the moment he had been waiting for and, indeed, the purpose of his travel to India. Eager to test his vaccine in an endemic setting, he spared no time in reaching the location.

On his visit to the locality the very next day, Haffkine realized that each household faced equal exposure to the infection. However, persuading people to accept vaccinations – a concept they hadn't even heard of – proved difficult.

Undeterred, Haffkine saw a great opportunity. By convincing some individuals in each household to be vaccinated while others remained unvaccinated, he could compare outcomes directly.[4] With unwavering support from Simpson and his team, Haffkine began engaging with the community, using his negotiating skills to build trust. In a few days, inoculations slowly commenced.

Gradually, as more and more people got vaccinated, the campaign gained momentum. When analyzed after two months, the results were promising enough to convince the authorities to support prolonged trials.

With a small grant from the Calcutta Corporation, a bacteriological laboratory† was set up to bolster the vaccination drive. From March 1894 to August 1895, cholera cases and fatalities from across the city were meticulously recorded, with Simpson and Haffkine personally visiting locations frequently to verify the data.

The data was encouraging, to say the least. Among 335 uninoculated individuals in the bustee, there were 45 new cases and 39 deaths. In contrast, there were only four new cases and four deaths among the 181 inoculated‡ individuals. Of course the numbers were

* Rod-shaped bacteria; in this context, it refers to the cholera-causing bacteria.

† A lab where scientists grow and study bacteria to understand diseases and find ways to fight them.

‡ When a small amount of disease-causing material is introduced into the body to help it build resistance to that disease.

still insignificant for any definitive conclusions on the efficacy of the vaccine in an endemic situation.

As news spread about the success of Haffkine's cholera vaccine, requests to conduct vaccination campaigns poured in from across British India. Buoyed by the interest, Haffkine began preparing for a large-scale drive to eradicate cholera across the subcontinent. But soon an unexpected setback struck: Haffkine contracted malaria,* caused by another organism, the Plasmodium parasite.† By this time, it had been almost 30 months since he'd first landed in India from the lab of Louis Pasteur in Paris in March 1893.

* A disease caused by a parasite transmitted through mosquito bites, leading to fever and chills.

† The tiny organism that causes malaria when it infects red blood cells.

3

THE BIRTH OF INDIAN VACCINES

TOWARDS THE END OF THE NINETEENTH CENTURY, WHILE THE world grappled with outbreaks of plague* and cholera, Louis Pasteur's laboratory in Paris emerged as the hub of groundbreaking research aimed at preventing epidemic diseases.

In 1880, Pasteur made a landmark discovery: injecting chicken with the live bacteria prepared in the laboratory could protect them from future attacks of cholera. He postulated that introducing aged, weakened bacteria into the body in advance could prevent new infections. Over the next six years, he extended the same principle for combatting other deadly diseases, such as anthrax† and rabies in humans. This innovation came to be known as the 'live attenuated' vaccine.‡

Pasteur's lab marked the beginning of a period of renewed hope in the fight against pandemics. It promised a path to control diseases that had plagued humanity for centuries. It was a leap forward since Edward Jenner's discovery of the cowpox vaccine over a century earlier in England, which earned him the title 'Father of Immunology'.

---

* Refers to bubonic plague, a deadly infectious disease spread primarily by fleas that live on rats.

† A disease caused by *Bacillus anthracis*, a bacteria found in soil, mostly affecting animals but can infect humans through skin, inhalation or consumption.

‡ A vaccine made using a live but weakened version of the germ that causes a disease, designed to trigger immunity without causing illness.

Jenner had famously tested his hypothesis that a mild, prior cowpox infection could render a person immune to smallpox. On 14 May 1796, he inoculated eight-year-old James Phipps with pus scraped from the cowpox blisters of his milkmaid who had contracted the disease from her herd. Phipps had developed only a mild fever and uneasiness but not a full-blown infection.

After observing Phipps for a few days, Jenner injected himself with variolous matter.* As he had anticipated, no infection occurred, even after days of waiting. To ensure the correctness of his findings, he repeated the experiment multiple times, with no signs of smallpox. He extended the trial to twenty-three additional individuals, including his own son, to further ascertain his findings. The outcome remained consistent.

Terming this ground-breaking discovery a 'vaccine', Jenner presented his findings to the Royal Society of London for Improving Natural Knowledge, the United Kingdom's national academy of sciences. However, the Royal Society refused to publish Jenner's findings without a thorough peer review.

It was only when Jenner supplemented his paper with data from twenty-three further experiments and engaged in elaborate discussions and debates about his new method of vaccination – contrasting it with the prevailing practice of variolation,† which involved injecting people with raw substance from smallpox pustules‡ – that it was published.

The British government formally recognized vaccination as an effective method of disease prevention through the Vaccination Act of 1840. The Act endorsed vaccination and banned variolation, nearly two decades after Edward Jenner's death. Thus, when Pasteur

* Infectious material taken from someone with smallpox, used in early forms of vaccination called variolation.

† An old method of protecting against smallpox by deliberately infecting a person with a small dose of the virus to create immunity.

‡ Small, inflamed, pus-filled blisters that appear on the skin during infections like smallpox.

reported his findings on cholera from Paris, Jenner's technique had already received the British government's stamp of approval. The difference was that Pasteur's work focused on controlling cholera – another devastating pandemic that had ravaged many parts of the world for over a decade.

Pasteur had first shot to fame with his doctrine of spontaneous generation,* which proved that microorganisms could not develop in sterilized, sealed flasks but would thrive when exposed to air. For this discovery, he had received the Alhumbert Prize from the French Academy of Sciences in 1862. He had also documented pasteurization – treating milk and wine to avoid bacterial contamination – and postulated germ theory,† positing that diseases could be prevented by killing or stopping germs. This theory laid the foundation for modern clinical medicine.‡

Among those inspired by Pasteur's work was Waldemar Mordecai Wolff Haffkine, a young Russian researcher born in Odessa (present-day Ukraine) in 1860. Soviet Odessa was a prominent centre of biological research and intellectual activity until the end of the eighteenth century. The city was also the birthplace of N. F. Gamaleya, the first Russian virologist; Selman Waksman, the inventor of Streptomycin; and Elie Metchnikoff, who first proposed that white blood cells defend against bacteria.

Haffkine's early life was fraught with challenges. His mother died before his seventh birthday, and he relied on his elder half-brother for financial support. To make ends meet, he tutored students while pursuing his education. In 1879 he was admitted to the Novorossiysk University of Odessa, where he studied under Elie Metchnikoff and earned a Doctor of Science degree in zoology in 1884. Fascinated by Metchnikoff's research, Haffkine joined his mentor's laboratory.

Haffkine's early political engagements significantly influenced his

* The outdated belief that living things could arise from non-living matter without reproduction.

† The idea that many diseases are caused by tiny organisms (germs) that invade the body.

‡ The part of medicine that deals with the actual care and treatment of patients, as opposed to lab research.

later professional trajectory. During his university years, he actively participated in the Narodnaya Volya (Will of the People) party, a prominent force in the Russian revolutionary movement. As a leader in student protests against newly implemented university policies aimed at quashing political radicalism – particularly by prohibiting student assembly and petition for grievance redressal – Haffkine was at the centre of political activism.

In 1879, Haffkine was arrested, marking the initiation of a police dossier that would follow him for years. Accused of disloyalty to the government, he endured eight years of constant police surveillance while in Russia. After the assassination of Czar Alexander II in St Petersburg on 1 March 1881 by members of Narodnaya Volya, the government launched mass crackdowns. Subsequently, rumours of Jewish involvement in the assassination led to widespread pogroms across Russia. In response, Haffkine and his fellow students in Odessa organized and led the First Jewish Self-Defense to protect the community. This act led to another arrest, on charges of possessing a pistol.[1] In February 1882, he was charged with treason and spent one month in prison. His release came through the intervention of Professor Metchnikoff.

By 1888, disillusioned by the oppressive climate, Haffkine decided to leave Russia.[2] He moved to Switzerland, a common destination for Jews at the time, as the opportunities for advanced scientific research in Odessa were limited. Haffkine joined the Geneva Medical School as an Assistant in Physiology.[3] It was during this period that he was charmed by Pasteur's research, which beckoned him to Paris in 1889 to work under the renowned biologist until he left for India four years later.

Metchnikoff had already moved to Paris after Pasteur – impressed by his cell process theory of 'phagocytosis'* as a means of protection against infections – had invited the former to head one of the

* The process by which certain white blood cells 'eat' harmful germs to protect the body from infections.

laboratories at the newly set up Pasteur Institute. Haffkine requested his mentor-professor for a position at the Pasteur Institute.

Initially, all Metchnikoff could offer him was the position of librarian, which he readily accepted. It allowed Haffkine access to a lot of reading material even as he spent the rest of his time in Metchnikoff's lab working on how microbes adapted to adverse conditions. It wasn't long before Pasteur noticed Haffkine's potential.[4]

In 1890, a position opened up when another researcher Alaxandre Yersin left the lab for Saigon (Thailand) in the Indo-China region. Pierre Roux, one of Pasteur's closest collaborators and a co-founder of the institute, quickly inducted Haffkine into his team, where he began working on diseases like diphtheria, cholera, rabies and tuberculosis. On 1 October 1890, Haffkine was appointed as *préparateur*[*] of technical microbiology in the Laboratory of Physiological Chemistry at the École Pratique des Hautes Études (Physics and Chemistry section, under Pasteur's supervision). His focus soon shifted to the *Vibrio cholerae*.

Haffkine's growing expertise in microbiology coincided with ongoing global efforts to understand cholera. In 1883, German bacteriologist Robert Koch had travelled to India and Egypt, two perennial hotspots of *Vibrio cholerae*. Koch had collected samples and isolated the bacteria from infected people – a step that provided Haffkine with a starting point for his research. His research was also guided by Koch's Postulates,[†] the four steps necessary to confirm the causative agent of a disease.

Building on Jenner's work from a century ago and Pasteur's achievements with the chicken cholera vaccine, Haffkine launched his research to develop an effective vaccine against human cholera. He initially followed a technique similar to that of Spanish researcher

---

* A junior researcher or lab technician responsible for preparing experiments and supporting scientific studies.

† A set of four steps used by scientists to prove that a specific germ causes a particular disease.

Jaume Ferran Clua, who had tested the vaccines in Barcelona in 1885, administering *Vibrio bacilli* collected from cholera patients. But due to variability in bacterial virulence* and absence of any data to conclude its efficacy, Clua's methods were soon discontinued.

Drawing from Jenner and Pasteur again, Haffkine theorized that inoculating people with bacteria which had attained an increased, fixed state of virulence through animal passage† could protect them from infections. In his lab, he observed that repeated passages of cholera bacilli through the peritoneal cavity‡ of guinea pigs led to bacteria with increased (exalted) virulence. He determined that thirty-nine passings were sufficient to reach the heightened virulence. It could be further transformed into an attenuated state by exposing the exalted culture§ to aeration¶ at a higher temperature. The difference between attenuated culture and exalted culture was that the potency of the latter dissipated after two weeks whereas the former remained stable for a longer time. Developing an attenuated state** of bacteria therefore became critical to advance the research.

Haffkine was working in his lab on developing an attenuated state of bacteria late at night when he first observed the transformation firsthand. Fearing this phenomenon might not recur, he rushed to Yersin's house a few yards away, woke him up and urged him to rush to the lab. Recently returned from Saigon, Yersin reluctantly walked over to Haffkine's lab to observe the process. Haffkine explained the reason to summon him at this late hour: 'The phenomenon so long

---

* The strength or severity of a germ in causing disease.

† A lab technique where germs are passed through animals repeatedly to change their behaviour or strength.

‡ The space inside the abdomen that holds the stomach, intestines and other organs.

§ A lab-grown version of bacteria that has become more powerful or deadly after being altered.

¶ The process of exposing something to air, often used in labs to change how bacteria behave.

** A weakened form of bacteria or virus that's still alive but not strong enough to cause disease, used in vaccines.

sought for, once demonstrated to a qualified observer, becomes a scientific fact.'[5]

Haffkine documented every observation and conclusion in his research diary. In May 1892, he wrote, 'The general aspect of these results, which can be indifferently applied to all laboratory animals, allows us to believe that a subcutaneous injection,* first of attenuated microbes and then of exalted microbes, will preserve man from an attack of the disease known under the name of Asiatic cholera.'[6]

Pasteur had always strongly supported Haffkine's work. A story of note is when the Prince of Siam visited the Pasteur Institute in November 1891. During his visit, the prince evinced keen interest in the research on cholera and asked about the work being done at the institute.

Pointing to Haffkine, Pasteur responded, 'Yes, we are studying cholera. Here is the person who has been working on it. Here is the person who is now very near, nearest of all, to this discovery. It is possible that a remedy will be found soon. We even hope that it will be this year. This gentleman is the nearest to the discovery.'

Haffkine felt embarrassed since his research hadn't concluded anything at all. But that was Pasteur's way of encouraging his researchers and pushing them to deliver.

The Prince was overwhelmed by Pasteur's response and said, 'If you find a remedy, Siam will erect a statue of you.'

'Let it be a golden statue,' retorted Pasteur.[7]

With mounting pressure and no concluding results yet, Haffkine began to spend long days and nights in the laboratory. By December 1891, his efforts paid off as he was able to isolate cholera bacteria from the intestine of rabbits.

Haffkine began by using an attenuated strain of the cholera bacteria. He grew it in a controlled environment and altered the strain to reduce its harmfulness while preserving its ability to stimulate an immune response. This strain served as the first vaccine for humans.[8,9]

---

* An injection given under the skin, but not into a muscle or vein.

For the second one, Haffkine needed a more virulent strain of the bacteria. He initially isolated cholera bacteria from a patient's excreta but found it was not as potent. To enhance its virulence, he passed the bacteria through a series of guinea pigs, selecting animals based on their resistance to the bacteria. The process continued until the strain reached its maximum virulence. Haffkine closely monitored the bacterial purity through microscopic examination and culture.

The attenuated strain derived from this enhanced version served as the first vaccine, inducing immunity with minimal harm. The process involved careful cultivation, controlled transfers and meticulous testing to ensure both safety and effectiveness.*

Soon, Haffkine began to contemplate moving his research from animal to human trials. Since he believed that live vaccines provided stronger immunity, Haffkine developed two distinct live cholera vaccines: one attenuated (weakened) by growth at 39°C with aeration, and the other with enhanced pathogenicity† through repeated animal passage.

Confident in the vaccine's potential to protect humans, he moved to human trials by early 1892. He first tested the vaccine on himself, followed by three of his close aides. The four of them became the first humans to be inoculated with the cholera vaccines, all with the permission of Dr Roux.

The trial began on 18 July 1892 with subcutaneous injections in his left flank with the attenuated vaccine. This caused symptoms like malaise, temperature elevation and local pain accompanied by mild swelling. Once the pain subsided, the enhanced vaccine was administered in the right flank, resulting in elevated temperature and local pain, though without swelling. Subsequently, the three volunteers were inoculated with both vaccines, experiencing similar reactions. Haffkine presented the results to the Biological Society of Paris on 30 July 1892, concluding that both the anticholera vaccines,

---

* How well a vaccine intervention works in the real world, considering factors like adherence, side effects and other real-world complexities.

† The ability of a germ to cause disease in the body.

which had proved effective in animal experiments, could be safely administered to humans and posed no health hazards.[10]

At the end of his report he suggested that people could become immune against cholera six days after vaccination. Subsequently, he sent a report to the *British Medical Journal* describing how he had conducted the animal and human trials, his observations and the methods of producing the vaccines.[11,12]

Haffkine is today recognized as a pioneer in conducting controlled field trials,* his live vaccine having proved effective in challenging conditions. Despite shortcomings, Haffkine's contributions laid essential groundwork for future vaccine development.

His rival was Jaume Ferran i Clua, a Spanish medical practitioner and bacteriologist. Ferran was known for introducing vaccination for cattle against anthrax and had headed the Municipal Bacteriological Laboratory of Barcelona since 1886. His primary focus was preventive inoculation, which led to his work on vaccines against diseases such as cholera, typhoid, diphtheria, plague, tuberculosis, tetanus and rabies.

Modern science writers cautiously credit Ferran's role in demonstrating the potential for active immunity against cholera, viewing his approach as injudicious. Some even argue that Ferran's work may have caused more harm to science than good.[13] Among his contemporaries, scientists such as Gamaleya – who pioneered research on vaccines and microbiology – dismissed his work and sought to distance it from Pasteur's research.

Tensions between Ferran and Haffkine came to a head in July 1892, when Ferran vehemently contested Haffkine's claims of developing Pasteurian† protective vaccines against cholera. Ferran, who was known for defending the superiority of his research, launched a critique of Haffkine's findings. Three months later, he

* Scientific studies where one group gets the treatment and another does not, to fairly test if the treatment works.

† Refers to followers of Louis Pasteur's methods or principles, especially regarding vaccination and microbiology.

submitted a note to the French Society for Biology, challenging the originality of Haffkine's discovery.[14]

Ferran even sarcastically congratulated Haffkine for 'having demonstrated the truth of the conclusions described in my notes of 1885' and encouraged him 'to pursue with ardor his studies applying them to man, without any fear, because, since many thousands of people were vaccinated in 1885, the harmlessness of cultures of the comma bacillus is beyond discussion.'[15]

Despite Ferran's criticisms, Dr Auguste Chauveau, president of the French Society, acknowledged Ferran's role in cholera vaccination while rejecting his protocol of mass immunization. In 1893, after Haffkine acknowledged Ferran's work, the latter responded with strong displeasure. He accused Haffkine of dismissing his contributions and reasserted his claim as the true developer of the cholera vaccine. Ferran asserted that his human-adapted strain of the cholera bacillus was superior to Haffkine's guinea pig-adapted isolate and questioned the efficacy of Haffkine's methods, particularly those implemented in India.

Despite their heated exchanges, which played out through publications in the *Bulletin de l'Institut Pasteur*, Ferran acknowledged Haffkine's significant achievements in cholera vaccine research and vaccination, emphasizing the need for recognizing each scientist's contributions in advancing the field.

On his part, Haffkine credited Ferran with demonstrating the possibility of such experiments, while emphasizing that Ferran's subsequent attempts failed to convince skeptics about the feasibility of a cholera vaccine. He disparaged Ferran's method as 'variolation' instead of vaccination. In a lecture delivered to the Conjoint Board of the Royal Colleges of Physicians of London and Surgeons of England in December 1895, Haffkine remarked, 'It is the difference between vaccination and variolisation that distinguishes the method which I have applied in India from that tried in Spain by Dr Jaime Ferran in 1885.'[16] Eventually, the dispute concluded with both Ferran and Haffkine receiving the prestigious Breant Prize from the French Academy of Sciences, which recognized their individual achievements.

Upon proving that his method could prevent cholera in human beings, Haffkine began toying with the idea of testing it on a larger human population. However, he had no idea how to proceed.

Cambridge fellow E. H. Hankin, a chemical examiner and bacteriologist at the North West Frontier Province of British India, remarked that the existing evidence indicated Haffkine's method of inoculation did not cause serious health disturbances and could be safely practised on humans. He also noted that its ability to confer immunity against cholera in various animals, such as guinea pigs and pigeons, raised hopes for its effectiveness in humans.[17]

Desperate to conduct fields trials for his vaccine, Pasteur initially sought permission to test it in Russia in 1892. But his request was denied. He then approached the Prince of Siam who had earlier visited the Pasteur Institute in Paris to carry out trials in Siam. To facilitate this, Pasteur entrusted the task to a French resident in Indo-China, Hirman (no second name).[18]

Hirman conveyed the news to Lord Frederick Dufferin, the former Viceroy of British India and then the British Ambassador to France. Pasteur also sent word to Lord Dufferin, who liked the idea of carrying out trials in his former territory. Given that cholera was rampant in the region and colonial authorities placed little value on Indian lives, Lord Dufferin suggested Bengal, the hotbed of cholera, as the ideal location.

Later that year, he organized a meeting in London for Haffkine to meet with Lord John Kimberley, the Secretary of State for India, to present the potential success of vaccination experiments and their advantages.

The meeting took place soon after. Lord Kimberly was impressed with Haffkine's arguments but imposed one condition: the vaccinations had to be administered voluntarily, with no forced injections.[19] Haffkine agreed.

This set Haffkine onto a new path in his life, which led him to India in March 1893.

4

FROM CHOLERA TO PLAGUE

WHEN HAFFKINE RETURNED TO INDIA, AFTER HIS BRIEF sojourn in Europe because of a malarial attack and a visit to Louis Pasteur who was on his deathbed, the ground situation on the disease front had drastically changed. In the winter of 1896, a plague epidemic broke out in the subcontinent, and Haffkine had to quickly shift his focus from cholera to plague. He resumed his work on anti-plague vaccines, picking up from where he had left off at the Pasteur Institute in Paris before leaving for India. Two years earlier, Alexandre Yersin, Haffkine's colleague at the Pasteur Institute, had rushed off to Hong Kong during an outbreak where he successfully identified the agent causing the plague: a gram-negative bacillus,* later named *Yersinia pestis* after him.†

When he landed in Calcutta in late 1896, the British government directed Haffkine to Bombay to help control the crisis. On 8 October, he was appointed a member of the coveted Indian Civil Service.[1] Packing his belongings, he left for Bombay, where he set up the first camp at the Grant Medical College. After he was allocated some space to work, he quickly put together a makeshift lab using the room and accompanying corridor. With the help of a local clerk and three support staff, he resumed his work.

* A type of bacteria that doesn't retain a certain stain in lab tests (gram stain).

† The bacterium that causes the plague. Named after Alexandre Yersin, who discovered it during an outbreak in Hong Kong.

The first breakthrough came in December: Haffkine successfully vaccinated rabbits in the laboratory by injecting the animals with the heat-sterilized cultured broth* of plague microbes. Encouraged by these results, he decided to put his own life at risk and injected himself with the vaccine on 10 January 1897.[2] Save for some mild side effects, such as some pain at the injection site and a slight increase in body temperature for two days, he experienced no adverse side effects.

As Haffkine prepared for large-scale testing, an outbreak was reported at the Majesty's House of Correction in Bombay's Bycullah area. He was rushed to the prison to vaccinate some 154 willing inmates. The results were encouraging, especially when the conditions of the vaccinated men were compared with the remaining 191 inmates.

Soon after this success, accolades followed. The vaccine received praise for generating reasonable protection for vulnerable populations and proving effective as a prophylactic option. In 1897, in the Birthday Honours List of Queen Victoria, Haffkine was named Companion of the Order of the Indian Empire (CIE). With the honours conferred on him, Haffkine applied for and became a naturalized British citizen.[3]

Meanwhile, demand for the vaccine surged across Bombay, and within three months nearly 11,000 people from affected areas were vaccinated. To meet the increased demand, Haffkine's laboratory also had to be shifted to larger facilities twice in succession. In 1898, it moved to Khushru Lodge, a bungalow owned by Sir Sultan Shah, Aga Khan III, the head of the Khoja mussulman community. Aga Khan not only funded the modifications needed for Haffkine's use but at his insistence, half of the Khoja *mussulman* population of Bombay – almost 12,000 individuals – received prophylactic inoculations.†[4]

By this time the facility was known as the Plague Research

* A nutrient-rich liquid used in labs to grow bacteria for study or vaccine production.

† A medical treatment or vaccine given in advance to prevent disease rather than cure it after infection.

Laboratory. It was staffed with one officer from the Indian Medical Service, four medical professionals deputed from the Secretary of State for India, four local medical staff, three clerks and six last grade employees. Soon after the shift, Haffkine received a request from Baroda, where the Black Death* had spread from Surat to a village named Undhera, meaning darkness. With a population of 1,031 people, this tiny village turned out to be a testing site for further validating the results obtained from the Bycullah Prison trials.

The following year, the laboratory would shift again, this time to the Old Government House in Parel. The new facility offered sufficient space for large-scale production – lakhs of doses of injections. Soon it expanded to over fifty employees.

More accolades followed. The University of Edinburgh awarded Haffkine the prestigious Cameron Prize for Practical Therapeutics† in 1900 for saving thousands of lives with prophylactic vaccinations against cholera and plague. A year later, the British government made him Director-in-Chief of the sprawling Bombay Plague Laboratory. Under his leadership, the laboratory commercialized the production of an anti-plague vaccine for both domestic use and export. In the following years, the Bombay Plague Laboratory went on to produce millions of doses of plague vaccine.

Despite being at the pinnacle of his career, something was troubling Haffkine. The British government's Indian Plague Commission had just been empowered with a new member. With this aggressive new member, the Plague Commission began to unravel many aspects of the plague – including the 'recipe' of Haffkine's plague vaccine.[5]

* Another term for the bubonic plague, historically used to describe the devastating medieval outbreaks in Europe and Asia.

† The branch of medicine concerned with the treatment and cure of diseases.

5

THE BOMBAY PLAGUE

IN 1896, THE DISEASE BROKE OUT IN BOMBAY. CHARACTERIZED by swollen lymph nodes under the armpits and groin – known as buboes – it was swiftly classified as the bubonic plague. The first cases in the city, home to nearly 800,000 people, were reported in a densely populated port locality.

Mandvi, with approximately 33,000 residents packed into approximately 1,600 *chawls* (small houses in rows) primarily accommodating port workers, was the most overcrowded area in the city. Poor ventilation, damp floors, shared water taps and toilets and grain storage on the ground floors made it an ideal breeding ground for rodents. It was therefore no surprise when the plague took root there.

The disease was believed to have been brought to the city by travellers headed on a pilgrimage to Nasik, some 160 kilometres northeast of Bombay. It likely came from the Himalayan region, where the plague had been endemic for a while due to the closeness to Chinese territories. Two years earlier, 80,000 people had succumbed to the disease in Canton, China in a matter of weeks. Another theory, though less likely, suggested it may have come via merchant ships carrying goods from Hong Kong.

There were also reports of monks from the Himalayas visiting Mandvi while staying at a temple in Walkeshwar, a few miles away – an act possibly contributing to the outbreak.[1] From Mandvi's slums and chawls, the disease quickly spread to wealthier areas, affecting

Bombay's elite, the rich and the British.

The city administration swung into action quickly. A committee with officers from the British Indian Medical Corps was formed, with Walter Charles Rand, an Indian Civil Services officer, appointed as its commissioner. Medical officers were dispatched to the affected areas, which were isolated to curb further spread of the disease. Travellers were screened at the railway station and prevented from leaving the city, and eventually, the army was deployed to manage the escalating emergency.

During this time, Alessandro Lustig, an Austrian-Italian pathologist,* arrived in Bombay with a curative serum.† Soon the city became a hub for testing various plague vaccines. Haffkine was also summoned, pausing his ongoing cholera field trials in Calcutta.

While Haffkine had spent years developing the cholera vaccine, the high point of his research career became his efforts with the plague vaccine and subsequent field trials in India. Ironically, this very success would later jeopardize his research career, temporarily discrediting his achievements.

Efforts to discredit Haffkine's work on the cholera vaccine were not new. Research in this field had started long before he was involved. In 1884, Spanish researcher Jaume Ferran i Clua had demonstrated a workable vaccine. To persuade the authorities of its effectiveness, Ferran had drunk a few drops of *vibrio cholerae* after vaccinating himself. He submitted his findings to the Academy of Medicine in Barcelona and the Academy of Sciences in Paris. The latter never published his work, instead praising the research of Gamaleya, who in 1888 conducted animal trials using heat-killed bacteria on doves and guinea pigs.[2] Gamaleya's work was likely known to Haffkine and may have influenced his research in 1892 with devitalized bacteria‡ killed by heat or chloroform.

---

* A medical expert who studies the causes and effects of diseases.

† A liquid containing disease-fighting substances (like antibodies) used to treat someone already infected.

‡ Bacteria that have been killed or rendered inactive, used in vaccines to safely trigger the immune response without causing disease.

Around the same time, one of Haffkine's collaborators, Georgi Tamamcheff, who was also researching devitalized bacteria, found that the immunity generated from devitalized microbes was comparable to live vaccines. However, Haffkine rejected his findings, believing that the live vaccines offered superior immunity.

German bacteriologist Wilhelm Kolle had also developed a devitalized cholera vaccine,* claiming it was as effective as Haffkine's live vaccine since it induced comparable levels of agglutinating antibodies.[3] However, Haffkine refused to link agglutinin† levels to immunity against infectious diseases, having observed cases of typhoid fever where patients with high levels of antityphoid agglutinins‡ in their bloodstream succumbed to the illness.[4]

Yet another British bacteriologist was working on devitalized vaccines: Almroth Wright, later known as Sir Almroth Wright. Haffkine had an ongoing rivalry with Wright, especially over the latter's claim to be the pioneer of vaccination with devitalized bacteria. Wright had introduced the technique of vaccination for typhoid fever, but Haffkine found this unacceptable as this would have stripped him of his achievements.

In 1893, Wright had expressed high regard for Haffkine's work, acknowledging it in a publication on the typhoid vaccine. A decade later, in 1904, he changed his narrative, presenting an entirely different sequence of events that had led to the development of his typhoid vaccine.[5]

By 1899, Wright had been inducted as an expert member of the India Plague Commission (1898–1902). The commission was set up in 1898 to examine the origin of the plague outbreaks in India, investigate the mechanisms through which it was transmitted, assess the effectiveness of the curative serum and preventive vaccination and

---

* A vaccine made from bacteria that have been killed or inactivated so they can't cause disease but can still trigger immunity.

† Special immune proteins that cause bacteria or viruses to clump together, helping the body to eliminate them.

‡ Specific antibodies produced by the body to fight against typhoid bacteria.

evaluate the therapeutic value of Haffkine's plague vaccine.[6]

Led by Calcutta-born British professor Thomas Richard Fraser, who later became the president of the Royal College of Physicians of Edinburgh in 1900, the commission conducted an exhaustive study. It held over seventy meetings across British India, and two in London, where the members addressed nearly 27,000 questions.[7] They concluded that Haffkine's vaccine was effective against plague infections and reduced mortality.* With Wright's influence in the commission, the report also criticized Haffkine's data as 'inaccurate'. It further described the determination of the immunizing dose as inadequate, the method of vaccine preparation crude and suggested that the vaccine could have been contaminated by extraneous microbes.[8]

Some of these findings, appearing like accusations, cast a shadow on the scientist's painstakingly built reputation. This report would come back to haunt him a few years later when an unexpected tragedy struck a vaccination drive being carried out by Haffkine's team in Mulkowal, a village in the northwestern province of Punjab.

* Mortality refers to death caused by a disease; morbidity refers to how often people get sick from it.

6

THE MULKOWAL TRAGEDY

DESPITE EFFORTS BY THE BRITISH ADMINISTRATION, THE plague started to spread to the hinterlands. This sparked a mass exodus from the urban areas as people fled to their villages in search of refuge. In response, the Bombay municipal administration deployed medical teams to physically inspect people for buboes at various checkpoints. However, these physical examinations, particularly involving women, would soon lead to widespread unrest and accusations of outraging modesty.

By the turn of the nineteenth century, Punjab had become a hotspot for the disease, with more and more cases being reported from the region. The Punjab administration sought Haffkine's help to arrest further spread.

Haffkine's team began the vaccination drive in Punjab in October 1902, after administering almost half a million doses that year across British India. The team operated by travelling with the vaccination materials from the Plague Research Laboratory in Bombay to designated areas, inoculating a couple of villages before returning to the laboratory for resupply.

On 30 October 1902, one such vaccination camp was held in Mulkowal (current-day Mullowal), in Sangrur district, about 130 kilometres away from Chandigarh. The local administration had widely publicized the event, drawing a large crowd from nearby areas. Some had travelled by ox carts, while most others had walked to reach the venue. The drive began at 9 a.m. and by afternoon, the team had vaccinated 107 people.

The vaccinations, carried out in the open air, were being overseen by British doctor A. M. Elliot. As per protocol,* shortly before the drive started, a 'Plague Manual' was handed out to the inoculators. It outlined the safety conditions thus: 'The opening of bottles of prophylactic and the infilling of syringes are the chief duties of the compounder† ... If there is great press of work, the duty of actually opening the bottles may be entrusted to any intelligent person, care being taken to see that he observes the above instructions carefully.' It then continued to state: 'The compounder, in proceeding to open a bottle, must shake it well, then dip its neck in carbolic lotion, 1 in 20,‡ and then, with a pair of dissecting forceps,§ which when not in use are to be kept in the carbolic lotion, of remove the cork.'[1]

The camp proceeded without incident, save when a compounder, while administering vaccines, dropped a pair of forceps on the ground when trying to open a bottle. Accounts differ on what happened next. Some suggest he picked it up quickly and hurriedly dipped it in carbolic lotion before removing the cork of bottle number: 53-N. There was another account which indicated that since he dropped the forceps, he used a different instrument to open the bottle.

No unusual developments were observed for the next couple of days. As 3 November dawned, however, an unsettling development overshadowed the vaccination drive of 30 October: A growing number of individuals, who had eagerly participated in the drive now found themselves afflicted with lockjaw,¶ associated with tetanus.**

* In clinical trials, the detailed plan for how a clinical trial will be conducted, including what is tested, how and on whom.

† A medical assistant or technician who prepares and sometimes administers medicines under supervision.

‡ A disinfectant solution made by diluting carbolic acid (phenol) with water, used to kill germs. '1 in 20' means one part acid to twenty parts water.

§ Small tweezer-like tools used in surgeries or medical tasks to hold or pick up objects.

¶ A painful condition where jaw muscles tighten and can't open, often linked to tetanus.

** A serious infection caused by bacteria that affects the nervous system and causes

This unforeseen outbreak spread slowly, with the number of affected individuals increasing steadily each day.

In just a week to ten days, the village was plunged into a state of disarray. A staggering nineteen individuals, seemingly healthy days ago, died mysteriously. Panic descended upon the community, casting doubt and fear over the vaccination efforts.

The incident marked the first-ever 'adverse event' in the history of vaccination. The Australian Bundaberg tragedy – where twelve children had died following diphtheria vaccinations – would occur much later in 1928. Other fatal events had occurred in Dallas, Texas in 1919; Baden, Austria in 1923; Concord and Bridgewater, Massachusetts, in 1924, and Russia and China in 1926.[2] In Kyoto, Japan, 68 out of 606 children died after receiving diphtheria vaccinations in 1948. Later in 1955 the infamous Cutter incident in the US infected nearly 250 children with polio from the polio vaccines that were supposed to protect them.

As news of the Mulkowal disaster circulated, criticism mounted against Haffkine, his research and the vaccination campaign. Discontent was widespread, and voices of condemnation grew louder.

A commission was set up to investigate swiftly: it found that Haffkine had introduced a change in the vaccination sterilization process,* using heat instead of carbolic acid to expedite production – a method previously successful at the Pasteur Institute for years.

Criticism persisted, questioning Haffkine's methods and judgement. The commission's verdict pointed to bottle 53-N, suggesting the contamination had occurred at the Plague lab in Bombay. Haffkine now faced imminent repercussions. He was relieved of his directorial duties at the lab and placed on leave from the Indian Civil Service, a tumultuous turn of events for the once-celebrated scientist.

Caught in controversy and realizing his defence lay in London, he

---

muscle stiffness and spasms.

* A method used to make equipment or substances completely free of germs and bacteria.

promptly left India to clear his name. Two years after his suspension, the black death peaked in India, with a death toll of 1,143,993 people in 1904, rising above 1.3 million a year mark by 1907.[3]

Nevertheless, Haffkine's vaccine remained the 'main line of defence'. Later, the Government of Punjab would acknowledge that Haffkine's vaccination did help reduce new disease outbreaks among the inoculated to about one-fourth and the mortality to one-twelfth, and at least 10,000 lives have been saved by Haffkine.

7

ROSS AND THE RESCUE MISSION

IN AUGUST 1897, BRITISH SCIENTIST RONALD ROSS DISCOVERED the malarial parasite inside an Anopheles* mosquito's gut – a finding that earned him the Nobel Prize.

Two years earlier, at his laboratory in Hyderabad Ross had embarked on his study. He raised twenty adult mosquitoes from collected larvae and conducted a unique experiment – inducing them to feed on the blood of a malaria-stricken patient named Hussein Khan, compensating the latter with a modest fee of 8 annas. Four days later, Ross dissected the insects and discovered the malarial parasite. He identified these mosquitoes as 'dappled-wings', later recognized within the Anopheles genus.

Ross was born three days after the Indian Mutiny of 1857 in Almora, British India, a scenic town perched upon a ridge in the Kumaon Hills. He was the eldest of a bustling brood of ten, and his father Sir Campbell Claye Grant Ross was a general in the British Indian Army. His forebears had been linked to India for three generations.[1] At eight, Ross moved to England, leaving his Indian homeland behind. And it was while living with his aunt and uncle on the serene Isle of Wight that his inquisitive mind truly flourished.

Ross returned to India in 1881 to join the Indian Medical Service

---

* A group of mosquito species that are known to spread malaria to humans. Only female Anopheles mosquitoes transmit the disease.

with a clear aim: to study malaria. At his first posting in Calcutta, he delved into research on mosquito-borne transmission of malaria, a subject he had encountered during his studies. In 1912, he moved to London, where he became a physician for tropical diseases at King's College Hospital.

During his time in India, Ross had formed a friendship with Haffkine, though they rarely met. Ross worked in Bangalore and Hyderabad, while Haffkine was based in Bombay. Following the Mulkowal tragedy, Haffkine had undergone a gruelling four-year investigation that concluded in 1906. Despite significant evidence suggesting that the vaccine contamination with tetanus organisms had occured due to negligence at Mulkowal, the investigating committee held Haffkine responsible.

Investigations by the British Indian government, along with studies conducted by London's Lister Institute, traced the contamination to Bombay, speculating the omission of carbolic acid in the process as the potential cause. Ross and other supporters of Haffkine condemned this claim, contending that carbolic acid was irrelevant and that the contamination occurred when an assistant at Mulkowal accidentally dropped forceps on the ground and then used the non-sterile instrument to open bottle 53-N. They pointed out that if the contamination had indeed occurred six weeks earlier in Bombay, as the government claimed, the bottle would have emitted a noticeable odour. Yet the medical officer at Mulkowal had reported the bottle as odourless upon opening.

Thanks to the Lister Institute report, Haffkine was facing increasing pressure and humiliation for his alleged involvement in the disaster. In December 1906, Haffkine sought Ross's counsel, eager to hear his perspective and of other prominent figures who could influence the British empire and the Liverpool School of Tropical Medicine, where Ross was a professor.

Ross, known for his tenacity and loyalty, agreed to assist. With Haffkine's encouragement, he suggested pursuing rectification through both medical and general press.

Within the month, Ross took action. He wrote a letter in the *British Medical Journal*, decrying the disgraceful treatment meted out to Haffkine.[2] Ross also contemplated the possibility of mobilizing a group of prominent medical personnel to advocate for Haffkine and even arrange a delegation to meet with the Secretary of State for India, John Morley.

The first of his four impassioned missives, which he called 'hot letters', was published in the *London Times*.[3] He made a compelling case for Haffkine's vaccine, comparing it to Edward Jenner's smallpox vaccine. Meticulously outlining the chronology of the Mulkowal incident, he launched a rigorous critique of the Government of India for its baseless position and demanded reparations for the injustices inflicted upon Haffkine. His fiery critique demanded justice, sparking public outrage and solidarity. A week later, *Nature* published his blistering rebuke of authorities' mishandling of the incident, backed by Haffkine's evidence.

When responses to his *Times* letter justified further action, Ross penned another missive, lambasting systemic British incompetence and India's plague unpreparedness. He stressed Haffkine's singular effectiveness against the epidemic, declaring, 'The entire narrative arouses our deepest indignation,' while citing his own struggles with bureaucratic obstinacy during malaria research.

Haffkine, now stranded in London awaiting bureaucratic decisions, thanked Ross for amplifying his plight through the press, noting widespread attention to their campaign. Though grateful, he doubted parliamentary intervention would yield meaningful results, resigned to hollow official responses.

In another letter to the *Times*, Ross asserted that Haffkine's laboratory had no connection with the tragedy in Mulkowal. While Indian newspapers denied that Haffkine faced any punishment, Ross argued otherwise: Haffkine had been on half-pay for two years and received no pay at all for one year, losing opportunities for salary, advancement and recognition that his contributions deserved. Ross regarded this as a severe and unjust form of punishment.

Escalating his pitch, Ross pointed out that even after the erroneous verdict had been convincingly debunked, the authorities hesitated or refused to offer proper amends. He demanded that the government either fully reinstate Haffkine or settle its debt to him through a reasonable royalty for the millions of doses of his life-saving vaccine that had been administered.[4]

Despite Ross's efforts, the India Office remained unyielding. On 5 June, it informed Haffkine that the Secretary of State would not reopen an inquiry into a matter they considered exhaustively examined.

In the meantime, Haffkine confided to Ross that the evidence clearly proved his innocence, but the government was unwilling to accept it. Resigned to his fate, he decided to leave the Indian service. Ross, disheartened by the India Office's 'incorrect' conclusion, agreed that Haffkine was justified in resigning from a government that had treated him with such ingratitude and injustice.

In June 1907, both men received copies of the Parliamentary Return of Papers, a comprehensive 108-page document detailing the Mulkowal incident. For the first time, the entire account was accessible to the scientific community, presenting an opportunity for a decisive statement. Recognizing this, Ross joined William Simpson, a founder of the London School of Tropical Medicine and the first medical officer of Calcutta, along with eight other prominent scientists, in drafting a joint letter to the *Times*. This document presented a measured analysis of the Mulkowal tragedy, dismantling each charge one by one. In conclusion, the letter expressed a hope that the Government of India would either exonerate Haffkine or initiate a new and more authoritative inquiry.[5] It worked.

Later that summer, the India Office extended an offer of employment to Haffkine. In September, he responded to the Secretary of State reiterating that the Mulkowal incident should not have been attributed to the Bombay laboratory. While addressing the offer indirectly, Haffkine pointed out that he had faced censure and punishment. His primary concern was to clear his name. He requested that the government absolve him of responsibility for the accident and reinstate him under the earlier terms. This, he argued, would allow him to accept the position he was being offered.

By November 1907 the Secretary of State acknowledged Haffkine's stance. In turn, Haffkine accepted the offer of re-employment but with key clarifications. He insisted that his unaltered salary should not be seen as a reprimand and highlighted that a significant consensus absolved him of the blame for the Mulkowal incident.

Though the resolution reinstated Haffkine, it fell short of restoring his position as Director of the Bombay Laboratory, which he had founded. Nevertheless, it marked an end to his prolonged ordeal.

8

HAFFKINE'S HUMILIATION

UPON ARRIVING IN CALCUTTA, HAFFKINE RESUMED HIS research from where he had left off in 1905. He quickly realized the Indian government was unwilling to involve him in public health initiatives. Although frustrated, he focused on fine-tuning his vaccine against cholera and completing the research on the plague vaccine.

For nearly two years, Haffkine occupied himself with routine administrative work. In April 1909, he wrote to L. C. Porter, the Secretary to the Government of India, emphasizing his experience in developing a devitalized anti-cholera vaccine in 1892. He hoped to remind the decision makers of his value to vaccine research.

Fearing the government's concerns about him deploying live microbes on humans in trials,* Haffkine changed his proposal. He suggested focusing his expertise on devitalized plague vaccine and advancing large-scale production and trials of the devitalized anti-cholera vaccine.[1]

The government responded months later, rejecting his request to conduct any kind of vaccination campaign.[2] Unofficially, this reluctance was attributed to fears of unrest, particularly in light of the disastrous Bilibid Prison incident in Manila, Philippines, in 1906. In the Bilibid case, thirteen prisoners had died after receiving

* Microorganism, like a bacteria or virus, that are still active and capable of causing disease.

contaminated plague vaccines, sparking riots in the prison. But unlike the Mulkowal incident, the Manila case was quietly swept under the carpet. The British scientist responsible, Richard Pearson Strong, did not face any career setbacks and went on to become the first professor of tropical medicine at the Harvard School of Public Health.[3]

The official response to Haffkine's proposal did not acknowledge them either. Instead it referenced the 'fair measure of success' of a devitalized vaccine in Japan in 1902 and cited a 'general hesitancy' among the public towards voluntary inoculation. It emphasized ordinary sanitation measures as a sufficient form of protective strategy. Haffkine was 'encouraged' to continue his laboratory investigations but cautioned to adhere to the conditions of his engagement, limiting him to pure research and barring him from field trials. He was also strongly advised against privately corresponding with field health officers about his vaccine.[4]

By now it was clear Haffkine had been set on a tight leash by the British masters; his activities were closely watched, his communications scrutinized, his autonomy restricted. But undeterred, the scientist kept petitioning the authorities for research support and permissions.

In February 1911, he appealed to the government again, reiterating that he had demonstrated the preparation of devitalized vaccines long before. He reminded them of the successful human trials of his anti-cholera vaccine in Paris and its proven efficacy during the 1900 cholera outbreak in Naghpour Central Jail. He still got no response. Once again, Haffkine wrote to Porter, this time requesting an expansion of his laboratory staff – one medical officer and one technician – to advance his research on the devitalized vaccine.[5]

Porter's response reiterated the prohibition on human trials while expressing scepticism about the research. Haffkine was offered temporary assistance for laboratory work to perfect the devitalized cholera virus, but the response explicitly stated that the vaccine could not be administered on humans until a report on the experiments was submitted with its results corroborated by other researchers.[6]

Haffkine faced his final defeat when he lost control over the production and distribution of his anti-plague vaccine. His attempt to regain influence through the introduction and field tests of a new cholera vaccine also proved unsuccessful. By then, it had been seven years since he had first arrived in India after being exonerated. Dejected, he decided to seek retirement in 1915, just after crossing fifty-five, the minimum legal retirement age, not only from the service of the British government in India but also from any scientific activity.

Until his retirement, he continued to seek opportunities to conduct field trials for his newly developed devitalized anti-cholera vaccine. These efforts subjected him to many humiliations – a bitter experience for a researcher who had developed two life-saving vaccines, conducted trials across the country and played a key role in containing a pandemic to a great extent.

While Haffkine was away from India since 1902 after his suspension, the production of a devitalized anti-cholera vaccine became the principal activity of the Bombay Plague Institute, overseen by W. B. Bannerman, who succeeded Haffkine as director.

In 1911, Bannerman was replaced by W. G. Liston, an ex-assistant of Haffkine's, whom he suspected of playing a role in his downfall. Liston's tenure ended in 1913, and in 1925, the Bombay Plague Laboratory was renamed the Haffkine Institute.[7] However, by that time, Haffkine had been gone from India for over a decade.

When he left the second time, Haffkine's departure was deeply painful. He believed his British bosses did not trust him because of his Soviet origins, and his association with the Narodnaya Volya and Russian student politics.

It was clear that the British military hierarchy, whose medical officers wielded influence in public health, had fallen out with Haffkine. Over time, the military's control over anti-plague measures began to decline. Because of Anglo-Russian differences, he was also accused of being a spy. Russian writers cautioned Christians to be wary of him, citing his Jewish background.

The growing antisemitism of the era exacerbated his plight,

rooted in centuries of prejudice across Europe. During the Black Death of the 1340s, Jews had been accused of causing the bubonic plague pandemic by poisoning wells – a baseless claim that ignited widespread violence.[8]

By the twentieth century, calls for annihilation of Jews had reached a fever pitch, exploited by leaders like Hitler and Mussolini. Haffkine, therefore, prudently decided to pack his bags to France, not Britain. in 1915. He settled in Boulogne-sur-Seine, a quiet suburb of Paris, before he shifted to Lausanne, Switzerland, a year before his death.

On 26 October 1930, Haffkine died a quiet and solitary death. He left his modest wealth to fund Jewish schools, reflecting his later years' dedication to religious education.

Haffkine's trajectory was less fortunate than that of the British-born scientist J. B. S. Haldane, who in 1961 arrived in India, offering his scientific acumen and his *Journal of Genetics* to a young republic. Haldane's support was a triumph for India as it sought to redefine science in a post-colonial era. In contrast, Haffkine's illustrious public health career was curtailed at fifty-five, largely because of the inoculation accident at Malkowal while he was the director of the laboratory responsible for manufacturing and distributing the vaccine.

Nevertheless, the scientific community acknowledged Haffkine's contributions to the cholera and plague vaccine. He was considered the architect of the controlled human testing of an acceptable cholera vaccine and for convincing the medical world that protective inoculations were safe and effective. Decades later, the World Health Organization recognized Haffkine 'as the first to define the principles of controlled field trials and, moreover, to use them.'[9]

When news of Haffkine's death reached the Haffkine Institute on 26 October 1930, the institute and Grant Medical College in Bombay closed their doors in his honour. The media hailed him as a saviour of humanity, placing him alongside Jenner, Pasteur and Joseph Lister, forming the trinity of modern medicine.

PART II

BUILDING BLOCKS
(1931–1960)

9

SAHIB SINGH SOKHEY

THE BURMA CAMPAIGN, PART OF THE SOUTHEAST ASIAN THEATRE of World War II, was a brutal military campaign where the Allied forces – the British Empire and the Republic of China, with support from the United States – fought against the invading might of the Japanese Army. Backed by the Thai Phayap Army and two collaborationist independence movements, Japan invaded Burma and soon seized control over Rangoon. In 1942 and 1943, the international Allied forces, stationed in British India, launched several offensives, seeking to reclaim lost territories. The forces of the British Empire swelled to around a million – land and air troops – and at its peak, faced an unseen, formidable enemy in the impenetrable jungles of Burma – snakes.

Infested with highly poisonous cobras and vipers, these forests turned out to be killing fields for the advancing British and Allied troops. Unfortunately, there were no proven or efficient anti-venom remedies to treat the reptile-bitten soldiers, making matters worse. It was then that the British government reached out to a medical officer who had joined the Indian Medical Service as Lieutenant in 1913 and served in the World War I in France and Mesopotamia, Sahib Singh Sokhey.

Sokhey was heading the Haffkine Institute in Bombay. He began developing a potent polyvalent antivenin* at his Serum Department,

* Anti-venom treat that works against multiple types of venomous snakes.

capable of providing protection against the bite of four venomous snakes – Indian cobra, Russell's viper, Indian saw-scaled viper and common krait. Unlike the existing antivenin, which only safeguarded against cobra bites, the refined polyvalent antivenin was freeze-dried,* allowing it to retain its efficacy indefinitely, without any deterioration. Sokhey's anti-venom proved invaluable for the British and Allied forces and after a visit to a snake farm in Bangkok, he started a similar farm at the institute.[1]

Sahib Singh Sokhey hailed from a family of traditional craftsmen who had played a leading role in the construction of the Golden Temple in Amritsar. He did his schooling from Central Medical School and Government College, Lahore, going on to secure an honours degree in physics and chemistry from the University of Punjab. Sokhey then joined Edinburgh University, where he completed an MBBS degree in 1911 and an MA in Economics in 1912. During his time in the UK, Sokhey actively engaged in local political activities, shaping his outlook in alignment with Western intellectual traditions. He joined the Indian Medical Service as a lieutenant in 1913.[2]

In 1923, Sokhey received the Rockefeller Fellowship and began his postgraduate studies in the US, Canada and England. He sharpened his skills in clinical biochemistry while studying at Harvard and Trinity College, Cambridge.[3] It was in these renowned institutions that Sokhey's dedication to and aptitude for sound scientific thinking found a fitting environment.

In 1925, after twelve years of service with the Army medical corps and serving in World War I, Sokhey, now a major at the IMS,[4] embarked on a new chapter at the Haffkine Institute, formerly known as the Bombay Plague Laboratory. With a grant of ₹73,000 from the

* A way to preserve medicine by removing water, so it lasts longer and can be stored easily without refrigeration.

Indian Research Fund Association (IRFA) and ₹15,000 from the Bombay Government, he set up a biochemistry department as he strongly believed that '[i]t is practically impossible to practice modern medicine without the aid of biochemical analytical work.'[5]

Picking up from the work of Haffkine, Sokhey began focusing on a pressing issue – the refinement of the plague vaccine. In a year's time, the young Biochemistry Department, with its stellar work, had started looking more promising. Having served as the officiating director on multiple occasions, Sokhey secured the permanent director position in 1932, becoming the first Indian to assume the role. Thereafter, he served with distinction for an unprecedented seventeen years, including a two-year extension, and finally retired in 1949.[6]

To focus on the plague, he created an Entomology[*] Department in 1938, headed by eminent Cambridge-trained entomologist Dr R. V. Deobhankar. Two years later, a Serum Department was instituted to produce tetanus, diphtheria, dysentery and gas gangrene antitoxins[†]; tetanus and diphtheria toxoids[‡]; and polyvalent antivenin. The same year, a Chemotherapy Department too was established to conduct research on synthetic drugs.[7]

The Pharmacology Department, maintained by the IRFA, was integrated with the institute in 1943 and began drug testing and biological standardization.[§] This would eventually become the Drug Control Organization, the pharmaceutical regulatory system of the country. Under Sokhey's leadership, advancements were made in the manufacture of plague and cholera vaccines, one such advancement being the introduction of the casein-hydrolysate liquid medium.[¶][8]

---

* A branch of science focused on studying insects.

† Medicines used to treat a dangerous infection where tissues die due to lack of oxygen and release deadly toxins.

‡ Germ toxins that have been made harmless but still teach the body to defend itself – used in vaccines.

§ A process to make sure medicines and vaccines are consistently effective and safe.

¶ A nutrient-rich liquid made from milk protein, used to grow bacteria for making vaccines.

In the meantime, the institute was emerging as the main vaccine factory of the country, serving almost 300 million people. The vaccine production kept increasing and by 1947 it was producing nearly 50 million doses, ten times the quantity that was being produced when Sokhey had taken over as the full-time director in 1932. However, his biggest contribution was redesigning the plague and cholera vaccines to make them more efficient.

At the time of his joining in 1925, Sokhey had been inundated with complaints from all over the country regarding the toxicity of the plague vaccine. He identified several issues, including the lack of proper staff training, crude production methods and erratic standardization and quality control of vaccines. Armed with this knowledge, he embarked on the laborious task of redeveloping the plague vaccine.[9]

Sokhey discovered that repeated subculturing of plague bacteria in blood agar could render the organism avirulent,* moving away from the conventional method of passing bacteria through rats. Since bacteria lose their ability to cause strong responses over time when grown in artificial media, they were injected into a live rat, allowed to multiply within the animal and then extracted from the infected tissues or blood. This finding led to the development of a live plague vaccine, the efficacy of which proved to be superior to the traditionally killed vaccine.[10]

The techniques Sokhey developed for the plague vaccine were applicable to the cholera vaccine as well. Using white Swiss mice as test subjects, he devised a mouse protection test† to assess the cholera vaccine's effectiveness. He also employed a similar approach to compare the efficacy of the cholera vaccine, prepared in a casein hydrolysate medium with the standard agar-grown vaccine.[11] The cholera vaccine, produced in the liquid medium, demonstrated improved efficacy and was subsequently manufactured in large

* A microorganism that is alive but no longer causes disease – safe to use in vaccines.

† A lab test using mice to check if a vaccine works by seeing if it protects them from a disease.

quantities using the equipment and system designed for the plague vaccine.[12]

During 1938–39, the Indian National Congress was looking for experts for a National Planning Committee covering various issues under the leadership of Subhas Chandra Bose. This was soon after the British had promised India independence in order to secure Indian support in World War II. After defining the composition of a national plan, the Committee decided to work on detailed plans in specific areas. Twenty-nine sub-committees, organized into eight groups, were formed to address various aspects of national life. In this dispensation, Sokhey was the natural choice to head the health sub-committee.

Though the sub-committees commenced their work in 1939 after some unexpected delays, everything went awry when World War II broke out in September of that year and Bose disappeared from India to work against the British from outside the country. The work of the committees halted until the end of the war in 1945, although some of the final and interim reports, already prepared by sub-committees, were considered during plenary sessions of the parent committee in 1940. Due to the arrest and imprisonment of the new committee chair Pandit Jawaharlal Nehru towards the end of that year, the Committee's work had to be temporarily suspended. The report would eventually be ready and released in 1947, the year India gained independence.[13]

Sokhey's fascination with planning, as an enthusiastic admirer of the Soviet Union, came in handy while preparing the report, as did his rational approach for determining tasks, allocating priorities and managing resources for the collective benefit of the nation. Back then participating in such a committee was nearly considered a violation of service rules for government officers yet Sokhey dared to defy convention.

Sokhey firmly advocated for the drug and vaccine industry to remain exclusively in the public sector, devoid of profit motives – a perspective shared by Jawaharlal Nehru, as can be derived from many of his speeches. This brought him closer to the tallest leader of the time,[14] Mahatma Gandhi, whom he admired for his non-dogmatic and non-fanatical views. He always cherished Gandhi's visit to the Haffkine Institute, when they had demonstrated the measures undertaken by the institute to control plague. He disapproved those who exploited Gandhi's name for personal gain and harboured contempt for many high-ranking politicians for their lack of understanding of economics and ignorance of global developments.[15]

In 1945, when the British Indian government established a committee on fine chemicals, drugs and pharmaceuticals, Sokhey was inducted as a senior member.[16] Along with other experts like K. Ganapathi, he provided details on the production of vaccines, anti-toxins and sera, in addition to sharing comprehensive information on the manufacturing processes of sulpha drugs,* mepacrine (atebrin),† penicillin‡ and vitamin A concentrate from shark liver oil.[17]

By the time of India's independence from the British, Sokhey had elevated the Haffkine Institute to a globally renowned medical research institution and vaccine factory. However, his journey was about to take a significant turn. In 1949, Dr Brock Chisholm, the director general of the World Health Organization (WHO), after spending three days with Sokhey in Bombay, was so impressed by the accomplishments of the institute and the visionary plans of its director that he offered Sokhey the position of Assistant Director General for Technical Services with a focus on epidemiology,§ biological standardization and health statistics at WHO Geneva.

However, Sokhey was faced with a dilemma. The biggest challenge in accepting the Geneva position was bringing Prime Minister Jawaharlal Nehru on board. He succeeded by outlining his vision of leveraging his new role to build world-class projects and institutes in

---

* Or Sulphathiazole; early antibiotics used to treat bacterial infections before penicillin became widely available.

† A drug used to treat malaria and sometimes other parasitic infections.

‡ The first widely used antibiotic, discovered in 1928, that treats many bacterial infections.

§ The science of studying how diseases spread and affect populations.

India. True to his word, Dr Sokhey played a pivotal role in initiating and finalizing the establishment of a penicillin factory at Pimpri and a DDT factory to aid pest control, with support from WHO and UNICEF.

In 1952, when Dr Sokhey returned to India after completing his term, he was honoured with a nomination to the Rajya Sabha by the Indian Government. He was recognized as one of the top healthcare and medical research experts in the country. Subsequently, he chaired the Pharmaceutical and Drugs Committee of the Council of Scientific and Industrial Research (CSIR), laying the groundwork for a significant public sector drug project, which would later emerge as the Indian Drugs and Pharmaceuticals Limited (IDPL), the country's most extensive initiative in drug manufacturing in its time.[18] Although his advocacy for a National Microbiological Laboratory did not fully materialize, it did eventually integrate with the National Biological Laboratory.[19]

In the 1950s, the Haffkine Institute faced a significant obstacle when it endeavoured to produce sulphathiazole, an antimicrobial with powerful curative properties. A foreign firm held a patent* on the drug, posing a challenge to the institute's plans. The institute sought a compulsory license, a provision under which the Government can issue a license notwithstanding the patent rights held by any company. The case then proceeded to the High Court in Calcutta and as the legal proceedings unfolded, it became evident that the Indian Patent Act had flaws that were detrimental to national interests.

Sokhey refused to accept the status quo and took a proactive stance. He wrote to the Government of India, urging a revision of the Act in a way that would better align with the nation's needs. This initiative led to the formation of the Patent Enquiry Committee, with Sokhey serving as a member. The committee was tasked with a thorough examination of the provisions of the act and proposing necessary changes.

---

* A legal right given to inventors or companies to exclusively make and sell their invention for a certain period.

The interim report submitted by the committee suggested amendments to Sections 22 and 23 of the Indian Patent Act, specifically addressing the issue of compulsory licenses. Despite continued challenges and resistance from foreign patentees and their local supporters, it was only in 1970 when a comprehensive revision of the Indian Patent Act of 1911 was carried out, marking a major breakthrough after twenty-five years of efforts.

Sokhey, a staunch advocate for the complete abrogation of the Act, played a pivotal role in pushing for reforms. The resulting 1970 Patent Act, while not fully aligning with Sokhey's position, represented a compromise between opposing viewpoints, ultimately shaping the landscape of new patent regulations in India.[20] It would further be reviewed comprehensively only in 2005 to align with the TRIPS Agreement of the World Trade Organization (WTO).

It would be accurate to suggest that the history of the Haffkine Institute and India's vaccine research from 1925 to 1949 is essentially the story of Sahib Singh Sokhey. His influence continued over the institute and India's medical research even after his retirement, although this time as a mentor and strategist. Under his leadership, the Haffkine Institute rose to the pinnacle of medical research in the country.

In many ways, Sokhey was the unique hero of a rapidly transforming India, someone who was deeply invested in building a strong healthcare foundation for an emerging independent nation.

Perhaps the greatest tribute to the legacy of Sokhey was the award-winning American novelist Louis Bromfield featuring him in two of his novels, *Night in Bombay* and *The Rains Came*. The latter was even adapted as a Hollywood movie with the same title in 1939 and then again as *The Rains of Ranchipur* in 1955.

10

SMALLPOX: A BIG CHALLENGE

LONG AGO, A DEADLY SCOURGE, MARKED BY FEVER AND PAINFUL pustules, ravaged the Indian subcontinent. Known as smallpox, it claimed thousands of lives wherever it appeared. On average, three out of ten infected died, while survivors bore permanent scars all over their bodies.

In Sanskrit, smallpox is known as *masurika,* a term drawn from the lentil, whose shape and orange hue mirror its telltale pustules. Many Indic languages adopted derivatives of this name – *chechak* in Hindi, for instance.

The deadly impact of smallpox is documented in ancient medical texts of Charaka and Sushruta. The ancient Indian physician Vagabhat describes the chilling progression of the disease in *Ashtangahrdaya Samhita,* a Sanskrit text on Ayurveda: 'He on whose body the masurika, appearing like coral globules, breaks out then swiftly vanishes, dies quickly.'[1] Around the same time, the Christian physician Ahrun from Alexandria wrote the first Western treatise on smallpox, clearly identifying the disease.[2]

In the Indian subcontinent, where myth and mysticism often intertwine, smallpox acquired a unique position. Each village had its own local deity, placing their idol beneath an ancient tree. Among these deities, one reigned supreme: Sitala, the goddess of smallpox, whose name paradoxically meant 'cool'. In southern India, she went by the name Maariyamma (Mother of Diseases), a maternal figure associated with the final embrace of death.[3]

Sitala or Maariyamma and her counterparts were believed to protect communities against smallpox. Survivors attributed their recovery to the goddess's benevolence, while those who died were thought to have faced her wrath. For Hindus, smallpox was more than a medical malady; they considered it a divine message, a sign of the wrath of the goddess. To appease her, they performed fervent rituals, including animal sacrifices, pleading for her divine intervention to get reprieve from the relentless scourge. People credited her for the decline in deaths, even while seeking and accepting modern medical aid.[4]

Smallpox is considered to have first appeared around 10,000 BCE, almost alongside the first agricultural settlements in Africa. Anthropologists argue that it spread to India through ancient Egyptian merchants and migratory routes.[5] Evidence of smallpox is visible on Egyptian mummies over 3,000 years old, while the earliest written records of similar disease date to fourth-century China and seventh-century India.

By the sixth century, burgeoning trade with China and Korea introduced smallpox to Japan. The seventh-century Arab expansion carried the disease to the shores of northern Africa, Spain and Portugal, leaving a trail of suffering in its wake. By the eleventh century during the Crusades, a time of religious zeal and conquest, smallpox was entrenched in Europe.[6]

Fast forward to the fifteenth century, Portuguese colonization led smallpox to western Africa, unwittingly introducing smallpox to this new frontier. The transatlantic slave trade and European settlers in the sixteenth century imported smallpox onto new lands. The Caribbean, Central and South America bore the brunt of this calamity. By the seventeenth century, it reached the shores of North America, and in the eighteenth century, explorers from Great Britain introducing smallpox to a previously unscathed territory, Australia.

Smallpox was both endemic and seasonal, mostly spreading

during the hot season stretching from February to June. The virus could survive outside the human body for several years: it spreads more during drought seasons and recedes when there is increased atmospheric humidity.

One of the earliest methods used to control smallpox was variolation, a crude technique to induce immunity in people who had never been exposed to the virus. The term derives from the virus that causes smallpox, *variola*. This practice probably originated in the Middle East or China, where it was first observed that individuals who survived smallpox seldom got infected again.

Variolation involved exposing someone who had never been infected to material from smallpox sores (pustules), either by scratching it into a small cut on their skin or by making them inhale it. Usually, individuals afterwards develop symptoms of smallpox, such as fever and a rash. George Washington is known to have used it to protect his army during the War of Independence against Great Britain.[7]

However, it wasn't until the end of the eighteenth century that a reliable prophylactic measure was introduced. In 1796, Edward Jenner came up with the cowpox vaccine as a powerful preventive measure, using lymph from infected calf. This was when efforts to prevent smallpox marked the first large-scale state-sponsored medical interventions around the world.

Haffkine, in a lecture before the Conjoint Board of the Royal Colleges of Physicians of London and Surgeons of England in 1895, described the origin of smallpox vaccine. He noted: 'The practice of inoculation against smallpox was originated from the observation that there are mild and severe epidemics of the disease, and that people affected in mild years remained immune in severe years.'[8] This observation would later lead to the development of vaccines to generate herd immunity.*

---

* When enough people in a community become immune to a disease, either through vaccination or past infection.

He also made a clear distinction between the term 'vaccine' and the matter used for variolation: 'The Eastern practice of inoculating [with] smallpox virus against smallpox is variolation. On the other hand, the substance cultivated under conditions intended to keep the morbid agent at a given and fixed state of virulence, permitting the use of it with safety and sure measurement, such as Jenner's calf lymph,* or Pasteur's rabies emulsions, is a vaccine.'[9]

This speech offers one of the earliest accurate explanations of vaccine. Although Haffkine did not sway into research on smallpox viral vaccines, maybe because he was focused on bacterial vaccines, he was keenly observing the smallpox research – treatments and modes of prophylaxis.† He encouraged clinicians and researchers working on smallpox, both while he was at the Pasteur Institute in Paris and in India.

By the nineteenth century, the most common form of vaccine was humanized lymph, initially produced by vaccinators and later at designated spots called 'depots'. The production process involved collecting pustular material from a cow or a buffalo that had been inoculated with smallpox matter. Human beings were 'operated on' with this artificially induced vaccinifier, often travelling with vaccinators to serve as a source of fresh lymph or milked for vaccine matter that was stored for deployment by touring officials at a later date.[10]

In March 1801, the Government of India requested the authorities in Constantinople (Istanbul) to send the smallpox 'vaccine matter' to Bombay. However, the challenge lay in safely transporting the vaccine matter across thousands of kilometres. The only viable option was through land routes via Constantinople, Vienna, Baghdad and Bussora, and from Bussora (Basra) to Bombay by sea.

It wasn't until September 1801 that the request was fulfilled, and the 'precious cargo' began its journey. The solution was to send the 'vaccine matter' through human carriers, individuals inoculated with smallpox vaccine matter who would carry the live virus within their bodies.

---

* A fluid taken from a cow or calf infected with cowpox, used to create a vaccine for smallpox.

† Preventive treatment taken to stop a disease before it happens.

After several unsuccessful attempts, the vaccine matter was successfully produced in Baghdad in early 1802, sourced from a person previously vaccinated in Constantinople and brought there for this purpose. A set of people were vaccinated with the 'vaccine matter' in Baghdad to be human carriers. These newly vaccinated carrier individuals started their journey from Baghdad, covering around 2,100 kilometres by road to reach the port in Bussora. Between Baghdad and Bussora, they encountered numerous setbacks as the vaccine pustules healed, rendering them non-infectious. Nevertheless, active carriers with unhealed pustules set sail for Bombay, traversing approximately 3,400 kilometres or 1,800 nautical miles across the sea.[11]

The ship carrying this most 'precious cargo' finally landed in Bombay in June 1802. The first recipient was a three-year-old baby girl named Anna Dusthall, who was vaccinated in Bombay in June 1802. Although of European ancestry, the origins of her mother remain shrouded in uncertainty. As Professor Michael Bennett puts it in his book, *War Against Smallpox*: 'All vaccinations in the subcontinent came from this girl.' In the following week, the torch of immunity was passed on to five other children in Bombay, as they received the pus taken from Dusthall's arm. This gave rise to the entire stock of vaccine virus in use across India.

The vaccine then traversed the length of India's eastern coast. In the port-city of Madras, thirteen-year-old John Cresswell from Port Jackson in Australia was vaccinated. He then became a carrier – a journey that led him to Bengal by November 1802, marking a significant milestone.[12]

Europeans readily embraced the vaccine. In one year, approximately 11,100 individuals had been inoculated. The local populations, however, especially Hindu communities, expressed reservations about the vaccine due to its bovine origins,* as cows held a revered status in their culture. Also, in some cases, parents of vaccinated children

* Coming from cows or related to cattle.

refused to allow them to become carriers, adding further complexities to the expansion programme.[13] Nevertheless, the vaccine continued to travel, transferred arm-to-arm across territories in India, including Hyderabad, Cochin, Tellicherry, Chingleput and ultimately, the royal court of Mysore.

At the time, in Mysore, the twelve-year-old Devajammani was on the precipice of a life-altering union with Krishnaraja Wadiyar III, the newly anointed ruler of the southern kingdom. Soon Devajammani found herself enlisted for a monumental cause – to champion the smallpox vaccine. Unbeknownst to her, her role was immortalized in a nineteenth-century painting – three half-smiling royal women striking a casual pose with Devajammani's right hand pointing to the injection site on the left hand – commissioned by the East India Company to rally support for the vaccination programme, creating the first-ever vaccine promotion campaign.[14]

While the names of many who ensured the vaccine's supply and propagation went unrecorded, unlike Devajammani's case, the responsibility passed through the hands of many 'unexceptional bodies.' Among these were three 'half-caste' children who played a pivotal role in re-establishing the supply in Madras, and a young Malay boy who served as a dedicated ferryman, ensuring the vaccine's safe arrival in the bustling city of Calcutta. These often-overlooked contributions of marginalized individuals, who played essential roles in the successful distribution and propagation of vaccines during such crucial public health efforts, would only come to light much later. At a time when untouchability was at its peak among upper castes, most had no hesitation in receiving vaccines that had been transferred from lower-caste children.

This shift in attitudes towards vaccination highlights a broader transformation in colonial health policies. With the advent of vaccination, the British stance on variolation shifted dramatically. By the mid-nineteenth century, variolation was condemned as 'a murderous trade.'[15]

Vaccinating the vast population of Indians proved challenging.

British administrators acknowledged the potential to build human resistance to smallpox by introducing milder forms of smallpox 'poison' but consensus on the matter was difficult to achieve. Debates about the vaccine's efficacy often centred on constitutional predispositions and climatic factors believed to influence the virulence of the smallpox virus.[16]

The public response to vaccination was labelled 'resistance' due to perceptions of irrationality and superstition. Among Hindu communities, the Brahmins who controlled temples feared vaccination would bring down the importance of gods and goddesses and thereby, their influence on people. There was also a deep-rooted concern about introducing a bovine disease into their healthy children. Translating the concept of cowpox to the locals was a more persistent challenge. Sanskrit scholars were enlisted to find terms that resonated with the community, which hinted at diseases far more menacing than cowpox. Alarm also grew that cowpox might wreak havoc among cattle.

A more pressing dilemma loomed. The most effective method to administer the vaccine was an 'arm-to-arm' technique, wherein the initial recipient was inoculated by applying the vaccine to their arm using a needle or lancet. A week later, when a cowpox pustule formed at the vaccination site, a physician would incise it and transfer the pus onto another person's arm. At times, the lymph from a patient's arm would be painstakingly dried and sealed between glass plates for transportation, but more often than not, it did not survive the arduous journey intact.

Progress was slow and uneven. Across vast stretches of the nation vaccination efforts only gained momentum well into the 1850s, and it wasn't until the 1880s that its impact became unmistakably evident. This ushered an era in which smallpox became a minor contributor to mortality in India.

Regional examples, such as Oudh (modern-day Uttar Pradesh) and Berar (present-day North Karnataka) vindicate the intricate connection between the expansion of vaccination and the decline of smallpox.

Notwithstanding its introduction in 1802, vaccination took nearly seven to nine decades to fully proliferate across the subcontinent. Once established, however, mass primary vaccination significantly reduced smallpox mortality.

Ironically, during this period, specifically from the 1870s to 1890s, India endured severe blows to its population due to devastating famines and epidemics. Yet, this medical intervention went undeterred. After a prolonged and arduous battle spanning most of the nineteenth century, smallpox was restrained. Yet it vigorously resurfaced several times in the twentieth century. As late as 1958, it claimed over 150,000 lives in India.

In 1959, WHO initiated a global plan to eradicate smallpox. The effort faced significant challenges, including a lack of funds, personnel and limited international commitment, coupled with a shortage of vaccine donations. As a result, smallpox outbreaks persisted through the 1960s across South America, Africa and Asia.

A turning point came with the Global Intensified Smallpox Eradication Programme in 1967, ushering in a renewed commitment to the cause. Laboratories in many countries where smallpox remained endemic could now produce a greater quantity of high-quality freeze-dried vaccines. The success of these intensified efforts was also bolstered by key developments, including the bifurcated needle, a robust case surveillance system and large-scale vaccination campaigns.

In India, the National Smallpox Eradication Programme (NSEP), launched in 1962, initially aimed to vaccinate the entire population within three years. But it failed due to insufficient coverage and accessibility. By 1964, the government shifted its strategy to focus on high-risk regions like Bihar, Uttar Pradesh, Madhya Pradesh and West Bengal. Despite these efforts, in 1974, the country faced a severe smallpox epidemic, creating significant challenges in vaccinating its 600 million people.[17]

By this time, smallpox had already been eliminated in North America and Europe over a decade ago. The campaign focused on the disease-prevalent regions in South America, Asia and Africa. By 1971, South America had been declared free of smallpox, followed by Asia in 1975 and ultimately Africa in 1977, marking a monumental triumph in the global fight against the disease.[18]

India's 1974 smallpox epidemic affected 188,000 people and resulted in 31,000 deaths. While media reports portrayed it as the worst outbreak in history, even worse than the epidemics of 1875 and 1967, this claim is debatable due to improved reporting standards. Strangely, it coincided with the intensified anti-smallpox campaign, which shifted from mass vaccinations to search and containment. The states of Bihar and Uttar Pradesh were hit the hardest, accounting for about three-quarters of the total cases.[19]

In 1975 three-year-old Rahima Banu from Bangladesh became the last person in the world to naturally contract *variola major*, marking the end of active smallpox in Asia. She was isolated at home under a twenty-four-hour guard, with a house-to-house vaccination campaign conducted within a 1.5-mile radius of her home. The last person to naturally acquire smallpox caused by *variola minor* was Ali Maow Maali, a hospital cook in Merca, Somalia, who fell ill in 1977 after accompanying smallpox patients in a vehicle. Initially misdiagnosed with malaria and then chickenpox, he was later confirmed to have smallpox and recovered completely. A year later, the last person to die from smallpox became Janet Parker, a medical photographer at England's Birmingham University Medical School, who fell ill with a rash but wasn't diagnosed with smallpox until nine days later.

In India, the last smallpox case was reported in 1975 in Karimganj, a village in the Cachar district of Assam. The patient had contracted the disease in the Sylhet district in Bangladesh, before travelling to India. The final case where the disease was acquired in the country involved a nine-year-old boy from Pachera in Bihar's Katihar district.[20]

Now that the smallpox virus has been eradicated globally, routine vaccinations are no longer required. However, vaccine stocks maintained in key laboratories to address sudden outbreaks. Modern smallpox vaccines contain the *vaccinia* virus, not the variola virus matter. It offers protection but in rare cases can present serious, and potentially fatal, side effects. Since eradication, it has been used to safeguard researchers working with variola and related viruses. Recently, a newer, third-generation vaccine with safer strains was developed for high-risk groups, but its effectiveness remains uncertain since it has not been used on humans yet.

By the early 1980s, remaining stocks of the smallpox virus were destroyed or secured in two laboratories: the Centers for Disease Control and Prevention in Atlanta, Georgia, United States, and the Russian State Centre for Research on Virology and Biotechnology in Koltsovo, Novosibirsk Region, Russian Federation. No other laboratory has been officially granted access to the virus since.[21]

A debate continues over whether to retain or destroy these last samples. Proponents of destruction highlight the risk of accidental release in retaining the samples, while opponents argue for their scientific and research value, particularly in studying smallpox virus variants in the natural world. The real threat remains the re-emergence of the virus as a bioweapon.

11

TYPHOID MARY

IN 1906, GEORGE SOPER, A RESEARCHER IN NEW YORK, uncovered a unique case in the battle against typhoid fever in New York. He was able to trace a series of outbreaks to a single individual.

Typhoid, a bacterial infection that typically spread through food and water contaminated by *Salmonella* Typhi, was rampant in New York at the time, and had caused around 639 reported deaths that year. Soper's investigation revealed that thirty-seven-year-old Irish cook Mary Mallon, employed in various wealthy households, had been unwittingly transmitting typhoid through her cooking. What set Mallon apart was her lack of symptoms, making her the first known healthy carrier* of typhoid.

After four months of investigation, following a trail of twenty-two infected people, Soper located Mallon working in a Park Avenue brownstone. On being confronted with evidence and asked to provide urine and stool samples for further analysis, Mallon surged at Soper with a carving fork.[1] Because of her lack of symptoms, Mallon resisted providing the samples. She was eventually apprehended with the help of the New York police. Quarantined on North Brother Island, Mallon was soon labelled 'Typhoid Mary' and prevented from moving around freely.

---

* A person who has a disease-causing germ in their body but doesn't show any symptoms, yet can still spread the disease to others.

Mallon did not believe she was a carrier, most likely never understanding the word's meaning, and felt that she was being unfairly treated, so much so that she refused the only cure to her condition – a gallbladder removal. She went on to sue the New York City Department of Health in 1909, a case that ignited a heated debate about personal autonomy versus public health in times of crisis. She was released in 1910 on the condition that she would cease to cook; however, Mallon stealthily returned to her old job under a fake identity and caused another outbreak in 1915. Permanently isolated at North Brother Island, she spent her years in quarantine reading and working in the laboratory, where she died of a stroke in 1938.[2]

The legacy of 'Typhoid Mary' taught the medical world about the challenge of addressing carriers in disease outbreaks and shaped the concept of 'superspreaders', asymptomatic* individuals who could transmit disease at a large scale, prompting changes in public health responses worldwide. In 1913, Soper declared, '[s]ince "Typhoid Mary" was discovered, the whole problem of carriers in relation to infectious diseases has assumed an immense importance, an importance which is recognized in every country where effective public health work is done.'[3]

A few decades prior, research on vaccines to control typhoid had gathered steam in Europe. The research primarily followed the concept that the dead virus and bacteria could be used to induce immunity against their live virulent counterparts, a pathbreaking invention towards the end of the nineteenth century. It formed the basis for the methods employed, on a gigantic scale, to protect humans against cholera, plague and typhoid.

Besides Haffkine from India, others who worked relentlessly on this concept were A. E. Wright, D. Semple, R. Pfeiffer and W. Kolle. Wright assumed the role of pathology professor at the Army Medical

* A condition where a person shows no symptoms despite being infected with a virus or bacteria.

School in Netley, England in 1892. Between 1892 and 1902, he established a highly productive research group with a strong colonial character. Many of its members, like Semple, George Lamb, William F. Harvey and Lyle Cummins, were British nationals being trained to join either the Indian Medical Service (IMS) or the Bacteriological Department of the Government of India. Breaking away from the Pasteurian practice of using attenuated (weakened) live viruses, the group focused on using killed viruses* as vaccine material as they found them to be safer and more effective in inducing the formation of antibodies.[4]

Wright had been collaborating with F. Smith to develop an agglutination test† for Brucellosis or Malta fever, when during an experiment, Wright accidentally infected himself. He soon shifted his focus to typhoid prevention and treatment. Wright's research had groundbreaking results and the initiation of the anti-typhoid vaccination in 1896 is widely attributed to him, despite having other strong claimants. His persistent efforts, undeterred by the myriad challenges he faced, culminated in the first large-scale vaccination campaign against the typhoid fever in the British and Indian armies.[5]

Wright observed in his work that individuals administered with an anti-typhoid vaccine exhibited heightened bactericidal power‡ in their blood a day after the inoculation. He also noted increased phagocytic response in patients a day after they were administered a staphylococcus vaccine. In numerous cases, he observed an increased opsonic power§ of the blood within an hour of administering patients with a tubercle vaccine.[6] Around the same time, Richard Pfeiffer, who

* Viruses or bacteria that have been completely destroyed so they can't cause disease but can still help the body learn to fight them.

† A test used to detect disease-causing germs by mixing blood or serum with a substance that causes the germs to clump together if they're present.

‡ The ability of a person's blood or immune system to kill bacteria.

§ The ability of the immune system to mark bacteria so that other immune cells can easily destroy them.

was working at the Robert Koch's Institute for Infectious Diseases in Berlin, was expounding a diagnostic agglutination test for typhoid fever. He would soon jump into the fray of typhoid vaccine research.

As early as 19 September 1896, Wright presented a paper that reported the use of oral calcium chloride* for managing local side effects following the subcutaneous injection of *typhoid bacilli,* citing two experiments – the first titled 'Horse – Typhoid Vaccination', involved injecting live bacilli into a horse, and the second pertained to 'two officers of the Indian Medical Service undergoing typhoid vaccination with dead bacilli.'[7] In fact, the *Lancet* published it within eight days of the completion of the horse vaccination study, and two weeks after the completion of the dead bacilli experiment.[8]

By the time Wright was conducting his initial experiments with typhoid vaccination, the method of heat-killed typhoid vaccines was reasonably well-established, with Haffkine having suggested that preventive inoculations against typhoid fever should be based on the Pasteurian system (use of live attenuated microorganisms).

During this period, the swift publication of experimental data to claim precedence over pioneering research was commonplace, as was research rivalry. For instance, when Richard Pfeiffer and Wilhelm Kolle of Robert Koch's Institute for Infectious Diseases, Berlin published a paper in November 1896 on their investigations into vaccination against typhoid, they did not mention Wright's paper but referred to the work of others, even acknowledging an earlier work by E. Fraenkel and M. Simmonds.[9]

In retaliation, Wright and D. Semple, through an article on vaccination against typhoid fever published in the 30 January 1897 edition of the *British Medical Journal,* took the rivalry one step further by praising Haffkine for proposing the application of the effective cholera vaccination method, used in India, for the prophylaxis of typhoid fever. They added that they had, since then, dedicated their

---

* A salt-like substance used in medicine and research, sometimes to reduce pain or swelling after injections.

attention to developing anti-typhoid vaccination using the Haffkine method.[10]

They also mentioned that their 19 September 1896 paper was shared with Professor Pfeiffer, insinuating that he had likely learnt about the method from their work. Approximately two months later Professor Pfeiffer, in collaboration with Dr Kolle, published a paper on two cases of typhoid vaccination wherein they expounded the method of inoculation adopted by them – the same method that Wright and Semple had previously used and reported. This would eventually lead to the controversy over who invented typhoid vaccination.[11]

Wright's claim was subsequently accepted, primarily because the British Army approved the typhoid vaccination in 1914, at the beginning of the World War I. However, further evaluations conducted by researchers concluded that it was, in fact, Richard Pfeiffer and not Almroth Wright who provided the first account of human typhoid vaccination.[12]

This story highlights how the apparent superiority of the English over Germans, easy access to English journals like *BMJ* and the *Lancet* and above all, being persistent and at times forceful had helped Wright to establish himself as the inventor of the typhoid vaccine, despite Pfeiffer being the first to break ground with his all-important research.

In 1902, when Wright visited India as part of the British Plague Commission, he used the occasion to test the efficacy of the typhoid vaccine in some of the garrisons in British India. The observations he made from these tests convinced him that the vaccine did confer immunity. Subsequently, he used this vaccine in the South African War as well; however, the results were confusing since typhoid and paratyphoid fever were not properly differentiated back then.[13,14] The skewed results also stemmed from the fact that Wright's vaccine targeted *Salmonella Typhi* bacteria specifically, and not the other forms.

It is noteworthy that while the existence of paratyphoids had been acknowledged by 1896, it wasn't until 1902 that they were formally categorized as paratyphoids A and B. It was only in 1901–02 that Aldo Castellani initiated experiments on vaccines combining typhoid and paratyphoid components.[15,16]

By 3 May 1905, Semple, who had collaborated with Wright at the Army Medical School in Netley on typhoid vaccine research, had set up the Central Research Institute – initially known as the Pasteur Institute for North India – in Kasauli, located in present-day Himachal Pradesh.

In 1909, Semple wrote a scientific memoir, *An Inquiry on Enteric Fever in India,* from Kasauli which contained his findings regarding the role played by typhoid carriers in spreading the fever in India. A note of the memoir that appeared in *JAMA* the same year stressed that detecting and isolating individuals harbouring typhoid bacilli was key to preventing typhoid fever among the British troops in India.[17]

Typhoid fever was a considerable threat in India, particularly to the British troops stationed there, and therefore the Indian Government was well advised to institute an inquiry into it.[18] This was the reason Semple was sent to India by the British Government to launch an investigation. He started his typhoid research in India first with British Indian Army troops and later with the elites of Calcutta and Bombay.

From his research and fields trials, Semple published a preliminary note on the vaccine therapy for enteric fevers, in the *Lancet* on 12 June 1909. In this note, he delved into the early stages of exploring vaccine-based treatments for enteric fever, emphasizing on the significance of this novel therapeutic approach.

Semple believed that typhoid fever, characterized by both general septicemia,* where bacteria or their toxins get into the bloodstream and spread throughout the body, and localized foci, specific areas

* A serious condition where bacteria spread through the blood, causing infection all over the body.

where an infection starts and stays initially during the multiplication of microorganisms, could potentially benefit from the principles of curative vaccination. He argued that since these principles had proven successful in addressing other septicemic diseases and localized infections, there was no inherent reason why they should not be applicable to typhoid fever as well.[19] He suggested that when bacterial elements were introduced subcutaneously through vaccination in appropriate doses, tissues prompt the generation of protective substances.

In 1908, Semple helped establish the Naini Tal Enteric Depot, where convalescents were screened for carrier status, a step that would go a long way in creating the precedence for mobile bacteriologic units of World War I. As a result, by 1915, India had a 'carrier-free Army.'[20] He would go on to develop his own carbolized dead vaccines to prevent typhoid in India. Around this time, experiments on oral administration of dead typhoid bacilli as vaccine were getting attention in the US, with the work of James Carroll at the laboratories of the US Army Medical School.[21]

Efforts to develop immunity against typhoid fever through vaccines date back to 1896. However, it wasn't until the 1950s that scientists rigorously tested the effectiveness of these vaccines. There were two types of injectable vaccines, one using acetone and the other using heat-phenol. Both vaccines had an efficacy rate in the range of sixty to ninety per cent for three to five years. Despite the popularity of oral vaccines, they had not been consistently proven to be effective under strict scientific conditions. Live oral vaccines made from modified, non-harmful versions of the bacteria appeared to be more promising. Notably, the Ty21a, a capsular polysaccharide* vaccine showed a ninety-five per cent protective efficacy in a three-year trial in Egypt, outperforming previous vaccines.[22]

Due to their strong adverse reaction upon administration, whole

* Long chains of sugar molecules found on the surface of some bacteria. The body can learn to attack bacteria by recognizing these chains.

cell vaccines are no longer recommended and have been replaced by weak antigen*-strong protein† carrier conjugate vaccines,‡ virulent (Vi) polysaccharide vaccines and attenuated vaccines. Notwithstanding, a whole-cell heat-phenol or acetone inactivated vaccine is still used in many developing countries. WHO recommended replacing it with the conjugate vaccine, the Vi polysaccharide vaccine or the Ty21a oral vaccine, the only vaccines available through the prequalification programme§ of the organization. Currently, there are three types of vaccines with demonstrated safety and efficacy – a conjugated Vi polysaccharide vaccine that is bound to a carrier protein, a non-conjugated Vi polysaccharide vaccine and a live attenuated Ty21a vaccine.

However, it is crucial to understand that vaccination, while creating immunity to typhoid, is not a guarantee against infection. The risk of infection depends on the bacterial load to which one is exposed. Even those with immunity should maintain good personal and food hygiene to ensure complete protection against typhoid.[23] It is the only way one can ensure complete protection against the disease – the same lesson that the world learned a century ago from the case of Typhoid Mary.

---

* Any substance – chemicals, bacteria, viruses or pollen – that the body's immune system does not recognize and produce antibodies to fight against.

† Proteins are made up of chemical 'building blocks' called amino acids, which are used build and repair muscles and bones and to make hormones and enzymes.

‡ A type of vaccine where parts of a bacteria are combined (conjugated) with a carrier protein to improve immune response.

§ The process by which WHO evaluates and certifies that a vaccine meets international safety and efficacy standards.

12

SEMPLE VACCINE: DEAD OR LIVE?

IN THE LATE NINETEENTH CENTURY, A SHADOW LOOMED OVER humanity – an acute encephalitis* known as rabies, caused by a vicious virus that spared neither animals nor humans. To fight this invisible enemy, the foremost medical scientist of the time was called to action – Louis Pasteur.

In 1884, while working at the École Normale's Laboratory of Physiological Chemistry, Pasteur delved into the mysteries of rabies. Through a series of rigorous experiments, he soon pinpointed the central nervous system as the virus's primary battleground. Pasteur attempted attenuation by passing the rabies virus through rabbits, not once or twice, but multiple times, in a process that aimed at taming the viral agent. After several passing, he removed spinal cord material from rabbits and left it to dry in a moisture-free and sterile environment for various lengths of time. The tissues thus obtained were ground up and suspended in a sterilized broth, which was then tested as a vaccine to tackle rabies.[1]

This was the first live attenuated viral vaccine to be derived from desiccated brain tissue, inactivated using formaldehyde.† It was also the first vaccine ever produced to confront the deadly rabies virus, for which there is no effective treatment even today, and the mortality rate of full-blown infections is 100 per cent.

---

* Swelling or inflammation of the brain, often caused by a virus.

† A chemical used to preserve or inactivate viruses in vaccine preparation.

Pasteur then vaccinated dogs. Almost fifty dogs did not develop rabies. In July 1885, despite inconclusive results from post-exposure* dog vaccination experiments, Pasteur took on the momentous task of treating a human patient, Joseph Meister. The boy, who had been bitten fourteen times by a rabid dog just sixty hours earlier, received a series of thirteen inoculations over a ten-day period. Pasteur administered rabies virus injections derived from progressively less attenuated strips of spinal cord, each dried for shorter periods.

Meister never developed rabies. In October of the same year, Pasteur was presented with another case of Jean Baptiste Jupille, a shepherd boy who had valiantly intervened in a dog attack. This gave Pasteur another opportunity to successfully use his vaccine. Despite concerns about the safety of the vaccine, which contained highly virulent virus, the medical community swiftly embraced Pasteur's treatment method for what was once considered an inevitably fatal infection.[2]

Pasteur's ground-breaking work paved the way for a new era in medicine, where humanity stood a chance against the relentless assault of this fearsome virus. However, the work had only begun, and the job of continuing this crucial task was left to Semple who had just moved to India in search of a typhoid vaccine. In India, Semple improvised the typhoid vaccine he had developed with Wright by carbolizing the vaccine to make it more effective. Seizing the opportunity, he shifted his focus from typhoid to rabies and began developing an indigenous vaccine, adopting a similar technique as Pasteur's attenuated method.

In order to ensure that the rabies-exposed humans were saved from further damage, Semple began experimenting with serum treatment prior to administering the new vaccine. In 1904, Semple treated almost 200 patients in Kasauli with antirabic serum as a preliminary to the usual vaccine treatment, with very positive

* Giving a vaccine after someone has been exposed to a disease, like a rabies vaccine after a dog bite.

outcome. Even though it wasn't clear whether the results were due to the serum treatment or from the vaccine, he continued this line of treatment for a long time.[3]

By 1911, Semple had shifted his focus from serum therapy and began working on a more traditional anti-rabies vaccine. It is likely that he realized serum therapy was ineffective on its own. Consequently, he developed a carbolized vaccine,* using brain cells from rabbits that were deliberately infected with rabies and then euthanized.[4]

Semple's innovative carbolized anti-rabies vaccine represented a unique convergence of Pasteurian method and British research on germs while simultaneously diverging from both traditions. He moved from the traditional Pasteurian dry-cord-attenuated vaccine to carbolized dead vaccine, which prioritized safety and ease of transport in tropical climates over adhering to Wright's principles of opsonins† and vaccine therapy.

Semple focused on three key aspects that ensured his vaccine's success. First, safety was paramount – since it was a dead vaccine, there was no risk of causing the disease it aimed to prevent. Second, the vaccine's stability allowed it to maintain effectiveness when it was transported to distant locations within India. Third, the production process could be standardized, enabling centralized production at a single Pasteur Institute for distribution throughout India.[5]

With the ground-breaking development of his new anti-rabies vaccine, Semple challenged the relevance of live vaccines, proving unequivocally that dead vaccines were both safe and effective. This marked a significant shift from the Pasteurian logic that advocated for the ubiquity of live vaccines. In the tropical climate of India, where bacteriological research was traditionally confined to Pasteur Institutes built by the British and suitable only in hill stations, Semple's carbolized dead vaccines introduced a transformative shift.

---

* A vaccine preserved using carbolic acid – an early method of making vaccines safe.

† A type of protein that tags microbes to help immune cells to attack them.

Aside from their suitability in tropical climates, dead vaccines became crucial for another reason: the decentralization of vaccine treatment in India. Semple's vaccine, stored in hermetically sealed ampoules,* could maintain its quality during long journeys, thus facilitating its widespread distribution and use across the country.[6] By 1923, carbolized anti-rabies vaccine reached various centres in north and south India, impacting both awareness and treatment of the disease.

In 1924, the opening of a railway centre at Allahabad marked a major distribution revolution, supplying Semple's vaccine for antirabic treatment in north India. It was soon followed by similar centres in Lahore and Rawalpindi a year later. In Western India, the Bombay Bacteriological Laboratory implemented a policy to bring antirabic treatment closer to those in need.[7]

In two years, the Pasteur Institute in Coonoor in South India reported a decrease in rabies-related deaths and an increase in patients at local centres, indicating the positive effects of vaccine decentralization.[8] Since the arrival of Semple's vaccine in 1907 through 1924, the Pasteur Institute in Coonoor treated 30,253 persons, of whom only forty-five people succumbed to the virus. It was observed that in most fatal cases, either there was a delay in starting the vaccine treatment or the virus had unusually brief incubational periods.†[9]

Therefore, it wasn't surprising that Semple's antirabic vaccine gained widespread popularity and acclaim, not just in India but globally. The Director General of the IMS asserted that Semple's discovery had revolutionized rabies treatment in India.[10] The *Lancet*, in its 1911 July despatch, praised the vaccine as both safe and efficient, deeming it an ideal solution for a unique and diverse landscape like India.

Around the same time, a similar transition from live vaccines to

---

* Small, airtight glass containers used to store vaccines safely.

† The time between being infected with a virus or bacteria and showing disease symptoms.

dead anti-rabies vaccines was also happening in Europe. The primary motivation for the shift was that Pasteur's live vaccine method was being severely critiqued by the medical community, after it was found that a form of rabies – 'laboratory rabies' or *rage du laboratoir* – was seemingly being induced by the vaccine itself during the laboratory preparation.

In fact, since the days of Meister, Pasteur's anti-rabies methods had been facing intense criticism from scientists and anti-vaccinationists who argued that his vaccines caused more harm than good.[11] In 1886, researcher Michel Peter had presented a comprehensive account of 'laboratory rabies' to the scientific community, detailing eleven cases where patients had died from the 'poison' of Pasteur's vaccine. He suggested that Pasteur's live vaccines carried rabies germs, coining the term 'intentional inoculation with M. Pasteur's "laboratory rabies"'.[12] Peter's presentation challenged the core tenets of the Pasteurian vaccine, implying that scientists had failed to 'control' the living microorganisms, as Pasteur had claimed.[13] Consequently, 'laboratory rabies' became symbolic of the shortcomings of Pasteur's method, used by both scientists and historians to describe patients who had died exhibiting signs of paralysis after undergoing the Pasteur treatment.

The apprehension regarding live vaccines, especially in the case of rabies, stemmed from the presence of nerve cells in the vaccines that posed a risk of neurological complications. These concerns regarding the administration of live nerve cells and the occurrence of 'laboratory rabies' became a focal point of discussion at the First International Rabies Conference, organized by the League of Nations in Paris in April 1927. The Conference saw participation from directors of prominent anti-rabies institutes and the delegate representing British India was John Taylor, the director of the Pasteur Institute in Rangoon, Burma.

The conference marked the pinnacle of success of Semple's vaccine, with discussions centering on global anti-rabies treatment methods and associated accidents. Taylor's presentation at the event included statistics from all Indian Pasteur Institutes – around 170,000 cases, surpassing those of any other country – with many cases displaying more severity than that of other countries. Taylor demonstrated that paralytic accidents were significantly reduced with carbolized dead vaccines. This revelation positioned the dead carbolized vaccine of Semple as a newfound hope for Europe.

Even within the core Pasteurian group, the Indian antirabic experience garnered high praise. A. C. Marie, a professor at the Pasteur Institute in Paris, deemed Semple's method to be the 'most significant.'[14] Paul Remlinger, director of the Pasteur Institute in Morocco, who had extensively analyzed post-vaccinal paralytic* cases in Pasteur Institutes all over the world, found Semple's method to be the safest and considered the elucidation of this fact the most crucial lesson from the conference.[15] The conference affirmed that dead carbolized and etherized vaccines were most suitable for widespread production amid the increasing adoption of anti-rabies vaccination globally.[16]

Taylor reported the deliberations and the increased global acceptance of Semple's dead vaccine to Edward J. Turner, the Under Secretary of State for India in London, who forwarded it to Delhi, recommending the Government of India publish a summary of it in Indian medical journals.[17] J. D. Graham, the Public Health Commissioner (PHC) for India, wrote to the India Office in London, advising against the immediate publication of the report in India, apparently 'in view of certain local factors.' Graham subsequently emphasized that despite the endorsement from Europe, the carbolized dead vaccine was not yet considered definitive in India.

There was one more reason for Graham to take this position. The new director at the Pasteur Institute in Kasauli, John Cunningham, was more aligned with the thinking of Pasteur. A Scottish physician who had joined the IMS in 1905 and worked in various laboratories in India, Cunningham joined the Pasteur Institute in Kasauli as its

* Paralysis that occurs after receiving a vaccine.

director in 1926. Fellow IMS officer Anderson G. McKendrick had introduced Cunningham to etherized vaccines, who soon convinced its potency over Semple's carbolized dead vaccine. He began conducting comparative tests with both etherized live and carbolized dead vaccines, in an effort to discredit the latter.

Contrary to the decision in Paris, Cunningham was experimenting with live vaccines attenuated by ether, claiming that the Indian Pasteur Institutes faced far more severe cases than those in Europe and therefore, needed a more potent live vaccine. He defended his project by invoking the old Pasteurian doctrine while asserting that India must exercise scientific autonomy from European trends.[18]

This development had immediate implications for the Government of India's anti-rabies vaccination policy. The ongoing decentralization of rabies treatment had to be halted as Cunningham insisted that all patients be sent to Kasauli to facilitate large-scale experiments. This revealed the conflicting political interests in vaccination policy in India, with the India Office in London urging the Government of India to discontinue ongoing efforts to centralize all rabies vaccine research, in order to have a safe vaccine at the earliest. Cunningham's approach, on the other hand, raised concerns about the possibility of increasing mortality since vaccines were not available locally.[19]

Scientific opinion in India largely supported the Semple vaccine, and directors of other Pasteur Institutes were skeptical of Cunningham's experiments.[20] Despite their reservations, the elite group in Shimla, comprising influential medical personnel of the Government of India, decided to stop the decentralization of vaccines in light of Cunningham's experiments, underestimating the fear of paralysis associated with live vaccines that had taken hold of European scientific opinion.

They decided against opening any new centres in the plains till Cunningham came out with the final outcome from the experiments with live vaccines. They foresaw that the upcoming conference in Paris, influenced by a strong Pasteurian legacy and lobby, would strongly endorse the etherized live vaccines advocated by Cunningham.[21]

Soon after Cunningham began his experiments with etherized vaccines, he received a report of a suspicious death involving a British subaltern named Norman, who had been treated with the carbolized vaccine. He also found documented cases of post-vaccinal paralysis. Troubled, Cunningham expressed his concerns to Graham and then following his advice, began conducting large-scale experiments with ether-attenuated virus and advocated for centralizing vaccination in his Kasauli laboratory.

Cunningham was skeptical of the evidence supporting the early success of the carbolized vaccine in Indian institutes. Unable to locate original records of Semple's experiments in Kasauli, Graham provided him with Semple's confidential notes from 1911–12, which mentioned 'paralytic complications from time to time.' Cunningham was surprised to note that even one per cent carbolized vaccines of Semple caused paralysis. Based on this evidence, he argued that the carbolized vaccine was not the ultimate solution for antirabic treatment.[22]

To build his case of live vaccines further, he highlighted recent work with etherized vaccines by scientists such as Alivisatos, Hempt and Busson in Europe, which showcased better results. Since the nature of the etherized vaccine was live, it needed to be prepared daily in the laboratory and therefore, he advocated for the need to keep the treatment centralized.[23] In fact, he was wary that a decentralization policy might turn the Indian Pasteur laboratories dispensable and strove to retain its status as ground-breaking and experimental.

In January 1927, Cunningham's experiments with etherized vaccines faced a significant setback when a soldier named Kalyan Singh developed severe paralysis that led to his death after receiving the treatment at Kasauli. Cunningham identified similar cases and reported them to Fleming; however, he cautiously avoided directly linking them to the dreaded 'laboratory rabies.' Instead, he suggested that the paralysis was caused by the presence of foreign nerve tissue, attempting to justify the incidents by claiming that occurrences were common in all anti-rabies treatments.

This series of cases had severely shaken Cunningham's confidence in the ether vaccine. Consequently, he proposed a strategic retreat, recommending the use of his live ether vaccines only for severe cases in Kasauli.[24]

As the Paris Rabies conference in February 1927 approached, Cunningham sought McKendrick's support and shared a crucial revelation: the virus strain he had been using in Kasauli was so weak that it died when it was immersed in ether, unlike the attenuated strains used by Hempt and Alivisatos in Europe. He had been working with a nearly dead etherized vaccine, not a live attenuated vaccine.[25]

This meant that he couldn't really extol the advantages of a live etherized vaccine, not only because his own strain was effectively dead, but even this non-viable form had been found to cause paralysis. Cunningham found himself in an ambiguous position at the time of the Paris conference. He chose not to provide the details of his experiments, hoping that the conference would favour the new European etherized vaccine which would allow him to continue his research.[26]

At the Paris Conference, McKendrick faced the daunting task of navigating between the traditional Pasteur approach that favoured live vaccines and the emerging support for dead carbolized and etherized vaccines. The conference highlighted a clear division between the two camps, where the central debate was framed as 'living versus dead', as McKendrick mentioned in his communication with Cunningham. The discussions indicated a clear preference for dead vaccines, encompassing both carbolized and etherized varieties, when the fear of paralysis associated with live vaccines became evident. Even Pasteurian scientists like Hempt had shifted to dead vaccines to avoid post-vaccination paralysis. McKendrick noted that Remlinger was also caught between conflicting perspectives and reflected a sense of inner turmoil. Despite encountering paralysis cases with dried cord vaccines* in Morocco, he faced pressure from Pasteurian hardliners in Paris who advocated for the original method.

McKendrick celebrated the setback to Pasteur's original dry cord method. Upon returning from the conference, he highlighted the unique opportunity for India to contribute significantly to the evolving understanding of dead vaccines, whether etherized or carbolized. He discussed his views on India's prominence in the context of rabies with Cunningham and encouraged him to consider the international impact of their research. 'Rabies may not be economically as important to India as, say, Malaria. But regarding Malaria, India is a small unit, regarding Rabies India [sic] stands out prominent. Think that over,' McKendrick urged Cunningham.[27]

Cunningham interpreted this as support for his research on the live etherized vaccine and remained steadfast in his belief in the potency of living vaccines. He was unable to experiment extensively with the living vaccine due to the Kasauli strain's weakness; however, he saw potential in contributing to the anti-rabies research, especially in the severe cases prevalent in India. This stance led him to adopt a position contradictory to the Paris resolutions of 1927.

Amidst his continued experiments, he received communication from European scientists expressing interest in the Semple vaccine. In August 1927, Carl Prausnitz, a German bacteriologist who was impressed by the discussions of the carbolized vaccine at the Paris conference, wrote to Cunningham about his decision to adopt the Semple method for his work. Prausnitz was surprised to discover that Cunningham had reverted to using live etherized vaccine, seeing as Hempt himself had shifted to a dead carbolized vaccine after detecting several cases of paralysis.

Cunningham shifted his allegiance to Alivisatos, favouring his method of using etherized vaccines for severe cases and rejecting dead carbolized vaccines of higher dosage. He argued that the

* An old type of rabies vaccine made using dried nerve tissue (usually from animals) infected with the virus.

unique conditions in India required a distinct vaccine, claiming that the Semple vaccine was better suited for European conditions. In 1928, Cunningham presented these findings at the Indian Rabies Conference in Calcutta, opposing the increase in carbolized vaccine dosage and advocating a combination of treatments. However, in February 1929, Cunningham abruptly left India and his deputy R. H. Malone replaced him.

Malone's first report in 1929, based on experiments conducted by him and Cunningham, demonstrated that Alivisatos vaccine (now considered a live vaccine) outperformed the five per cent carbolized vaccine, which, in turn, was more effective than the five per cent etherized-carbolized Hempt vaccine. Cunningham forwarded the report to Graham and dismissed any opposing opinion provided by the other directors. There was mounting pressure for decentralization with the carbolized vaccine in India at the time. In December 1929, the Rabies Committee examined an interim report that provided a comprehensive comparative analysis of Hempt, Alivisatos and Semple vaccines. In brief, the Kasauli research wasn't going in any productive way.

Antirabic research at the Pasteur Institute in Kasauli ceased in 1931 when Malone was transferred to Rangoon. The final report, authored by H. E. Shortt in the absence of Cunningham and Malone, clarified that the main variable in vaccines was the quantity of brain matter. The report emphasized that improved results were due to increased brain substance dosage, irrespective of the vaccine type or living virus presence. Soon antirabic vaccine research moved from vaccine type to dosage.

After a report published in 1934 highlighted the importance of higher brain substance dosage, the Semple vaccine was standardized with a five per cent sheep brain in carbolized suspension. By 1938, mass vaccination and decentralization had accelerated, with nearly 200 field units being supplied with the Kasauli vaccine. A year thereon, the Kasauli Pasteur Institute closed entirely and transferred all its routine work to the Central Research Institute (CRI) in Kasauli.

Gradually, the Semple vaccine with a higher dosage of brain matter replaced all other forms. Reports from the Pasteur Institute in Coonoor highlighted the history of the evolution of the Semple vaccine, transitioning gradually from Pasteur's dried cord vaccine in 1911 to the final standardized five per cent sheep brain carbolized Semple vaccine that came to be extensively used by 1940. This period witnessed increased decentralization and widespread adoption of the standardized vaccine.[28]

In the 1940s, Semple's vaccine became widely celebrated for antirabic treatments globally.[29] As William J. Webster, assistant director of CRI, Kasauli observed in 1943, 'Semple's vaccine is now in general use all over the world and has, to a large extent, replaced vaccines of other types.'[30] Meanwhile, researchers Umeno and Doi created the first vaccine to be used for mass vaccination of dogs based on the Semple vaccine. Contrary to the previously accepted inactivated vaccines for use in humans, live attenuated viral vaccines were developed for veterinary use. In 1948, a live rabies vaccine was introduced by Koprowski and Cox.[31]

The human rabies vaccine of the early twenty-first century was based on inactivated live virus and employed a technique of eliciting antibodies that could neutralize 'envelope glycoprotein', a type of protein that can be found on the surface of viruses, particularly enveloped viruses. These vaccines were expensive to prepare and carried the theoretical risk of transmission of live virus if not inactivated adequately. In one major incident in April 2004, leading manufacturer Aventis Pasteur was forced to withdraw several vaccine lots because a live strain of the virus was found in a batch.

Currently, there are two types of vaccines for rabies protection in humans – nerve tissue and cell culture vaccines.* Recently developed cell culture vaccines are not only more affordable but are also required to be given in a smaller quantity. Therefore, WHO recommends replacing nerve tissue vaccines with the safer and more effective cell culture vaccines at the earliest opportunity.

---

* A modern vaccine produced using cells grown in labs instead of animal brains or tissues.

13

THE KISS OF DEATH

IN THE LATE NINETEENTH CENTURY, TRAGEDY STRUCK THE royal household when Queen Victoria's daughter Princess Alice contracted diphtheria, a highly contagious bacterial disease that had previously claimed the life of her sister Anne at the age of thirty-five.

Four of Princess Alice's seven children and her husband, the Grand Duke of Hesse-Darmstadt, had also contracted the same disease. What perplexed the royal physicians and members of the court was the manner in which the disease had spread, seeing as none of the other sixty individuals residing in the opulent Grand Ducal household showed signs of infection. This curious phenomenon prompted a variety of speculation about the peculiar transmission of diphtheria, ultimately leading to a startling hypothesis.

There was speculation that the disease might be stealthily spreading through innocent acts, such as the tender exchange of a mother's kiss with her child. Both Princess Alice and her ailing child displayed no symptoms beyond a sore throat, creating an unwitting conduit for the transmission of this potentially fatal infection. An innocuous act of love had unwittingly become a silent accomplice in the spread of what ominously came to be known as 'the strangler', due the lethal grip of diphtheria on its unsuspecting victims within the court.[1]

Caused by *Corynebacterium diphtheriae,* diptheria thrives on close contact, typically through respiratory secretions* suspended in the air. The infection produces a toxin, destroying healthy tissue in the respiratory tract. This leads to a thick grey coating in the throat or nose, which can block breathing and swallowing, often causing death by suffocation. The insidious progression of the disease often leads to a fatal strangulation of the patient.[2] Beyond the throat, the toxin's reach extends to critical organs, jeopardizing the heart and other vital systems.[3]

If left untreated, the impact of diphtheria can be severe, with fatality rates ranging between 5 and 10 per cent. In vulnerable demographics, such as children under five and adults over forty, the statistics soared to over twenty per cent. Historical medical records trace the spectre of diptheria as far back as the early 1600s, with the disease gaining prominence as cities expanded, facilitating easier person-to-person transmission.

The late nineteenth century witnessed a surge in the diphtheria threat, and a corresponding increase in the mortality rate. Fuelled by the industrial revolution and burgeoning urban centres, the disease transcended class boundaries. While the infection presented itself predominantly among the impoverished, posing a particular peril to children, diphtheria did not discriminate based on class or age. The cause, spread and cure of this disease remained shrouded in mystery until the final decades of the nineteenth century.

The impact of diphtheria was reflected in the harrowing cases faced by physicians. For instance, one young girl, around five or six years old, became the fourth victim in a German farmer's family and eventually succumbed to the disease. Her case attracted considerable medical interest due to the detailed account provided by the treating clinician.

This poignant account, documented in the *Public Health Journal* in December 1927, served as a testament to the challenges faced by

* Tiny droplets from the nose or mouth (like from coughing, sneezing or talking) that can carry germs.

physicians in the battle against diphtheria before the development of its cure. There were various attempts to eradicate the membrane or combat the morbid condition; however, they had proved futile and the medical community was left helpless.[4]

In the history of this deadly disease, the earliest scientific breakthrough came in the early nineteenth century. During an outbreak, French physician Pierre Bretonneau made a significant contribution in the early nineteenth century by defining diphtheria based on clinical observations of throat membranes. He theorized that the disease is caused by bacteria, despite non-availability of microscopes to confirm it.[5] However, it wasn't until 1826 that the malady received its official name – *diphtérite*, derived from the Greek word for 'leather' or 'hide'.

The causative bacteria, *Corynebacterium diphtheriae* was identified by German bacteriologists Edwin Klebs and Friedrich Löffler in 1884, and thereafter came to be known as the Klebs–Löffler bacillus. They also noticed that the bacteria is usually harmless unless infected by a bacteriophage* that triggers the production of a specific toxin.[6]

Löffler's discovery of avirulent strains† of the bacteria in healthy individuals, identical to virulent strains causing diphtheria, pointed to the role of asymptomatic carriers in spreading the disease. Avirulent strains can transform into virulent forms when they come in contact with a bacteriophage having a particular gene.[7] Löffler also hypothesized that the bacteria released a soluble toxin‡ capable of causing damage beyond the respiratory tract.

In 1883, French physician, bacteriologist and immunologist, Emile Roux, along with Yersin, came up with a classical work on the causation of diphtheria by isolating diphtheria toxin (DT) from the bacteria obtained from the throats of affected children. They

---

* A type of virus that infects and can change bacteria – like a hacker taking control of a computer.

† Avirulent strains are mild and harmless forms of a germ; virulent strains are strong and dangerous ones that cause illness.

‡ A harmful chemical made by germs that can spread easily in the body through fluids like blood.

demonstrated the toxin's pathogenicity by injecting bacteria-free filtrates* into healthy guinea pigs, causing symptoms resembling human diphtheria. Roux concluded that targeting the newly discovered toxin could be a crucial strategy to combat diphtheria.

In 1890, Emil Behring of the Institute for Infectious Diseases in Berlin demonstrated that sub-lethal doses of diphtheria toxins or tetanus toxins injected into the body could initiate the production of blood substances that could neutralize the toxins. Behring also established the possibility of using the antitoxic ability of tetanus-immunized rabbit blood materials in other animals, thereby identifying these protective substances as antibodies.

This seminal research laid the foundation for serum therapy and passive immunization† against both diphtheria and tetanus, in addition to contributing to the understanding of humoral immunity‡ (antibody§ generation). This work earned Behring the first ever Nobel Prize for Physiology or Medicine in 1901.

Between 1891–92, reports of the first serum therapy trials with an antitoxin, prepared in sheep and horses, emerged. Clinical trials conducted in Leipzig, Germany and Paris demonstrated the efficacy of the antitoxin in reducing mortality rates among children. The experimental pursuit of the serum unfolded as a scientific competition involving heated debates between Roux and Metchnikoff, both from the Pasteur Institute in Paris, and Behring. These debates, in turn, played a crucial role in shaping the distinctive features of therapeutic experiments undertaken both in Berlin and in Paris.

---

* A liquid that has been filtered to remove solid parts – used here to test the effects of bacterial toxins without the actual bacteria.

† Giving someone ready-made protection like antitoxins or antibodies, instead of waiting for their body to make it naturally through a vaccine.

‡ Immunity involving antibodies produced by B cells that circulate in body fluids (humors), fighting off viruses and bacteria.

§ Also known as an immunoglobulin (Ig), an antibody is a Y-shaped protein produced by the immune system to identify and neutralize antigens, such as bacteria and viruses. They circulate in the blood and lymph, recognizing and binding to specific antigens, thereby triggering an immune response.

In 1894, two scientists, Anna Wessels Williams and William H. Park tackled the challenges of potency associated with antitoxin preparations by isolating Park-Williams No. 8, a highly toxigenic strain* later named after them.[8] This strain, documented by Lampidis and Barksdale in 1971 and Pappenheimer in 1984, is used to this day to produce diphtheria toxoid (DT).

At the same time, crucial research was ongoing in Spain, where Catalonian scientist Jaume Ferran i Clua had introduced a new vaccine that sparked considerable debate. He conducted trials on himself, his two children and two children of his friend Pere Aldavert, who would later become the president of the League of Catalonia. Tragically, three of the children fell seriously ill, and Aldavert's youngest son succumbed to the vaccine-induced complications. The ensuing controversy led to the formation of a Governing Committee, which accused Ferran of hasty experimentation with rabies and diphtheria vaccines in humans. As a result, the Commission decided to reduce Ferran's pay, mandate the use of the Pasteur method in rabies vaccine administration, and prohibit him from conducting any further vaccine trials on humans.

Nevertheless, in 1891, Ferran presented a report to the City Council, outlining the results obtained from applying the diphtheria vaccine. By 1894, he managed to prepare an anti-diphtheria serum, and the Hospital de Caridad in Cartagena was the first centre to administer it.

Meanwhile, in 1897, German researcher Paul Ehrlich pioneered a technique to standardize the potency of diphtheria antitoxin, the first international standard reference. Ehrlich's groundbreaking studies on toxin-antitoxin interactions laid the foundation for modern immunology. He showed how immune systems can specifically detect and neutralize harmful invaders using matching mechanisms, like a lock and key.[9] His seminal contributions to the field earned him the Nobel Prize for Medicine in 1908. In his Nobel Prize lecture, Ehrlich

* A version of a germ that produces a toxin capable of causing disease.

shared that these toxins exhibited a propensity to undergo changes, either spontaneously over time or under the influence of thermal conditions or specific chemicals like iodine.[10]

The widespread availability of the diphtheria antitoxin in 1895 earned it global recognition. Final validation came in 1898 from the Danish physician Johannes Andreas Grib Fibiger, who conducted a series of clinical trials to investigate the effects of the treatment on the mortality and morbidity of diphtheria patients. Soon, immunization campaigns kicked off in many parts of the world, including the United States. A toxin-antitoxin formulation, this vaccine demonstrated an eighty-five per cent effectiveness.

By the mid-1940s, the diphtheria toxoid was combined with tetanus toxoid[*] and whole-cell pertussis vaccine to formulate the diphtheria-tetanus-pertussis (DTP) vaccine combination. Subsequently, the DTP combination vaccine was adsorbed onto an aluminum salt[†] after researchers noted the heightened immunogenicity[‡] of diphtheria and tetanus toxoid in the presence of pertussis vaccine and the aluminum salt.

Toxoid vaccines are made by purifying bacterial toxins and neutralizing their toxicity by applying heat or with formaldehyde. This process maintains their ability to trigger an immune response, which then forms toxoids.[§] Vaccination with these toxoids produces antibodies that neutralize the toxin. However, it is essential to control the production to ensure that the toxins are detoxified without significantly changing their structure, so that the resulting toxoids are safe for use as vaccines.[11]

During the British rule, there was no noteworthy research in

* A vaccine designed to protect against tetanus, made from an inactivated toxin (toxoids) produced by the bacteria.

† A compound added to vaccines to help them work better by boosting the body's immune response.

‡ The ability of a vaccine to trigger an immune response in the body.

§ Inactive versions of toxins used in vaccines to help the body build immunity without causing illness.

India on diphtheria or tetanus toxoids that was reported in the *Indian Medical Gazette* or international medical journals, despite the prevalence of these diseases in the country. It could have been so because the British were more concerned about the lives of Europeans living in India, most of whom would have spent their childhoods in Britain. Childhood immunization to Indian subjects was never a priority for the colonialists. In the early twentieth century, even when the cholera and plague vaccinations were initiated by the British, those were mainly for their soldiers in their barracks, initially for the British officers and later extending to the Indian soldiers.

After independence, the Indian health ministry focused on rampant infectious diseases like tuberculosis and polio, and the historically virulent three – cholera, plague and smallpox. However, as early as in the 1950s and the 1960s, diphtheria and tetanus vaccines began to be imported to India for use by the elite classes in cities like Delhi and Bombay. Some of the global pharmaceutical companies who had set up their shops in India began distributing it in select hospitals. Many states began offering diphtheria, polio and tetanus (DPT), diphtheria and tetanus (DT) and tetanus toxoid (TT) vaccines under maternal and child health (MCH) services since the early 1970s.

In 1974, the WHO launched the Expanded Programme on Immunization (EPI), expanding its existing immunization programmes and extending them to various parts of the world.[12] Its goal was to immunize all children against diphtheria, pertussis, tetanus, poliomyelitis, measles and tuberculosis by 1990, and India decided to join the programme.[13]

In 1977, soon after eradicating smallpox, India launched its National Immunization programme, initially called the EPI by clubbing BCG, OPV, DPT and typhoid-paratyphoid vaccines. Thereafter, Indian vaccine manufacturing units began ramping up their operations to produce diphtheria, pertussis and tetanus (DPT), diphtheria and tetanus (DT), tetanus toxoid (TT), oral polio vaccine (OPV) in addition to smallpox, cholera and plague vaccines.

In 1978, the Central Research Institute, Kasauli developed its own version of DPT and began supplying it for national immunization programmes. The Pasteur Institute in Coonoor too followed suit and between these two institutes, India met the massive requirement for DPT vaccinations.

Initially, DPT was administered to children up to five years of age. Despite the original intention, the real integration of diphtheria, pertussis and tetanus vaccines with the EPI happened only in the 1981–2002 period. Thereafter, it came to be offered to children below two years of age and TT vaccine was offered to school children in their final classes of primary and secondary schools.[14]

When the World Health Assembly rallied for the global elimination of neonatal tetanus (NT)* and declared it a public health problem by 1995, India joined the programme.[15] In the 1990s, immunization for TT among pregnant women steadily increased, with sufficient immunity developed by the vaccinated mothers from the neonatal tetanus (NNT) to protect their newborn babies.[16]

With the development of effective vaccines and its widespread distribution covering almost a billion people, the vaccine requirements of India exceeded that of any other country. By the end of 1990, over 100 million doses each of DPT and TT vaccines were required annually. And India was meeting most of this demand on its own.

* A deadly disease affecting newborns, usually from unsafe delivery practices.

14

VACCINE RESEARCH AND EARLY INSTITUTIONS

IN JUNE 1897, POONA CITY (CURRENTLY PUNE) WAS ROCKED by a double murder, a gruesome killing of two high-ranking British officers. The head of the Special Plague Committee, W. C. Rand, who was also an officer in the Indian Civil Services, and his military escort Lt. Ayerst (no second name) were shot dead as they were returning from the diamond jubilee celebrations of the coronation of Queen Victoria.

The events that culminated in the June 1897 assassination had begun months earlier. In February 1897, the Plague epidemic was spiralling out of control in Poona, with one of the highest mortality rates. Panic ensued, causing half the city's population to flee. In response, a Special Plague Committee was hastily formed, chaired by Rand who enlisted European troops to combat the outbreak. The Government of India, on its part, passed the Epidemic Diseases Bill for 'better prevention of the spread of dangerous epidemic diseases.' The Epidemic Diseases Act (EDA) continues to hold sway till date and a wholesale revision was only attempted in 2022 after the Covid-19 epidemic.

The measures adopted by the British, however, were draconian and invasive. The committee forcefully entered people's homes, sometimes in the dead of night, to take the infected away. They even resorted to digging up floors because of a prevailing belief that the plague bacillus bacteria seeped into the floors of afflicted houses. To intensify control, they made it mandatory for the principal occupant of a building to report all deaths and suspected plague cases. Funerals were prohibited until deaths were registered, and the committee had the authority to designate specific grounds for plague-related burials.

This heavy-handed approach that commenced in early March of 1897 and continued through May came at a high cost. The estimated deaths caused by the plague crossed 2,000 in no time.[1] Unsurprisingly, these stringent measures fuelled public resentment against the regime. Bal Gangadhar Tilak, who lived in Poona, vehemently criticized these actions through his newspapers *Kesari* and *Maratha*.[2]

However, for the British, it was essential to protect the city. Poona was a bustling military town with an important military base, where a significant number of British soldiers and officers were stationed, along with their families. Infectious diseases were spreading like wildfire. Since the British population was constantly interacting with locals, it was necessary to protect the larger populace to protect their own people. In addition, the IMS included many British doctors who had pledged the Hippocratic oath – to serve everyone with integrity, humility, honesty and compassion – unlike the colonial bureaucrats and army officers.

As the need for public health initiatives became apparent, authorities began taking measures such as mass vaccinations and improved sanitary conditions. Yet, the implementation of these health strategies encountered many setbacks due to a clash of cultures and, at times, the imperious demeanor of colonial officers, which often ignited public discontent.[3] The growing public resentment culminated with the assassination of Rand and his escort Ayerst, who were shot by two revolutionary nationalists, the Chapekar brothers, on 22 June 1897.[4] Ayerst died on the spot and Rand succumbed to his wounds a fortnight later.[5]

These gruesome murders triggered a reassessment of public health policies across British India, thereby bringing in a delicate equilibrium between public health imperatives and the respect for individual rights. In the aftermath, the British government focused on strengthening public health and bacteriological research in the country as a strategic response.

The institutional momentum had been building for some time. Almost a decade earlier, in 1889, the establishment of the Imperial Bacteriological Laboratory in Poona had heralded a significant milestone in serotherapy.* The laboratory found its initial home within the premises of the College of Science, thanks to a generous donation of 5.5 acres of land. Under the administrative control of the Government of Bombay, the laboratory, led by distinguished bacteriologist Dr Alfred Lingard, commenced its journey. Lingard, with support from a clinical assistant and the superintendent of the Bacteriological Survey, was tasked with investigating diseases in domesticated animals across India. His mission was later extended to conducting biological research, both on-site and in the laboratory, to prevent and cure such diseases.[6]

During the laboratory's initial years in Poona, Lingard focused on studying surra, a fatal parasitic disease affecting horses, sheep and cattle. However, the challenging tropical climate hampered the smooth functioning of the laboratory, especially the preservation of the vaccine. Additionally, concerns arose about the presence of bovine blood in the laboratory, which was at odds with the religious sentiments of the Hindu students at the College of Science.

In 1893, much to the disappointment of the locals, a pivotal decision was made to relocate the laboratory to the hills and Muktesar (now Mukteshwar) in the Kumaon Hills in the north was chosen as the new site. The meticulous process of packing scientific instruments and laboratory fittings began in February 1895. By mid-May 1895, around thirty tonnes of goods were dispatched by rail to Kathgodam, which were then transported by bullock carts to Bhowalie, the closest point to Muktesar on the Kathgodam–Ranikhet road.

---

* A medical treatment that uses blood serum containing antibodies to help fight specific infections.

However, due to the insufficient number of porters, the transportation of goods to the laboratory site faced an unexpected delay. When news of the delay reached Poona, it sparked hope among a few civilian Europeans that they could appeal to the government to bring the laboratory back to Poona, given that it had not yet commenced operations in Muktesar. A petition was swiftly dispatched to Governor William Mansfield and was published in the *Bombay Telegraph and Courier* on 9 October 1895.

Despite the petition and the pressure from the media, the Governor stood firm, and the laboratory officially commenced its operations in Muktesar in 1896. Over time, it evolved into an integral part of the Indian vaccine research and development, with its major contribution being the production of vaccines for animal diseases rinderpest* and anthrax. A year after its opening, renowned bacteriologists Dr Robert Koch, Dr R. Pfeiffer and Dr G. Gaffky visited the centre and appreciated the work going on there. In time, it would undergo three name changes – in 1925, 1930 and 1936 – to finally become the Indian Veterinary Research Institute (IVRI) in 1947 after the country gained independence. Soon thereafter the centre shifted its headquarters from Mukteswar to Izatnagar in the current day Uttar Pradesh.[7]

In 1763, over a century before the establishment of the Poona Laboratory, the Bengal Medical Service had been formed with a team of forty surgeons to meet the needs of both civilians and armed services – a number that increased steadily.[8] On its initial success, the Bengal Medical Service was replicated in Madras and Bombay.[9]

In 1857, the Indian Rebellion led to the transfer of administration of India from East India Company to the Crown and different departments of civil services were developed. A year later, a separate

* A contagious viral disease that affects cattle and some wild animals.

civil medical department would be formed in Bengal. In 1869, the Public Health Commissioner (PHC) and the Statistical Officer would come under the Government of India.

The 1894 Indian Medical Congress made recommendations to conduct thorough research in bacteriology.[10] In 1896, all three medical departments – of Bengal, Bombay and Madras – were amalgamated to form the Indian Medical Services (IMS). The Army Medical Department, later called the Royal Army Medical Corps (RAMC), was formed under the IMS in 1898, responsible for providing medical care to the Royal Indian Army.[11]

This arrangement would continue until 1919, when the Montgomery-Chelmsford Constitutional Reforms led to the transfer of public health, sanitation and vital statistics* to the provinces – the first step in the decentralization of health administration in British India and subsequently in the Republic of India.[12]

The formation of IMS also resulted in the creation of several medical research laboratories across the British Indian territories, starting with the Imperial Bacteriological Laboratory in Poona in 1890. Two years later, another Bacteriological Laboratory came up at Agra and by 1896, the Plague Research Laboratory was established under the leadership of Haffkine in Bombay.

In 1900, the Indian Pasteur Institute meant for treating patients bitten by rabid animals was founded in Kasauli and later, Pasteur Institutes were established in Coonoor in 1907, in Rangoon in 1916, in Shillong in 1917 and in Calcutta in 1924. Around the same time, in 1903, the King Institute was established at Guindy on the outskirts of Madras to produce calf lymph and for general bacteriological study. These institutes began conducting research for the prevention and treatment of tropical diseases prevalent in the region.

Among them, the Pasteur Institute in Kasauli stood tall with its work on the typhoid vaccine and rabies vaccine, operating independently from the Central Research Institute (CRI) located

---

* Official data related to births, deaths, marriages and health conditions of a population.

nearby. It worked from a separate site in Kasauli from 1903 until 1936, when it was absorbed by the CRI. David Semple, who was the director of the Pasteur Institute from 1900 to 1905, became the director of CRI since its inception in 1906 and remained there till 1913. With the setting up of these institutes, laboratory research assumed critical dimensions in British India.[13] By 1905, a specialized cadre of science officers was formed from among the researchers involved in special projects. This came to be known as the Bacteriological Department, the first medical research organization in India.

In 1914, the expanding Bacteriological Department was rechristened the Medical Research Department, with the strength of its principal researchers reaching thirty. However, progress was interrupted due to the looming World War, as most researchers were drafted for the war, leaving a period of abeyance in research activities.

The Bacteriological Department had a tumultuous start with a plethora of challenges, such as administrative burden and a lack of trained resources for research in tropical diseases. To address these issues and to shape advancements in medicine and allied sciences by coordinating and funding research in university laboratories and medical schools[191], the Indian Research Fund Association (IRFA) was established in 1911. It was almost three years before the formation of the British Medical Research Council (MRC), a similar organization in England.

Along with IMS officer Sir Harcourt Butler, Sir Pardey Lukis, who also served as the inaugural editor of the *Indian Journal of Medical Research* and served as the Director-General of the IMS, played a pivotal role in establishing IRFA. Despite hoping for private contributions, it ended up receiving most of its funding from the exchequer of the Government of India. The key motives of the organization were to support research, disseminate knowledge and make efforts to prevent communicable diseases.[*14]

* Diseases that spread from one person to another, like malaria, tuberculosis or flu.

In 1913, the IRFA launched its flagship journal, the *Indian Journal of Medical Research*, marking an official beginning in the dissemination of scientific knowledge, two years after its establishment. The association played a crucial role in funding various medical research organizations, including the Nutrition Research Laboratories and the Malaria Institute of India.

While the IRFA laid the groundwork for medical research in India during this period, its expansion into substantial research activities occurred only after World War I. Initiatives such as the Beri-Beri Enquiry* and financial support to the School of Tropical Medicine, Calcutta laid the foundations for future institutions with a vision as well as purpose.

In 1923, the recommendations of the imperial Inchcape Committee† impacted the work of IRFA, leading to the closure of the Beri-Beri Enquiry. However, it organized the first All India Conference of Medical Research Workers in the same year, emphasizing on the importance of ongoing research programmes. Amidst a severe shortage of funds, significant support came from the Maharaja of Parlakimedi (located in current day Odisha) in 1926 that helped continue important research. The research on nutritional diseases that had been paused recommenced in Coonoor in 1925 and evolved into an institution named the Centre of Nutrition Research by 1929.

These important initiatives significantly transformed the landscape of Indian medical research that Ronald Ross had lamented about in the 1890s. By the 1920s, India's standing in the realm of medical research would considerably improve and soon, it would establish itself as a global leader in the treatment of tropical diseases.[15]

The Government of India Act, 1935 classified health activities into federal, federal-cum-provincial and provincial categories, ensuring that provincial governments gained increased autonomy.

---

* A project to investigate the causes of the disease beri-beri.

† A commission established in 1921 to advise the Crown on cutting government expenditure in British India, headed by Lord Inchcape.

The establishment of the Central Advisory Board of Health in 1937 aimed to coordinate public health activities, with the PHC serving as the Secretary. The year 1939 witnessed the enactment of the Madras Public Health Act, a pioneering step in public health in the country.

The Bhore Committee report of 1946 that reviewed medical research in British India recognized IRFA's contributions to research initiatives, despite its financial limitations. It also highlighted the lack of organized medical research in medical colleges, insufficient training facilities for scientific approaches and the negative impact of routine institutional work on medical research.[16]

Another notable development of the early twentieth century was the establishment of the Indian Science Congress in January 1914. The significance of modern medicine and medical research was highlighted in a series of presidential addresses delivered by key figures in the domain. In 1915, W. B. Bannerman, who assisted Haffkine in his research on plague vaccines, delivered the second address in Madras on 'The Importance of Knowledge of Biology to Medical, Sanitary, and Scientific Men Working in the Tropics.' In 1919, the sixth address was given by Sir Leonard Rogers in Bombay, who championed the use of hypertonic saline for treating cholera, centred on research on the disease, while the seventeenth address, 'The Science of Disease', was given by S. R. Christophers, who headed Central Malaria Bureau and CRI Kasauli, in Allahabad in 1930.[17]

As the East India Company, the British Raj had created a well-structured medical research and delivery establishment and kept improving it. Gradually, the imperial government's influence replaced traditional and indigenous therapies of Ayurveda and Unani prevalent in the region with practices of modern medicine.[18]

As Western education gained popularity in British India, prevalent attitudes towards new medical systems evolved. Consequently, the IMS and the Bacteriological Department/Medical Research Department garnered widespread acceptance by the late nineteenth century and firmly established themselves by the early twentieth century. This period also saw substantial improvements in medical and sanitary conditions, benefiting both the British population and the Indian residents of cities and large towns.

The IMS was successful in controlling epidemics such as plague and cholera as well as battling outbreaks of smallpox, leprosy and malaria. The work of IMS and the Bacteriological Department/Medical Research Department laid the foundation for a robust research and delivery system in modern medicine in India, many aspects of which continued beyond the departure of the British in 1947.

By then, the Indian Institute of Science – conceived and funded by J. N. Tata, and formally established in 1909, five years after his death – had been working on producing insulin, pancreatin, pepsin, vitamins and other proteins, many of which were handed over for commercial production. The appointment of Nobel laureate Sir C. V. Raman as the first Indian director of the Institute in 1933 led to the cultivation of penicillium and the preparation of penicillin, following Alexander Fleming's groundbreaking discovery of the antibiotic in 1928. The Tata Memorial Hospital in Bombay was then just six years old and it would be another five years before it established the Indian Cancer Research Centre, later called the Cancer Research Institute, as a pioneering institute for cancer research in the country.

CRI Kasauli was then producing Semple's typhoid vaccines for the Indian military as well as Haffkine's cholera vaccine for Punjab, Kashmir, the North West Frontier Province, Bengal, Assam, Burma (Myanmar) and other northern Indian regions. It was also making Semple's anti-rabies vaccine for northern territories like Punjab and the United Province (Uttar Pradesh), along with the defence department, and an anti-venom serum for the whole of India and the defence department. The Pasteur Institutes and the Haffkine Institute were producing and supplying one or more of these vaccines regionally, in addition to conducting research in medical science and vaccine development for some of the infectious diseases and challenges of the time.

In Calcutta, there were private companies like Bengal Chemicals and Pharmaceuticals Ltd. (BCPL), Bengal Immunity Ltd. (BI) and Smith Stanistreet & Co. Ltd. that were involved in the production of biologicals (vaccines and sera). Additionally, several firms, established during the war, produced biologicals under more satisfactory conditions than was the case earlier. While both state-supported institutions and private companies played important roles during critical times such as epidemics and the World Wars I and II, research was primarily conducted in publicly sponsored institutions. These institutions developed indigenous vaccines and sera against prevalent diseases like rabies, tetanus, diphtheria, pertussis (whooping cough), cholera, smallpox, typhoid and anti-snake venom.[19]

By the time of independence, the nation had established institutions such as the All India Institute of Hygiene and Public Health, the Medical Council of India and the Central Advisory Board of Health. Additionally, non-governmental organizations like the Indian Medical Association, Women's Medical Service, the All India Medical Licentiates Association and the All India Association of Medical Women also contributed to developments in medical research and healthcare landscape. However, it would take another two years after independence to re-designate the IRFA as the Indian Council of Medical Research (ICMR), with an expanded scope and responsibilities.

Post-independence, these promising institutions found themselves in desperate need for direction and focus for organizational and resource restructuring.

15

SOKHEY, HILL AND BHORE

IN 1943, AT THE HEIGHT OF WORLD WAR II, THE GOVERNMENT of India requested the Royal Society to send a capable representative to study and make recommendations on the reorganization of scientific and industrial research as part of the post-war reconstruction of India. The Royal Society had no better choice for this task than British Nobel laureate Archibald Vivian Hill.

Better known as A. V. Hill, he was a reputed scientist and strategist who had won the 1922 Nobel Prize in Physiology/Medicine for his research on the functioning of muscles in the human body. Heeding the request of the Royal Society, Hill visited India and toured the country from November 1943 to April 1944.

During this visit, Hill addressed the Indian Science Congress, presided over by Satyendra Nath Bose, an eminent scientist who had collaborated with Einstein on a new state of matter known as Bose–Einstein condensate (BEC).* Hill interacted widely with Indian Fellows of the Royal Society and deliberated on the admission of four new Fellows to the Society – Shanti Swarup Bhatnagar, Homi J. Bhabha, K. S. Krishnan and Birbal Sahni. Hill's discussions with Indian scientists and administrators eventually led to the proposal creating a structured institutional framework in India.[1]

---

* A special state of matter formed when certain particles are cooled to extremely low temperatures, making them behave like one single 'super-atom'.

Hill observed an unwarranted disconnect between the Indian scientific community and their counterparts in Britain, the British dominions and the US, hindering collaborative efforts. This resulted in the isolation of Indian scientists, limited access to latest scientific knowledge and subsequent underutilization of India's scientific and technical resources. His report pinpointed that practically no research work of any significance was happening in clinical medicine in Indian medical colleges, despite abundant clinical data.[2]

The report outlined a quadrilateral dilemma facing the country – population, health, food and natural resources. Hill assessed that the core issues were not primarily physical or technological but rather complex biological challenges, each interacting and often conflicting with the others.[3]

He listed eight institutes doing 'very distinguished work, particularly in tropical medicine*' – the Central Research Institute, Kasauli; School of Tropical Medicine, Calcutta; the Haffkine Institute, Bombay; the King Institute, Madras; the Malaria Institute of India, Delhi; the Drug Research Laboratory, Jammu and Kashmir, the All-India Institute of Hygiene and Public Health, Calcutta; and the Nutrition Research Laboratory, Coonoor. He recommended separate institutes for medical research in every discipline and that the existing research institutes be brought into closer contact with medical colleges.[4]

He strongly recommended establishing an advanced All India Medical Centre as the 'Indian John Hopkins' and cited the British Goodenough Committee's report to buttress this point.[5] This recommendation would eventually be implemented in the form of the All India Institute of Medial Sciences (AIIMS), established in Delhi in 1956.

Hill's key recommendation in the research space was setting up a centralized research organization along the lines of Great Britain's

* A branch of medicine that deals with diseases common in hot and humid regions, especially those caused by parasites and insects.

six research agencies – one each for medical, agricultural, industrial, natural resources, engineering and defence. By then, the Council of Scientific and Industrial Research (CSIR) had been established in 1942 under the eminent scientist Shanti Swarup Bhatnagar.[6] Therefore, Hill proposed notable changes in the affiliations of existing scientific organizations with the proposed central body. He recommended that current research institutions be integrated into the new framework in a gradual transition, considering the prevailing circumstances.[7]

The Report also proposed the creation of a consultative committee to advise members of the Viceroy's Executive Council for Planning and Development on general policy in relation to research and other special matters. On the basis of these recommendations, the Government of India would set up a Scientific Consultative Committee for Planning and Coordination of Research in 1945.[8]

Hill was confident that the systematic application of the scientific method would lay a strong foundation for India's progress, enabling the country to formulate a comprehensive national development plan. He believed this approach would also inspire international scientific cooperation with and goodwill towards India.

While Hill was working on a detailed blueprint for scientific research and science education in India, the government had appointed another Committee, under Sir Joseph Bhore, to survey health conditions and health organizations in the country, and to recommend changes for future development.[9] The Bhore committee, with experts from all realms of healthcare and health science, started its work in 1943 and would submit its report by early 1946.

The hurried formation of committees to address public health and healthcare research stemmed from a critical situation. Once regarded as one of the world's wealthiest regions, India was now contending with widespread poor health, low vitality and alarmingly short life expectancy. Chronic illnesses afflicted large sections of the population, further aggravated by recurring epidemics that exposed deep vulnerabilities in the country's health system.

Poverty, rooted in over two centuries of colonial exploitation and neglect, was identified as the primary cause of these issues. Providing for the people's basic needs was a challenge, leaving little for healthcare or education. Nearly half of the population did not live past the age of ten – life expectancy was around twenty-six years – and the death rate, as well as infant and female mortality, were alarmingly high compared to Western countries. The idea of physical training and a balanced diet seemed ludicrous amid widespread deprivation. Limited knowledge about health conditions among the underprivileged further hindered preventive measures, despite modern science offering solutions to scourges like smallpox, plague, cholera, malaria, tuberculosis, blindness and leprosy.

In urban areas, rapid industrial growth and overcrowding presented severe health challenges. Accustomed to open-air village life, migrants in cities like Bombay and Calcutta found themselves confined to cramped tenement chawls, lacking sunlight and ventilation, with air heavy from primitive cooking stoves fuelled by cow dung. Clean water and adequate sanitation were scarce, which inevitably compromised respiratory and gastrointestinal health. These conditions also fostered the spread of deadly communicable diseases, preventable by available vaccines.

Social customs further exacerbated public health issues. Widespread early marriages, mandated before puberty, imposed undue health burdens. Not only did they weaken vital bodily functions and reduce the body's resistance to diseases, early marriages led to frequent childbirth – a major contributing factor to increasing poverty and high infant mortality rates.[10]

The irony was that a nation where extensive and needless suffering had become so entrenched still held within it the potential for redemption through the strategic deployment of sufficient resources. The untold tales of anguish and the persistent grip of preventable diseases that cast its shadow over the Indian people – all of this misery could have been transformed into a story of resilience, health and prosperity, if only those in power had been willing to effect change.

In this unfolding tragedy, the required resources were not merely financial. A holistic approach was needed: educational resources to spread awareness about health, infrastructure for widespread healthcare accessibility and investment in research to continually advance preventive measures such as vaccines.[11]

The missed opportunity wasn't just statistic; it represented a collective failure to support the health of 340 million people. The tragedy persisted not due to a lack of solutions, but because British rulers were unwilling to prioritize them.

The British Government was aware of these appalling conditions and their tragic consequences. They were concerned about the increased mortality rate among Indian Army sepoys, whose health issues were indicative of those of the broader population. Following the 1857 uprising, a Royal Commission in 1859 assessed the sanitary conditions of the Indian Army and made specific recommendations for improvement. However, it wasn't until 1864 that Special Commissioners of Public Health were appointed to address these critical issues.[12]

However, their primary focus was on the three presidencies – Calcutta, Bombay and Madras – which limited their coverage on village sanitation problems. In 1888, a different commission highlighted the state of public health in villages and urged the local bodies to take measures for improving the health conditions in the overlooked areas.[13] The Plague Commission too in 1904 recommended strengthening of public health services* and establishing laboratories for research and production of vaccines and sera in large measure.[14]

The country was in dire straits by the waning years of the nineteenth century and the circumstances were well captured in the report of the sub-committee on national health headed by Sahib Singh Sokhey, published in 1947.

There was some speculation that Sokhey had drawn points and data from the Report of the Health Survey and Development

* Government-funded systems and programmes aimed at maintaining and improving the health of the general population.

Committee of Sir Joseph Bhore. The report contained a wealth of information and looked at all possible aspects of healthcare – medical research and education, environmental hygiene,* vital statistics, prevailing diseases, the health of women, children and industrial workers, nutrition, availability of drugs and vaccines, preventive healthcare and health administration.[15]

The Bhore Committee highlighted stark contrasts in healthcare expenditure, citing Great Britain's 20.4 per cent in 1934–35 and the United States' 13.8 per cent in 1938. The committee urged the Indian government to allocate a minimum of 15 per cent of its total expenditure to healthcare. The proposed plan recommended an annual per capita expenditure of ₹1.87 on recurring costs and ₹1.11 on non-recurring expenses, aiming not to exceed 1.33 per cent of the Gross National Product (GNP).†[16]

The committee's report highlighted the role of vaccines in healthcare, citing over thirty instances where prophylaxis was deemed crucial. It underscored that effective vaccine deployment could lead to herd immunity and even eradicate diseases like smallpox from the region. The report cited historical successes, noting that systematic vaccination efforts had nearly eradicated smallpox in the past. It also highlighted the increasing demand for the plague vaccine despite declining cases, as noted by the director of the Haffkine Institute. Stressing the government's duty to safeguard public health from epidemics, the committee recommended maintaining government responsibility for large-scale production of vaccines against cholera, plague, typhoid and rabies.[17]

With these insightful observations, two key points stood out that made the report potentially significant for Indians. First, the American lobbying organization Rockefeller Foundation showed an interest in impacting India's healthcare system through J. B. Grant,

---

* Practices that help keep the surroundings clean and healthy to prevent diseases (like sanitation, waste disposal, clean water, etc.)

† The total value of all goods and services produced by a country, used to measure a country's economic strength.

its representative on the committee. Foundation officials closely monitored the Bhore Committee deliberations and after the committee convened in April 1945, pertinent sections of the report were promptly sent to New York in preparation for implementing its recommendations.[18]

Second, the Bhore Committee predominantly endorsed Western medicine and marginalized indigenous medicine from the envisioned Indian medical system. When this was criticized, a Committee on Indigenous Systems of Medicine was established in 1948, chaired by Col. Sir Ram N. Chopra, IMS, Director of the School of Tropical Medicine, Calcutta. This initiative reflected the nationalist movement's support for indigenous medicine, a crucial step for extending medical care across the nation.

Interestingly, the Bhore Committee's deliberations were influenced by Sokhey's interim report of 1939, while the Sokhey Committee, in turn, drew extensively from the Bhore Committee's findings in preparing its final report in 1949.

These overlapping and hurried efforts by various committees reflected a late but notable attempt by the British to reform India's healthcare and medical research systems before the end of colonial rule. The most significant contributions during this period came from the Bhore Committee Report and the A. V. Hill Report. However, the real task of overhauling the system fell to the post-independence Indian administration, which relied heavily on the recommendations of the Sokhey Committee Report. The Hill Report, too, held considerable weight, as the well-intentioned advice of an eminent scientist respected across both Indian and British scientific circles.

Soon after independence, India's healthcare system underwent large-scale changes. Unfortunately, many of these reforms were shaped more by the growing influence of market forces than by a commitment to building a truly universal healthcare system accessible to all, regardless of financial means. While these changes did contribute to a decline in mortality rates, they failed to significantly reduce morbidity, leaving a large section of the population still grappling with chronic illnesses and poor health outcomes.

It would take another forty years – and a renewed policy vision – for more meaningful and inclusive reforms to begin taking shape in the country.

16

SUPREME SCIENCE COMMANDER

WHILE VISITING INDIA TO HELP THE COUNTRY REORGANIZE its scientific and industrial research post war, A. V. Hill delivered a message on the radio on 8 February 1944. He concluded it by suggesting, 'India requires a supreme science commander to plan and apply scientific research to India's development. This is unavoidably necessary if India were to prosper.'[1] In his message, Hill emphasized that true progress in human welfare requires a society to be dynamic, led not merely by politicians but by visionary leaders with a scientific temperament.[2]

The country already boasted a remarkable constellation of scientific talent; not just Indian-born British scientists like Ronald Ross, but also an inspiring generation of indigenous pioneers like C. V. Raman, Homi J Bhabha, Meghnad Saha, Vikram Sarabhai and Satyendra Nath Bose, who were shaping the future of science across diverse domains.

However, what India lacked was strong scientific leadership. The British administration had failed to cultivate indigenous scientific leadership, resulting in the absence of robust research institutions capable of driving innovation and supporting industrial growth.

In 1933, on a visit to Indian research organizations and universities, Sir Richard Gregory, editor of *Nature*, identified this gap and brought it to the attention of Sir Samuel Hoare, Secretary of State for India. He emphasized on the need for a research organization – similar to the Department of Scientific and Industrial Research (DSIR) in Britain – to harness the scientific capabilities of Indians for the development of the nation.[3]

Sir Gregory's concerns echoed those of other visionaries like C. V. Raman, Lt. Col. Seymour Sewell, and Sir Jnan Chandra Ghosh, who had earlier proposed the creation of an umbrella advisory board for scientific research in India. Initiatives were launched in Calcutta and Bangalore to establish a national institute for sciences and an Indian Academy of Science, respectively. At the 5th Industries Conference in 1933, the provincial governments of Bombay, Madras, Bihar and Orissa unanimously called for a coordinating forum for industrial research.[4]

Sir Hoare advised the Viceroy Lord Willingdon to support the idea of an Indian equivalent of DSIR. However, in May 1934, Willingdon told Hoare that the creation of such an institution in India wasn't necessary. Despite this rejection, a small concession was made with the creation of an Industrial Intelligence and Research Bureau under the Indian Stores Department, mainly to focus on testing and quality control.[5]

With the onset of the World War II, proposals emerged to abolish even the Bureau due to financial constraints. Sir Ramaswamy Mudaliar, Commerce Member in the Viceroy's Executive Council, took the lead in advocating for a broader and more structured scientific body. His efforts culminated in the establishment of the Board of Scientific and Industrial Research (BSIR) on 1 April 1940, initially intended as a two year initiative. The hunt for a distinguished person to head the organization ended in a promising young scientist – Shanti Swarup Bhatnagar.

Bhatnagar had made significant strides in applied chemistry* by developing a process to convert sugarcane bagasse into cattle feed, tackling industrial challenges for several companies like Delhi Cloth

* Chemistry used to solve practical problems, especially in industries – like making better fuels, medicines or materials.

Mills and Tata Oil Mills, and addressing a drilling issue for Attock Oil Company by using a local gum to prevent mud solidification in saline water. His success earned him a payment of ₹1,50,000 from Attock Oil Company, which he used to establish the Department of Petroleum Research at Panjab University, Lahore.

Bhatnagar's dedication was acclaimed, and his leadership bridged the gap between industrial applications across domains, from refineries to pharmaceuticals and vaccines. Bhatnagar assumed the role of Director of BSIR, with Sir Mudaliar serving as its first Chairman. One of the twenty committees soon formed under BSIR was meant for 'drugs', including vaccines.

Upon his arrival in Delhi, Bhatnagar faced the daunting task of establishing the necessary infrastructure for scientific and industrial research. Lacking a suitable laboratory in Delhi, he decided to set up the Board's headquarters in Calcutta.[6] Meanwhile, the Indian Research Bureau was suspended, and its staff was transferred to the new Department.

By the end of 1940, nearly eighty researchers were engaged under BSIR, and within two years, the organization developed numerous industrial processes at the laboratories. Bhatnagar soon persuaded the government to establish an Industrial Research Utilization Committee (IRUC) to translate research outcomes into practical applications. Following IRUC's recommendations, the Government agreed to create a separate fund from industry royalties* for further investment in industrial research. These efforts culminated in the formation of the Council of Scientific and Industrial Research (CSIR) as an autonomous body† in November 1941. CSIR officially began functioning on 28 September 1942, with the BSIR and IRUC serving as its advisory arms.[7]

---

* (In context of industrial research) Money paid to researchers or organizations when their inventions or processes are used commercially.

† An organization that runs independently, even though it may be funded or supported by the government.

The very next year, CSIR approved Bhatnagar's proposal to establish five national laboratories – the National Chemical Laboratory, the National Physical Laboratory, the Metallurgical Laboratory, Fuel Research Station and Glass and Ceramics Research Institute. In 1944 it received a grant of ₹10 million to augment these laboratories followed by the Tata Industrial House donating ₹2 million for specific research purposes.

These developments marked the beginning of nation-building in anticipation of the impending independence, under the leadership of a 'Supreme Science Commander', as envisioned by Hill. After India's independence, Prime Minister Jawaharlal Nehru took charge of CSIR, emphasizing the nation's commitment to scientific development, with Bhatnagar reporting directly to him to lead the development of India's scientific research infrastructure.

Although Bhatnagar was building CSIR in the 1940s, IRFA had held its first meeting as early as 1911. With achievements like the Beri-Beri Enquiry under its belt, IRFA's role expanded significantly after the World War II. Soon after independence, it was renamed the Indian Council for Medical Research (ICMR).[8]

Post-independence, India inherited two strong pillars of scientific progress: ICMR and CSIR. These institutions became crucial in driving research and development, spanning from industrial engineering to vaccine research. Together, they anchored applied research in the country, providing critical government funding, generating policy-relevant knowledge and nurturing pharmaceutical and biomedical innovation.

At the time, India's pharmaceutical market was overwhelmingly dominated and controlled by Western MNCs, who held between eighty and ninety per cent of market, primarily through imports. Nearly ninety-nine per cent of all patented drugs and vaccines in India were owned by foreign companies, resulting in some of the highest drug prices globally.[9]

Upon realizing that eight of the top ten pharmaceutical firms were subsidiaries of global companies, Bhatnagar, with ICMR, initiated efforts to set up state-owned pharmaceutical companies. The only government owned drug company at the time was the Bengal Chemical and Pharmaceutical Works, set up in 1930, the first public sector drug manufacturer in the country. Bhatnagar's efforts led to the creation of Hindustan Antibiotics Ltd. in 1954, which became the country's largest drug manufacturing company with support from the United Nations (UN) and UNICEF.

Around the same time the Virus Research Centre (VRC) came up in Poona, through a collaboration between ICMR and the Rockefeller Foundation, to focus on arthropod-borne viruses.* Eventually, the centre expanded its role to include the development and testing of vaccines for diseases like influenza, Japanese encephalitis and dengue, complementing the works of institutions like Haffkine Institute, Central Research Institute, Kasauli and the Pasteur Institute, Coonoor. In recognition of its growing mandate and critical contributions, the VRC was re-designated as the National Institute of Virology (NIV) in 1978.

During this transformative period, Bhatnagar emerged as a towering figure – an institution builder and true 'supreme science commander' steering India's scientific establishment as the nation transitioned from colonial rule to a sovereign republic. Amidst a constellation of brilliant Indian scientists, it was Bhatnagar who wielded the broadest influence across domains – from industrial research and applied sciences to atomic energy and vaccine development.

By the time Bhatnagar passed away due to a heart attack on 1 January 1955, he had already laid the foundations of a scientific renaissance in independent India. Under his leadership, twelve brand-new national laboratories, with a dozen more already in the pipeline, provided the country with a formidable infrastructure for scientific and industrial research. The foremost 'institution builder' of modern India, Bhatnagar created a wide spectrum of institutions, ranging

* Viruses spread by insects like mosquitoes and ticks, e.g., dengue or Japanese encephalitis.

from pure science research centres to application research institutes and public sector enterprises, giving shape to Nehru's vision of a scientifically driven nation.

Such was Nehru's faith in him that he was appointed the first Secretary of the Atomic Energy Commission and the inaugural chairman of the University Grants Commission – both positions that reflected his unmatched leadership across scientific and academic spheres. Therefore, it came as no surprise when, in 1958, CSIR instituted a coveted award for the best scientific minds of the country every year in his honour, known as the Shanti Swarup Bhatnagar Prize for Science and Technology.[10]

In 2024, the Bhatnagar Prize was renamed the Vigyan Yuva Shanti Swarup Bhatnagar Award. Even today, this prize stands as India's most prestigious recognition for excellence in science, an enduring tribute to the man who envisioned and shaped the nation's scientific destiny.

17

A VACCINE IN FOUR MONTHS

THE MONSOON SESSION OF PARLIAMENT IN 1957 WITNESSED an uproar over a subject that had been rarely discussed within the confines of India's highest policy making forum: the urgent need for a vaccine against influenza.

M Valiulla, the Congress member representing the Mysore constituency, raised a pointed question. Had the Pasteur Institute in Coonoor produced any therapies or vaccines to combat rapidly spreading influenza? What began as a routine query quickly snowballed into a heated discussion, as members across party lines joined in, pressing the Health Minister, D. P. Karmarkar, for answers.[1]

Just three months earlier, the Asian influenza* had entered Indian shores through Madras, triggering a swift and widespread outbreak. By May, the pandemic had surged across the subcontinent. Preliminary reports warned that the virus was unlikely to recede anytime soon. Over the next ten months, until February 1958, the outbreak infected almost 5 million people and claimed more than 1,000 lives.[2] Members of Parliament were worried that the toll would go further up, and the killer disease would continue to ravage the country. And for the first time, the question of vaccine development took centre stage in the Indian Parliament.

The story had been unfolding since May 1957.

---

* Or A/Asia/57 virus; a type of flu virus that caused a global pandemic in 1957.

On 11 May, the specialized Influenza Centre at the Pasteur Institute in Coonoor received information that the influenza outbreak in Southeast Asian countries, such as Japan and Malaya (current day Malaysia), was about to enter India. Fears arose when an approaching steamship named *S.S. Rajula* left Singapore on 9 May with 1,622 passengers and 200 crew members, and there was speculation that many people on board were probably infected with the deadly virus.[3] Sensing the looming threat, maritime and health authorities in Tamil Nadu swiftly intervened. The vessel was diverted to Madras, bypassing its original port of call in Nagapattinam. By the time *Rajula* sent word of its condition, 254 suspected cases of influenza were on board.

When it landed in Madras on the morning of 16 May, the steamer was first quarantined at sea and then a highly specialized medical team went in to investigate the severity of the situation. The team found forty-four cases, including four serious cases, and provided them with necessary treatment on board. Soon, an investigating team from Coonoor arrived to collect samples from the patients. Throat swab specimens were collected and taken to the Influenza Centre in Coonoor and were inoculated into chicken eggs intra-amniotically. The causative virus was isolated by 22 May and the isolated strain was sent to the World Influenza Centre in London, where it was identified as the A/Asia/57 virus.[4]

Unfortunately, four nurses who went into the steamship were found suffering from the same symptoms within forty-eight hours. This marked the beginning of the pandemic in India, following its progression through North China in January and Shanghai in February. Bombay reported its first cases on 21 May, while Calcutta reported 1,000 cases within two weeks, with the first two deaths on 1 June. It remained uncertain whether Madras, Bombay and Calcutta were independently affected or if Madras was 'ground zero' of the infection, spreading soon after to Bombay and Calcutta.

The remarkably swift and widespread dissemination of influenza across Asia in the initial months of 1957 suggested the potential presence of a novel strain or subtype. Researchers concluded that vaccines derived from older or mouse-adapted strains* might be ineffective. Therefore, acquiring etiological strains† became imperative for a new vaccine development.[5] A representative strain, identified as 'Par' and isolated in Malaya, was quickly acquired and brought to India. After being successfully established in eggs, the initial material was dispatched from Coonoor to the Armed Forces Medical College, Poona by 30 May for developing vaccine candidates. A vaccine was developed successfully and distributed to other vaccine production centres and laboratories across India for further replication and mass production.

To tackle the challenge of large-scale vaccine production, a committee chaired by the Director General of Health Services was constituted. It set a production target of 100,000 vaccine doses, with the Pasteur Institute, Coonoor successfully delivering 55,000 doses by 31 January 1958. However, the vaccine rollout faced a critical setback – by the time the initial batches became available in July, the first major wave of infections had already waned. As a result, the vaccine could not undergo a full-scale field trial during the peak of the outbreak, limiting its immediate public health impact.[6]

The development and production of the 1957 influenza vaccine – from procuring an etiologically strong virus strain to conducting field trails in less than four months – is still the record of producing a successful viral vaccine in India. The collaborative effort of the Pasteur Institute, Coonoor, Armed Forces Medical College, Poona and various other organizations and government departments under the leadership of Directorate General of Health Services was noteworthy in an era when mobility and communication were rudimentary, as was the technology.

The Pasteur Institute of India (PII), Coonoor has been at the forefront of vaccine development since its inception at the

* Virus strains that have been adapted to grow in mice for research.

† Specific virus or bacteria samples known to cause a particular disease.

very beginning of the twentieth century. Set up to produce anti-rabies vaccines, it quickly became a leader in vaccine and serum development in British India. Remarkably, in 1917, PII became the first institution in the world to introduce anti-rabies serum therapy. Therefore, when PII jumped into the fray to create a vaccine for influenza in 1957, it had experienced manpower and the required infrastructure to research and develop a vaccine in a brief period of time. Support from the Armed Forces Medial College, Poona also proved to be key.

Building on this momentum, PII soon found itself at the centre of another pivotal public health initiative. In 1963, amid growing concerns over the polio epidemic in India, the institute received a distinguished visitor – Albert Sabin, the Polish-American scientist who had developed the oral polio vaccine (OPV). During his visit to India in 1963 to identify a local institution to produce OPV, Sabin found PII Coonoor to be capable of developing and manufacturing OPV from his attenuated poliovirus strains. He then donated the strains to the institute and on his recommendation, Prime Minister Jawaharlal Nehru swiftly made resources available to produce OPV. The first consignment was released to the nation in 1968 by Dr Zakir Hussain, the President of India.[7]

Dr G. V. J. A. Harshavardhan, a key member of the PII team who worked closely with Sabin, recalls all going well with the Polio Vaccine Unit until 1975, when the unit was shut down abruptly for unknown reasons.[8] There were many conspiracy theories surrounding the move. One such theory suggested that in order to control its fast-growing population, India was resorting to measures both logical and illogical.

India soon began importing monovalent* polio vaccines. This shift was driven by pressure from elite sections of society, who were desperate to protect their children from the deadly scourge of polio. It was then that the Ministry of Finance recognized that relying on

* Vaccines designed to protect against one strain (type) of a disease.

imported polio vaccines was rapidly depleting the country's scarce foreign exchange reserves.

At the Pasteur Institute, after the initial disappointment passed, most of the 100-odd members of the polio vaccine project were moved to a new project to develop DTP vaccines. The project successfully culminated in the production of the DTP group of vaccines by 1981. A few years later, it also started producing measles vaccine.

In 2008, the entire vaccine production was shut down on the intervention of the Minister of Health and Family Welfare, Anbumani Ramadoss. The PII would go back to DPT vaccine production much later and build the capacity to produce 80–100 million DPT doses a year. It also set up BSL-2[*] and BSL-3[†] (Bio-Safety Level[‡]) facilities down hills in Coimbatore to manufacture viral, bacterial, conjugate and r-DNA vaccines.[§9]

In contrast, none of the other Pasteur Institutes – Rangoon, Shillong and Calcutta – ever matched the stature of Coonoor. Rangoon was no longer part of independent India, Shillong remained steeped in its legacy of having been established with the King Edward VII Memorial Fund to combat malaria and *kala azar* (black fever) among tea plantation workers, and PII Calcutta, set up in 1924, gradually lost its relevance after independence and was converted into a government hospital.

Besides the Influenza Centre, the PII Coonoor also created a centre in 1918 to research beriberi, caused by vitamin B1 deficiency. Within a span of seven years, this project expanded into a Deficiency Disease Enquiry and by 1928, emerged as the full-fledged Nutrition Research Laboratories. A decade after independence, it shifted

---

* Labs certified to handle moderate-risk microbes like hepatitis.

† Labs certified to handle dangerous pathogens that can cause serious diseases like tuberculosis.

‡ Safety classifications for labs based on the types of organisms they handle.

§ Vaccines created using genetic engineering techniques, by inserting one part of the genetic material of the pathogen into another organism (like yeast or bacteria) to produce a protein that acts like the virus or bacteria, prompting immunity.

to Hyderabad and, after yet another decade, was renamed to the National Institute of Nutrition (NIN).

The Pasteur Institute in Kasauli, operating independently from CRI, made significant contributions in typhoid and rabies vaccines. Established in 1903 at a separate site in Kasauli, it merged with CRI in 1936 and relocated to a new building on the CRI premises.[10] The institute has been at the forefront of development and production of indigenous vaccines and serums, and has played a pivotal role in public health by introducing several vital vaccines and serums to combat infectious diseases since its inception. Among its significant achievements are the development and manufacture of anti-snake venoms and sera in 1906, followed by breakthroughs in typhoid vaccine production in the same year, rabies vaccine in 1911, and a cholera vaccine in 1914.

With the integration of the Pasteur Institute, Kasauli, CRI doubled its efforts to expand its research potential by introducing critical interventions such as diphtheria anti-toxin in 1953, the tetanus anti-toxin* in 1954 and the rabies serum in 1955. The CRI also contributed to global health initiatives by developing the yellow fever vaccine in 1958 and the DPT vaccine in 1978. Its efforts extended to addressing emerging threats, which can be observed by the introduction of the Japanese Encephalitis (JE) vaccine in 1982 and the vero cell-based† JE vaccine in 2007.

Beyond its contributions to vaccine development, CRI Kasauli today serves as the national authority on quality control and the certification of all vaccines manufactured in India. Through stringent quality assurance measures, CRI ensures that vaccines produced in the country meet international standards.

Another vaccine research institute with a glorious history is the King Institute of Preventive Medicine. Established in 1897 as a public

* A serum used to neutralize toxins produced by the bacteria *Clostridium tetani*, which cause tetanus, a life-threatening infection.

† Made using cells from African green monkeys, which are used to grow the virus that is then inactivated (killed) to make the vaccine.

health laboratory named after the Madras Sanitary Commissioner, Lt. Col. W. G. King, one of the institute's earliest responsibilities was to manufacture smallpox vaccines developed by the Haffkine Institute. Soon after, it started a virology department and a tissue culture lab. The institute continued its original focus on vaccine production and bacterial disease control. It also strengthened its virology research and later diversified into yellow fever.

In 1948, the BCG Vaccine Laboratory was established in the campus of the King's Institute, Madras. The lab was solely responsible for meeting the entire BCG vaccine requirement of the country using the seed virus* procured from Copenhagen. In 1993, the lab replaced the seed strain with its own and by 2001, it was solely meeting the national requirement of tuberculosis vaccine for the Universal Immunization programme.

Throughout all of this, the Haffkine Institute in Bombay continued to produce vaccines for plague and cholera. In 1975, the Government of Maharashtra bifurcated the institute into two organizations – one to focus on research and training and the other to focus on vaccine and drug production. The latter was named the Haffkine Biopharmaceutical Corporation. In 1977, a subsidiary was formed – Haffkine Ajintha Pharmaceuticals Ltd. – to focus on the development and production of bacterial and viral vaccines for diphtheria, tetanus, whooping cough, plague, poliomyelitis and rabies.

Several vaccine research and production institutes were established across British India before independence, including labs in Calcutta, Hyderabad, Lucknow, Nainital, Bangalore, Trivandrum, Belgaum, Ranchi, Patna, along with institutions like PII and School of Tropical Medicine in Calcutta. After independence, public sector enterprises like Hindustan Antibiotics (1954) and Indian Drugs and Pharmaceuticals (1961) were set up to reduce dependence on imported medicines and boost domestic manufacturing.

Building on this public sector foundation, India's private vaccine

* The original virus sample used as a starting point to make large batches of vaccines.

industry began taking shape through early pharmaceutical companies in Bengal. Firms like Calcutta Chemicals, Standard Chemicals and East India Chemicals initially focused on bulk drugs, while pioneers like Smith Stanistreet Pharmaceuticals (1821), Bengal Chemical and Pharmaceutical Works (1901) and Bengal Immunity Ltd. (1919) gradually ventured into vaccine production, manufacturing cholera, typhoid, anti-rabies and anti-snake venom vaccines.

Founded by Indian chemist Prafulla Chandra Ray in 1892 with an initial capital of ₹700, Bengal Chemical Works aimed to foster indigenous enterprise and reduce reliance on colonial jobs. The company expanded across India but faced setbacks after Ray's death, eventually being taken over by the central government in 1977 and nationalized in 1980.

More than half a century after Ray's debut, another entrepreneur emerged in western India. In 1951, Indravadan Modi left his job as a chemist at a Mumbai firm to co-found Cadila Laboratories with his childhood friend Ramanbhai Patel. Starting operations in Ahmedabad from a rented bungalow with an initial capital of ₹25,000, the company achieved a turnover of about ₹125,000 in its first year. Meanwhile, Cipla, founded in Mumbai in 1935 by Khwaja Abdul Hamied as Chemical, Industrial & Pharmaceutical Laboratories, had already established itself. In 1937, Ranbir Singh and Gurbax Singh began a distributorship for the Japanese company Shionogi, eventually forming Ranbaxy, which changed ownership in 1952.

However, none of these pharmaceutical companies, except Biological E., seriously ventured into vaccine production. Established in 1953 by Raju and Raju in Hyderabad as Biological Products Private Limited, Biological E. became India's first private sector vaccine manufacturer. It entered the vaccine market in 1962 with DTP vaccines, challenging the dominance of government research institutes and public sector entities. One of the reasons why the company set its eyes on the vaccine market was the lack of a ready vaccine to prevent the influenza outbreak of 1957.

The public health crisis had exposed critical gaps in India's immunization preparedness and became a turning point. The early seeds had been planted for a private vaccine industry that would, in the decades to come, grow to play a pivotal role in India's healthcare landscape and spread its wings globally.

PART III

SAVING LIVES
(1961–1990)

18

TUBERCULOSIS AND THE BCG REVOLUTION

IN 1939, DR P. C. BHANDARI, AN INDIAN PHYSICIAN WHO WAS also a close friend of Jawaharlal Nehru, arranged a consultation for Indira Nehru with Dr Herbert, a well-known respiratory specialist in London. Upon examining her and performing an X-ray, Dr Herbert discovered a shadow on her left lung. He advised her to run X-rays every six months and to be 'very careful.'[1]

In early October, Indira developed a bad cold that rapidly transformed into a severe attack of pleurisy.* This resulted in fever that reached up to 103 degrees, rapid weight loss and severe chest congestion. She was moved to Bentford Hospital and her return to Oxford, where she was studying at the time, was cancelled. Her doctors advised her to go to a sanatorium in Switzerland as soon as possible. Though she had not yet been diagnosed with tuberculosis, the dreaded disease seemed the most likely culprit.[2]

To ensure the best treatment, rest and recuperation, Nehru wanted his daughter to go to Davos, the setting of Thomas Mann's novel, *The Magic Mountain,* which depicts a tuberculosis sanatorium. However, Mahatma Gandhi advised her to go to Dr Auguste Rollier's sanatorium in Leysin, Switzerland instead. She arrived there with her friend, Agatha Harrison, on 15 December 1939.[3]

---

* A painful condition where the lining around the lungs becomes inflamed, making it painful to breathe or cough.

At the time, tuberculosis (TB) was known as the 'white plague', an incurable disease that claimed at least a million lives every year in Europe alone, and accounted for one in every eight deaths in England and Wales.[4] Although Robert Koch isolated the tubercle bacillus, *Mycobacterium tuberculosis*, in 1882, the first antibiotic treatment for the disease was not developed until the 1940s. It would take equally long for an effective vaccine to be introduced, and it was nearly a century later that WHO recognized 24 March as World Tuberculosis Day.

During the early part of the twentieth century, when Indira Nehru was afflicted with tuberculosis, the very utterance of the word sent shockwaves among listeners. The prevalent manifestation of the illness was lung tuberculosis, commonly known as consumption or phthisis, and it primarily affected adults. The best available treatment for pulmonary tuberculosis* at the time was the 'open-air' method pioneered by Dr George Bodington in 1840. Bodington encouraged spending time outdoors so that patients could be exposed to fresh air, along with a regimen of rest, dietary therapy and light exercise.

Sanatorium cure, as it was called at the time, was gradually popularized as a recuperative method for TB. In 1854, it gained further recognition after Hermann Brehmer published his doctoral thesis titled, 'Tuberculosis is a Curable Disease'. In it, he reported that spending time in the Himalayan mountains had cured his TB. Brehmer later established an institution in the remote German village of Sokołowsko, located in present-day Poland, to treat TB patients with exposure to fresh air and good nutrition.[5]

A decade after Brehmer's initiative, French military surgeon Jean-Antoine Villemin demonstrated the infectious nature of the disease. He had observed that TB was more prevalent among soldiers stationed in barracks for extended periods than those in the field. He noted how healthy recruits from rural areas often developed tuberculosis within months of beginning their military service. To

---

* A type of tuberculosis that specifically affects the lungs.

test his hypothesis, Villemin conducted experiments by inoculating a rabbit with the purulent liquid collected from the tuberculous cavity of an individual who had died of TB.[6] Initially, the inoculated rabbit showed no signs of disease, but an autopsy* conducted three months later revealed that the animal had extensive tuberculosis. Villemin's work '*Cause et nature de la tuberculose: son inoculation de l'homme au lapin*' provided crucial evidence supporting the infectious nature of TB.[7]

The infectious nature of tuberculosis had long been a mystery, despite its presence throughout history. In fact, Mycobacterium genus, the causative agent of tuberculosis, is believed to have been present in Earth's environment for around 150 million years,[8] making tuberculosis one of humanity's most ancient diseases.[9] The earliest molecular traces of TB were identified in a fossilized Pleistocene bison using radiocarbon methods,† dated back 18,000 years. Traces of TB were found in human remains from a neolithic‡ settlement in the Eastern Mediterranean, dating back 9,000 years.[10]

Skeletal deformities that can be associated with tuberculosis were exhibited by Egyptian mummies from 2400 to 3400 BC.[11] In India and China, the earliest descriptions of tuberculosis date back around 3,300 and 2,300 years.[12] In Biblical texts, tuberculosis was referred to using the Hebrew term *schachepheth*, meaning a wasting disease.[13]

In ancient Greece, Isocrates was the first to propose that tuberculosis could be an infectious ailment while Aristotle highlighted its communicable nature and referred to it as the 'king's evil' in swine and cattle.[14] Ancient Greeks documented tuberculosis under the names phthisis or consumption, and Hippocrates detailed symptoms that closely mirrored the common characteristics of the tubercular lung lesions in Book I, *Of the Epidemics*. [15]

---

* A medical examination of a body after death to find out the cause of death.

† A scientific method used to find out how old something is by measuring the amount of carbon-14 left in it – often used with fossils or ancient bones.

‡ A time period around 9,000 years ago when humans began farming and living in settled communities.

In 1867, Theodor Albrecht Edwin Klebs was one of the earliest scientists who attempted to isolate the TB bacillus. Klebs cultivated tuberculous material on egg-white stored in sterile flasks. The culture quickly became turbid, revealing the presence of moving bacteria, that induced the disease upon being inoculated into the peritoneal cavity of guinea pigs. Robert Koch was the first to successfully isolate the tubercle bacillus using the methylene blue staining method,* as recommended by Paul Ehrlich. Koch identified, isolated and cultivated the bacillus in animal serum and replicated the disease by inoculating the bacillus into laboratory animals.[16]

On 24 March 1882, Koch presented his groundbreaking research to the Society of Physiology in Berlin, marking a significant milestone in the fight against TB. Koch would go on to win the Nobel Prize in Medicine in 1905 for his contribution to elucidating the infectious etiology of TB.

The decades following Koch's discovery would be marked by more in-depth research and breakthroughs in the study of TB. In 1907, Austrian paediatrician Clemens von Pirquet and French physician Charles Mantoux developed the tuberculin skin test,† which German physician Felix Mendel later also worked on. This came to be known as the Mantoux test and remains the simple standard test for latent TB infection to date.

Eight years after Koch's discovery, twenty-seven-year-old Leon Charles Albert Calmette, driven by a passion for scientific research in tropical diseases, joined the French Colonial Medical Service. He demonstrated such prowess in microbiology that Louis Pasteur handpicked him to head the Pasteur Institute in Saigon, Vietnam. Over the next two years at the institute, Calmette organized vaccination campaigns against smallpox and rabies and delved into researching snake venom. He was able to produce a polyvalent anti-

---

* A lab technique that uses a blue dye to highlight bacteria under a microscope so they're easier to see.

† A simple test where a small amount of a TB protein is injected under the skin to check if someone has been exposed to TB bacteria.

snake venom serum, a notable feat.

In 1901, Calmette was bitten by a venomous snake while in his lab, putting his life at risk. He swiftly injected himself with the serum he had developed and although he recovered, he lost the tip of his finger. Following this incident, Calmette's work expanded beyond snake venom research. During the savage plague epidemic in the Far East in 1894, he worked on developing an anti-plague serum, building on Haffkine's research in India. In 1895, he was transferred to the Pasteur Institute in Lille, France, where he served the next twenty-four years as its director. There, he made groundbreaking strides in TB research, collaborating with his colleague Camille Guerin.

Guerin studied veterinary medicine at the Ecole Nationale Vétérinaire d'Alfort, France under the directorship of Edmond Nocard. While studying at the school, Guerin was entrusted by Nocard with the task of delivering early samples of anti-diphtheria and anti-tetanus sera from Ecole Alfort to Émile Roux at the Pasteur Institute in Paris.

After graduating from Alfort in 1896, on Nocard's recommendation, Guerin joined the newly established Pasteur Institute in Lille as an assistant to Calmette. Guerin mainly helped with the preparation of vaccines and sera but his focus would shift to tuberculosis research by 1900.

In 1886, Calmette, observing Marfan's Law – which noted the rarity of pulmonary tuberculosis in individuals with a history of tuberculous neck lymph nodes – began working on a vaccine to artificially stimulate specific immunity to the tubercle bacillus.

Previous attempts to create such a vaccine had failed, as boiling or chemically treating tubercle bacilli proved ineffective. Live vaccines were deemed necessary, but injecting small doses of virulent human or bovine tubercle bacilli was too dangerous. Even experiments using bacilli obtained from turtles or attempting to attenuate the virulence by keeping the bacillus in leeches were unsuccessful.

However, a turning point came in 1908 at the Pasteur Institute in Lille, where Calmette and Guerin successfully cultivated tubercle bacilli on a medium of glycerine and potato.[17] After initial experiments, they added ox-bile to counteract clumping, leading to a surprising observation – subculturing (a microbiological cell culture made by transferring some or all cells from a previous culture to a fresh growth medium) lowered the virulence of the organism. This chance finding spurred their determination to develop a vaccine from the attenuated tubercle bacillus.[18]

By 1919, after developing about 230 subcultures, they finally arrived at a tubercle bacillus that didn't induce progressive tuberculosis when injected into various animals. In 1921, Calmette initiated the first human trial of the vaccine – later named Bacille Calmette-Guérin, shortened to BCG – by administering it orally to an infant at the Charité Hospital in Paris. The oral route was chosen because Calmette believed that the gastrointestinal tract was the natural infection route for the tubercle bacillus. Subsequent trials through the subcutaneous and cutaneous routes in infants elicited reactions such as redness or swelling. Such trials then were met with objections from parents, leading to the continued use of the oral method.

By 1924, 664 infants had been orally vaccinated with BCG, and mass production began at the Pasteur Institute in Lille. Calmette and Guerin confidently declared BCG a 'virus fixe'.[19] From 1924 to 1928, 114,000 infants were vaccinated without serious complications. In 1928, Guerin joined Calmette in Paris, taking charge of BCG preparation in the laboratory.[20]

The safety of BCG had been established, but questions arose regarding its effectiveness after Calmette and Guerin's statistics indicated a decrease in tuberculosis mortality among vaccinated infants. Although this decrease was initially seen as evidence of the vaccine's success, doubts emerged since the reduction could also have resulted from other factors, such as improvements in public health or living conditions, rather than the vaccine itself. In the 1940s, many studies supporting the efficacy of BCG emerged. With tuberculosis becoming a major health concern, BCG gained momentum, and its use was also encouraged by UNICEF and WHO.

In the 1950s, major trials in the UK and the US revealed that the UK's approach of using a Copenhagen strain of BCG for thirteen-year-olds who were tuberculin-negative was highly effective.[21] Meanwhile the Tice strain being used in the US on tuberculin negatives of various ages provided minimal protection.[22] Based on these findings, the UK recommended routine BCG for tuberculin-negative adolescents, while the US restricted its use to specific high-risk groups. The rest of the world, following Europe and WHO's lead, adopted routine BCG vaccination with various schedules, with Scandinavian countries being a strong votary. However, the results continued to vary across locations.

Two hypotheses surfaced to explain the varying results. One hypothesis attributed it to variations between different BCG strains used in vaccines, also because strains used by different manufacturers exhibited microbiological differences, potentially impacting immunogenicity, the ability to provoke an immune response. While there were over twenty genetically distinct BCG strains, more than ninety per cent of vaccines were from five strains: Pasteur 1173 P2, Danish 1331, Glaxo 1077 derived from the Danish 1331, Tokyo 172-1 and Russian BCG-I.[23]

Another theory stemmed from the US trials which linked poor results in specific regions to populations that had already been exposed to diverse environmental mycobacteria.[24] One of the regions that wasn't impacted much by this controversy was Asia. And more specifically India, a country in the midst of gaining independence from British rule.

At the time of independence, India was grappling with myriad challenges, with tuberculosis being one of the foremost focuses of the new Prime Minister, Jawaharlal Nehru. This may have been partly because his own daughter had suffered from the disease – an ordeal he had been a witness to – and partly because half a million lives in India were being lost to TB annually.

In May 1948, the new government declared that tuberculosis was reaching 'epidemic proportions' in the country. Therefore, an uncompromising crusade was launched against the disease, undeterred by budgetary limitations. One of the first steps taken was the establishment of a BCG vaccine laboratory at the King Institute in Guindy, near Madras. This collaborative effort, in partnership with vaccine-maker Staten's Serum Institute in Copenhagen, bore the crucial responsibility of manufacturing and supplying the BCG vaccine to the Indian population.

In 1948, BCG vaccination started for the first time in India. Soon after, a series of epidemiological surveys were conducted in Madanapalle in present-day Andhra Pradesh at the behest of the Government of India (GOI), as a prelude to the introduction of BCG vaccination on a mass scale.[25] This was a joint effort by the ICMR, the Union Mission Tuberculosis Sanatorium and WHO.

The survey was crucial because there was some skepticism regarding the effectiveness of BCG in tropical countries when it was deployed in the field, for two possible reasons. In tropical regions, a significant portion of the population had developed a naturally acquired, low strength tuberculin response of an unknown, likely non-specific, origin. Additionally, the effectiveness of BCG vaccinations in tropical areas could be compromised if the vaccine's efficacy deteriorated due to exposure to heat or light during transit and storage. The Madanapalle trials tried to address these challenges by analyzing the vaccine's efficacy in such conditions.

In 1960, an initial report of the Madanapalle trials disappointed the nation with its finding that the vaccine did not provide protection against tuberculosis. Though the number of tuberculosis incidences among the vaccinated were exceptionally small in the initial follow-up, subsequent follow-up assessments revealed a substantial increase in the number of cases.[26] However, it was concluded that BCG produced a significant reduction in the number of tuberculosis cases, though the degree of protection was only about 56 to 60 per cent.[27] This would turn out to be the first controlled trial of BCG vaccination on an Asian population.

Acting on the findings of the Madanapalle study, the GOI

took measures to create an advanced research institute dedicated solely to tuberculosis research, the National Tuberculosis Institute in Bangalore. The ICMR–National Institute for Research in Tuberculosis, Chennai, initially known as the Tuberculosis Research Centre (TRC), serves as a supra-national reference laboratory and a WHO Collaborating Centre for TB research and training.

In the 1960s, another study unfolded in the Chingleput region in Tamil Nadu. Based on a wider field trial using two BCG strains – Pasteur 1173 P2 and the Danish 1331 – each administered in two different doses. The region was specifically chosen for trials due to the mass exposure to environmental mycobacteria.

The trials, planned with the collaboration of the ICMR, WHO and the US Public Health Service, aimed to unravel the mysteries surrounding BCG's protective powers. A controlled trial in a northern Indian location with lower environmental mycobacterial exposure was also planned to compare outcomes. However, that did not happen due to some political unrest.

In 1963, another controlled field study was initiated that involved a larger population, spanning several years. By 1966, the project originally planned as a work of the National Tuberculosis Institute Bangalore became a separate project under the ICMR. The research protocol for a controlled field trial involving a placebo and two doses using two different strains of BCG was accepted by ICMR in 1968. Chingleput had been intentionally kept out of BCG vaccination trials earlier, to prepare for a larger study of this kind. The prevalence of tuberculosis in the region was almost 50 to 100 per cent higher than in Bangalore, a control location some 300 kilometres away.

The results, only made public in 1979 after seven and a half years of evaluation, surprised the scientific community. Contrary to expectations, neither of the two BCG strains demonstrated any significant shield against pulmonary tuberculosis. Individuals who were initially deemed tuberculin 'negative' exhibited a remarkably lower risk of the disease than anticipated. An even more confounding observation was that, shortly after vaccination, the vaccinated group remained more susceptible to contracting the disease than the control group, though the statistical significance of this observation remained uncertain.[28]

Despite two workshops organized by WHO that validated the trial's methodology, its results were not comprehensively presented. The absence of detailed data left researchers grappling with uncertainty about what transpired in the Chingleput trial. The unexpected outcome triggered a cascade of observational studies across different global populations, each probing the enigma of BCG's variable efficacy. The quest for a universally accepted explanation for this variation persisted, leaving the scientific community in a state of suspense regarding the true nature of BCG's efficacy.

One important takeaway from the evaluation was that incidence of TB could be less frequent among individuals initially non-reactive to tuberculin, especially those in younger age groups who could potentially benefit from BCG vaccination.[29] This translated to an increased efficacy of the vaccine among the younger population.

The study followed up on the entire population for fifteen years through surveys every thirty months, selective follow-ups every ten months and continuous detection of passive cases. Of the 109,873 tuberculin-negative individuals with a normal chest X-ray at intake, 560 TB cases emerged over the study period, less than 5.6 cases per thousand. Similar incidence rates in the three vaccination groups confirmed the absence of protective efficacy observed at the seven-and-a-half-year mark. It can be reasonably concluded that BCG offered no overall protection in adults and exhibited a low level of overall protection in children.[30] The fifteen-year findings demonstrated that, in a population with high infection rates and non-specific sensitivity, BCG did not offer any protection against bacillary pulmonary tuberculosis.

A series of unrelated studies were carried out simultaneously to assess changes in the tuberculosis situation in a population, particularly the prevalence of infection among children over different periods up to fifteen years. Following the initial tuberculin testing, additional rounds of tuberculin testing were conducted in some locations at intervals of ten and fifteen years for children whose ages ranged between one and nineteen years. One such study was in Chengalpet itself, where the fifteen-year vaccine trial was conducted.

The results of the study within Chengalpet aligned with findings from investigations conducted in other regions of the country. From 1961 to 1973 in the Tumkur district of Karnataka, similar prevalence rates were found among subjects up to nineteen years old over a twelve-year period. In a five-year study from 1974 to 1979, no decline in infections was noticed among children aged up to nine years in Doddaballapura taluk near Bangalore.[31]

A longitudinal study conducted in three taluks of Bangalore district reported fluctuating but stable infection rates over sixteen years, until 1977, among children aged zero to fourteen years.[32] A fifteen-year study carried out in Delhi from 1962 to 1977 too found no significant change in crucial epidemiological indices.[33] These multiple studies were used to conclude that there was no apparent alteration in the overall prevalence of the disease among children in the country.

The Chingelpet study established, for the first time anywhere in the world, the basic principles of double-blind randomized trials in which neither the participants nor the researchers involved knew who was receiving the treatment and who was receiving a placebo, thereby helping to eliminate any bias. The study's main outcome highlighted the inadequacy of the BCG vaccine in regions where tuberculosis was endemic.

Despite its long history and concerns about its efficacy, the BCG vaccine remains the only human vaccine against TB with solid evidence supporting its role in T cell generation as the primary mechanism of immunity. T cell responses are stronger, longer-lasting and offer greater cross-protection compared to humoral responses. As a result, modern vaccine development increasingly focuses on enhancing T cell-mediated immunity. Additionally, the regulatory mechanisms of T cells help prevent vaccines from triggering autoimmune diseases.

The BCG vaccine has been produced using two variants: the Copenhagen (Danish 1331) strain and the Pasteur 1173 P2 strain. In India, the Copenhagen strain was produced at the BCG Vaccine Laboratory in Guindy, Tamil Nadu until the laboratory developed its own BCG seed known as the Madras Working Seed Lot (MWSL), which was subsequently used to supply vaccines for India's national immunization programme.

Over time, private companies such as the Serum Institute of India in Pune and Green Signal Bio Pharma Ltd. in Chennai have taken over the production of the vaccine from the BCGVL. The Serum Institute of India began selling a live attenuated freeze-dried BCG vaccine under the brand name 'Tubervac', using the Russian strain.[34]

In the last few decades, drug-resistant strains* of TB emerged as a consequence of an increase in antimicrobial resistance (AMR). WHO reports the highest proportion of drug-resistant TB in Europe, with around twenty-five per cent of new patients and fifty per cent of previously treated patients experiencing drug resistance. Although TB predominantly affects LMICs, the number of cases has also been rising in some high-income nations since 2020, reversing the previous trend of gradual decline, thanks to AMR.[35]

In response to this emerging crisis, the Government of India has launched a plan to eliminate TB by 2025, establishing a TB Research Consortium under the ICMR to test and validate new drugs and vaccines. In parallel, WHO has set up the TB Vaccine Accelerator Council to facilitate the licensing and use of novel TB vaccines, working with funders, global agencies, governments and end users to overcome the challenges to TB vaccine development.[36]

In 2022, the Serum Institute of India developed the recombinant BCG (rBCG) vaccine† VPM1002 and sought emergency authorization‡ from the Indian regulator to use it on adults.

---

* Versions of the parasite that no longer respond to medicines that used to kill them.

† A recombinant vaccine is made by modifying the genes of a bacterium or virus in a lab to improve its effectiveness or safety.

‡ A special permission granted by a regulator to allow the use of a vaccine or medicine

VPM1002 is progressing through clinical trials as of 2025, with Phase 1 and 2b studies showing favorable safety and immunogenicity. The Phase III of 'PreVentTB' study, led by ICMR and involving over 12,000 adults, concluded in late 2024.

Additionally, other promising vaccine candidates are undergoing trials worldwide. MTBVAC, a live-attenuated Spanish vaccine derived from a human strain of *Mycobacterium tuberculosis*, is currently in Phase 3 trials in India and Phase 2b trials in South Africa, Kenya and Tanzania.[37] Meanwhile, the M72/AS01E vaccine candidate developed by GlaxoSmithKline (GSK) has entered Phase 3 trials across seven countries, following earlier Phase 2b results that demonstrated a fifty per cent reduction in the progression from latent to active TB in adults, indicating significant potential for disease prevention.[38]

Despite these advancements, WHO's 2024 TB report indicates tuberculosis claimed 1.25 million lives in 2023, with almost 10.8 million people infected worldwide. Alarmingly, 2.8 million infections and 315,000 deaths were from India.

---

undergoing trials during a public health emergency.

19

'COULD YOU PATENT THE SUN?'

IN THE SCORCHING SUMMER OF 1952, AS THE MERCURY soared above 100°F (38°C), a crippling disease gripped the American state of Texas. Swimming pools, cinema halls, bars and even bowling alleys were closed down and the streets were doused with insecticides, apparently to kill the transmitting vectors.*

Amid this growing panic and stifling heat, six-year-old Paul Alexander, who lived in a tranquil Dallas suburb, ventured out to play one afternoon, ignoring his parents' warnings. He returned in the evening with neck pain and a pounding head. A single glance at the boy's distressed face alarmed his mother, prompting her to send him to bed after retrieving his soiled shoes. Despite worsening symptoms a day later, the family doctor advised against hospitalization, citing the overwhelming patient load in the neighbourhood hospitals. Alexander's chances were better at home, he advised.

As the days passed, Alexander's condition deteriorated. Barely able to hold a crayon or perform basic functions, his parents rushed him to Parkland hospital, where he was diagnosed with poliomyelitis, a disabling disease caused by the poliovirus. Poliomyelitis, known popularly as polio, targets the motor neurons in the spinal cord, disrupting the communication between the body's central nervous system and muscles. This disruption ultimately leads to muscle

* (In genetic engineering) A DNA molecule used to carry a gene into a new cell.

weakness, making it challenging for an individual to breathe independently.

Overwhelmed by the sheer volume of polio patients, the hospital was struggling to accommodate patients. Left in a hallway on a gurney, barely breathing, Alexander was staring death in the eye until a kind doctor rushed him to the operation table and performed a life-saving tracheotomy* to clear the congestion in his lungs.

Alexander woke up three days later and found himself confined within a machine that echoed with wheezes and sighs. The machine, called an 'iron lung', is a cylinder-like canister that stimulated breathing in patients who were afflicted with respiratory paralysis.† With his body paralyzed, speech silenced and vision obscured by the fogged windows of the steam tent, he felt trapped. When the tent was finally lifted, he was met with the sight of other children encased in similar metal canisters surrounded by nurses in starched white uniforms. Rows of iron lungs, stretched endlessly in the hallway – a haunting tableau of the devastating impact of polio on young lives.[1]

Alexander did recover from the initial infection but was left severely crippled by polio, with near complete paralysis from the neck down. The iron lung became his lifeline, taking over the function of breathing as his diaphragm could no longer perform. Positioned flat on his back, Alexander's head rested on a pillow placed within the metal cylinder that enclosed his body from the neck down. A motor-powered set of leather bellows created a vacuum by extracting air from the cylinder, inducing negative pressure‡ to expand his lungs. The subsequent pumping of air back into the cylinder gently deflated his lungs, creating the consistent hissing and sighing sounds that sustained his life.

---

* A medical procedure in which a small hole is made in the windpipe (trachea) to help someone breathe when their airway is blocked.

† A condition where the muscles needed to breathe stop working, often caused by damage to the nerves from diseases like polio.

‡ A method of helping people breathe by creating suction around the chest, causing the lungs to expand like in natural breathing.

Alexander holds the Guinness World Record for living the longest time in an iron lung – over seventy years.[2] Despite the gradual availability of more modern ventilator machinery, he chose to stick to his 'old iron horse' that he had grown accustomed to.

Polio, caused by three serotypes* of the poliovirus, is a severe paralytic condition that attacked the central nervous system. The virus, in most cases, causes temporary or permanent paralysis and can even result in death. Poliovirus, an enterovirus† that infects the gastrointestinal tract, enters the body through the mouth. It spreads through direct exposure to an infected person, via oral-oral transmission through saliva or by consuming food contaminated with fecal matter, known as fecal-oral transmission. Commonly referred to as infantile paralysis,‡ polio predominantly affects younger children. Survivors face lifelong consequences, sometimes requiring leg braces, crutches, wheelchairs or artificial respirators like the iron lung.

Prior to the nineteenth century, most children were likely to be exposed to the virus before the age of one. However, antibodies passed from mothers to babies during pregnancy protected them from contracting the disease.[3] With advancements in sanitation, the chances of encountering poliovirus at an early age reduced. However, this meant children's immune systems were unprepared to defend against subsequent exposure to the virus later in childhood.

Polio's existence traces back to ancient times, as can be seen in ancient Egyptian depictions of children with characteristic withered limbs. Despite affecting children globally for centuries, the first clinical description was recorded in 1789 by British doctor Michael

* Different versions or types of the same virus, each with slightly different characteristics. For polio, there are three major serotypes.

† A group of viruses that usually enter the body through the mouth and live in the gut.

‡ An older term for polio, because the disease often affected children and could cause paralysis.

Underwood. It was not formally recognized until 1840, when a German physician named Jakob Heine identified it. The late nineteenth and early twentieth centuries saw frequent epidemics that turned polio into the world's most feared disease.

By the mid-twentieth century, the poliovirus annually killed or paralyzed over half a million children worldwide. Significant epidemics continued to leave thousands of victims, primarily young children, crippled and in some cases, dead. A major outbreak in New York City in 1916 led to over 2,000 deaths. In the US, polio swept the west each summer in the 1940s and '50s, causing over 15,000 paralysis cases annually. The worst US outbreak of 1952, in which Alexander was paralyzed, claimed 3,145 lives, disabling over 21,000 people.

Polio's unpredictability heightened its terror. The majority showed no symptoms, while thirty per cent experienced minor illness. However, four to five per cent faced serious symptoms, including extreme pain, fever, and delirium. Paralytic polio affected a small fraction of cases, with a five to ten per cent fatality rate. With no cure and escalating epidemics, the creation of a vaccine was a top priority.

Scientists began working on a vaccine in the US and Europe, and many high-profile individuals and organizations extended support and financial aid. One such organization was the National Foundation for Infantile Paralysis, set up by the US President Franklin D. Roosevelt, who himself was a victim of the disease at the age of thirty-nine and suffered significant physical disability.[4]

On 12 April 1955, a decade after President Roosevelt's death, Dr Thomas Francis Jr., who had supervised vaccine testing under Dr Jonas Salk at the University of Michigan, addressed an audience of 500, including 150 members of the press. An additional 54,000 physicians watched from movie theatres nationwide, while millions tuned in to the live national radio broadcast. The atmosphere in the auditorium was electric, with sixteen cameras capturing every moment. Eli Lilly, a major pharmaceutical company, invested $250,000 to broadcast the event, ensuring that even the most remote locations could witness this historic moment. Department stores set up loudspeakers to amplify the radio broadcast, judges suspended trials at the time of the address and people around the globe tuned in via the Voice of America radio station.

As the world waited with bated breath, Dr Francis proclaimed the groundbreaking news – the polio vaccine developed by Salk and his team had been a success. He uttered three words –'safe, effective and potent' –and this significant moment in medical history was received with thunderous applause. As Francis shared the results, revealing an eighty to ninety per cent effectiveness based on data from eleven states, the significance of the achievement sank in.

The trial, spread across sites in the US, Canada and Finland, was the largest in the history of medicine, involving 1.8 million children – over 600,000 received injections of either vaccine or placebo. Another million were observed as controls. More than 144 million separate pieces of data were collected and analyzed.[5] This breakthrough, made possible by tireless scientific efforts, marked the dawn of a new era in medicine. It would be described as 'the most significant biomedical advancement of the century.'[6]

The *New York Times* hailed the vaccine as a 'medical classic',[7] and Salk, when asked about improving effectiveness, expressed the tantalizing possibility of achieving 100 per cent protection from paralysis with the new vaccines and vaccination procedures.[8] In two days, when the details were published in the *Journal of the American Medical Association*,[9] the world witnessed a triumph over a relentless adversary, and hope had taken root in the form of a vaccine.

In 1954, Salk reported in the *American Journal of Public Health and the Nation's Health* that, through the correct administration of a properly prepared non-infectious vaccine,* the production of antibodies against polio could be triggered. In many cases, the concentration of antibodies in the bloodstream could be elevated to

* A vaccine made from a dead or inactivated virus that cannot cause disease but still triggers an immune response.

levels comparable to those present in individuals who had undergone a naturally acquired infection, he reported after running trials.[10]

With that, Salk became a hero in the US, and the rest of the world.

Born in 1914, Salk embarked on virus research during the 1930s as a medical student. One of his early contributions was to the development of flu vaccines during World War II. In 1947, he was heading a research lab at the University of Pittsburgh and secured a grant a year later to study the polio virus. By 1950, he had arrived at an initial version of the vaccine in his lab.

Salk's vaccine broke all three serotypes of polio virus that had been creating havoc. He used formaldehyde and injected the neutralized virus strains into a person's bloodstream, which triggered the immune system to create antibodies against poliomyelitis. Clinical trials involving 1.3 million American school children commenced in 1954. The vaccine's effectiveness and safety were confirmed by April 1955, initiating a nationwide inoculation campaign.

Soon after the announcement, the media questioned who would own the patent of the vaccine. Salk eloquently replied, 'Well, the people, I would say. There is no patent. Could you patent the sun?'[11] It is this embodiment of humanism, and not just his remarkable achievements, that has forever secured Salk's place in medical history.

Despite being the first to develop a polio vaccine, Salk neither won the Nobel Prize nor was offered a membership at the prestigious US National Academy of Sciences. Researchers who examined the Nobel Archives revealed that Dr Sven Gard, Professor of Virology at the Karolinska Institute, Sweden – who was also involved in polio vaccine research – was largely responsible for denying the prize to Salk. He may or may not have been influenced by pharmaceutical lobbies.[12]

Despite the media haunting his every step, Salk shied away from public attention even as he faced criticism from a section of his colleagues who viewed him as a 'publicity hound'. In 1962, he established the Salk Institute for Biological Studies in La Jolla, California, with initial funding from the National Foundation for Infantile Paralysis, which had been renamed the March of Dimes. Salk continued his research, focusing on multiple sclerosis, cancer and AIDS. In his later years, he dedicated himself to creating a killed-virus vaccine to prevent AIDS in individuals infected with the human immunodeficiency virus (HIV).

There is no denying that Salk's vaccine led to a significant drop in polio cases. It was popular till the arrival of Sabin's oral polio vaccine (OPV) in 1962, notwithstanding the tragedy caused by a defective Salk Vaccine produced by Cutter Laboratories, California which led to polio cases and fatalities.

However, not everyone was convinced that a killed-virus vaccine could effectively prevent polio. American researchers, mainly Herold Cox, Hilary Koprowski and Albert Sabin, were skeptical and explored alternate approaches. Foremost among these efforts was Sabin's work on developing a live attenuated vaccine for oral administration – a breakthrough that would soon lead to the advent of OPV, revolutionizing polio control measures.

Sabin began making big strides in his lab by utilizing techniques pioneered by Renato Dulbecco, an Italian–American virologist who won the 1975 Nobel Prize in Physiology. Sabin developed a vaccine consisting of attenuated strains of all three types of the poliovirus (trivalent) at the Children's Hospital in Cincinnati. He tested it on 10,000 monkeys, 160 chimpanzees and a few humans, including himself, his daughters and some young volunteers from the federal prison of Chillicothe, Ohio.

Sabin attenuated the virus by repeatedly passing the virus through non-human cells at sub-physiological* temperatures.[13] Once the attenuated virus in Sabin's vaccine was inside the human body, it replicated efficiently in the gut, where generally the poliovirus infects and replicates. However, it wasn't possible for the attenuated virus

* Less than that found in a normal physiology.

to replicate efficiently in the nervous system because of its reduced strength.[14]

Since a single dose of the vaccine contained three strains of attenuated virus, when it administered orally, it produced antibodies against all three poliovirus serotypes in nearly fifty per cent of people. Interestingly, after three doses, it provided immunity against all three poliovirus types in more than ninety-five per cent of the recipients.[15] Human trials were conducted in 1957 and a year later, the US National Institutes of Health (NIH) cleared the vaccine, disregarding the live vaccines of Koprowski and other researchers.[16] However, with the Cutter incident fresh in its memory and commercial interests, the US government did not approve large-scale field testing in its territory.[17]

As a result, subsequent testing of the vaccine happened in the Soviet Union and a few other regions. Sabin, being a person of Polish-Russian origin, facilitated the Soviet trials. From 1959 to 1961, millions of children, including 75 million in the Soviet Union alone (by another account, 15 million by July 1960), received Sabin's vaccine and he was honoured with the Soviet Union's highest civilian honour. Around the same time, Koprowski tested his vaccine in Northern Ireland and in and around Congo, while Cox tested his vaccine in Latin America.[18]

In contrast to Salk's injectable vaccine, the Sabin vaccine was administered orally, suspended in syrup or sugar cubes. Sabin asserted that his vaccine provided more potency and longer-lasting protection than Salk's. Furthermore, the oral administration made Sabin's vaccine more convenient compared to Salk's, which required multiple hypodermic injections for effectiveness. However, a significant drawback of the Sabin vaccine was the slight possibility of infection from the live virus that it contained.

By 1962, the Sabin vaccine received federal licensure and gained endorsement from the American Medical Association. By 1965, almost 100 million people in the US had received the vaccine, and many more in other countries.[19] The Sabin vaccine became the primary preventive measure for polio by the end of the 1960s.

Like Salk, Sabin too did not patent his vaccine and wanted it to be used as widely as possible. 'A lot of people insisted that I should patent the vaccine, but I didn't want to do that ... It's my gift to all the world's children,' he would say, refusing to exploit the vaccine commercially, making it very affordable to the poorest of the poor.[20]

Sabin's vaccine was deemed superior based on the veracity of outcomes. It provided longer-lasting immunity, eliminating the need for repeated boosters* and offered swift protection. It was more convenient to administer than the injectable Salk vaccine. More importantly, the Sabin vaccine helped in passive vaccination,† as it induced an active infection in the bowel, leading to the excretion of live-attenuated virus in fecal matter and thereby reaching municipal sewage systems, which in turn protected those who hadn't been vaccinated.

Over time, the Sabin vaccine replaced the Salk vaccine, and by 1968, Salk's vaccine was no longer administered in the US and in many western countries, with pharmaceutical companies ceasing its production altogether and opting for the Sabin vaccine instead.[21] Countries in Europe and Scandinavia continued the use of the Salk vaccine, despite the apparent advantages of the live-attenuated Sabin vaccine.

However, there was growing speculation that the live-attenuated virus strain in the Sabin vaccine could lead to paralytic poliomyelitis‡ in some people, especially adults – a condition that came to be known as vaccine associated paralytic poliomyelitis (VAPP). In response to multiple incidences of VAPP, in 1964, an advisory committee was appointed by the US Surgeon General to examine the occurrences between 1955 and 1961 (when only the Salk vaccine was used) and between 1961 and 1964 (when the Sabin vaccine prevailed). The findings revealed that fifty-seven of the eighty-seven reported cases of

---

* An extra dose of a vaccine given after the initial one(s) to increase or renew immunity.

† Unvaccinated individuals gain protection indirectly, through exposure to the weakened virus shed by vaccinated individuals.

‡ A severe form of polio that causes muscle paralysis, often in the legs.

paralytic polio in the United States since 1961 were deemed to have been caused by the attenuated poliovirus regaining its virulence.[22]

Therefore, by the mid-1960s, health officials around the world began balancing between the numerous benefits of the live-attenuated vaccine and the small but definite risks associated with it. The Salk vaccine was reconsidered by many researchers as it was relatively safer. Concerns about this risk led several countries, including Sweden, to prefer the Salk vaccine.

Notwithstanding these developments in the west, India was far behind in vaccine research, despite sporadic incidences of polio in many parts of the country. The only significant effort came from a Polio Research Unit established under the ICMR in 1949 and a handful of dedicated scientists conducting basic research in some of the laboratories.

While Western scientists were working to isolate the poliovirus, India launched its own virus isolation* efforts under the leadership of C. G. Pandit, the first director of the ICMR. In the early 1950s, while investigating a polio outbreak in the Andaman Islands, Pandit conducted experiments by inoculating monkeys with virus specimen obtained from humans and serially passing† it six times, but unfortunately, the strains were lost before its viral identity could be confirmed.

However, in the late 1950s, the Enterovirus Research Centre (EVRC) successfully isolated the virus in primary monkey kidney cell culture and confirmed its identity by neutralizing the virus with antiserum.[23] The Bombay-based unit worked on elaborate data collection, especially on the epidemiology of urban poliomyelitis and was later renamed Enterovirus Laboratory. In 1964, another centre came up at the Christian Medical College (CMC), Vellore in Tamil Nadu[24] that would go on to take over polio research, conducting

* The process of identifying and extracting a virus from samples (like blood or stool) to study it in the lab.

† The virus is transferred from one set of cells or animals to another, multiple times, to increase its quantity or study changes in it.

vaccine trials as well as polio surveillance for the next half a century till polio was completely eradicated from the country and over 1.4 billion people were saved from the disease.

The rigorous investigation and visionary experiments that led to the decline of incidence of polio were championed by a paediatrician turned epidemiologist from the CMC, Vellore – Dr Thekkekara Jacob John.

20

THE POLIO END GAME

IN THE WINTER OF 1967, IN VELLORE – LOCATED MIDWAY between Bangalore and Madras – Thekkekara Jacob John found himself faced with a medical mystery. In his out-patient department at the Christian Medical College he had noticed a few cases of children who, despite taking three doses of trivalent oral polio vaccine (tOPV, Sabin), were falling victim to the virus. He began passively investigating the case and assumed that it was possible that these cases indicated the failure of vaccines. Known in medical circles as 'vaccine-failure polio', such cases had not yet been documented in countries where tOPV was widely used, be it in North America or in Europe.

Polio was rampant in India at the time, with around 500 cases being reported daily on average. Armed with an MRCP in Paediatrics, a fellowship in paediatric infectious diseases and a post-graduation in microbiology from Denver, Colorado, John was drawn into the thick of it. He quickly shifted his focus from his clinical practice to the realm of public health and epidemiological studies, spending much of his time with local communities and civil society.

Soon after setting up the Enterovirus Centre in 1964, the Christian Medical College in Vellore carried out a longitudinal community survey in the area and found subclinical poliovirus infection* in 242

* An infection where a person carries the virus but does not show any obvious symptoms.

of 1,000 children below five years of age.[1] Another study in the nearby village helped establish that the prevalence of poliovirus was found to be higher in urban areas compared to rural communities.[2] These studies, along with research in places like Bombay, revealed that the country had a high prevalence of both poliovirus infection and paralytic poliomyelitis.

In fact, the incidence of paralytic polio in India was among the highest anywhere in the world, with a significant number of cases occurring in infants below six months of age. The findings suggested a high frequency of transmission, especially through respiratory means, contributing to the polio burden of the country.[3] Despite this dire situation, efforts to control polio received limited attention from the Government of India which was responsible for earmarking and devolving funds for its control and eradication.

Meanwhile, the government was focused on diseases like tuberculosis, malaria, leprosy and kala azar. This negligence continued for a while, despite the fact that IPV* had been available since 1955, and OPV since 1962, with demonstrated safety and efficacy. It was only in 1964 that OPV was introduced in the country, first in Bombay and then in Vellore.

However, OPV came with its own set of problems – it did not deliver the promised immunogenic efficacy† and vaccine efficacy, as was shown in the clinical studies. Despite being administered three doses of OPV, some children contracted the polio infection. These were the cases John began investigating in 1967.

Various reports of children developing poliomyelitis continued to come from other parts of the country as well, reflecting poor vaccine efficacy. In 1970, the first definitive study on the problem of low immunogenic efficacy of the OPV with standard potency was published by John, who had made it his life's mission to eradicate

---

* A polio vaccine made by using a killed form of the polio virus, ensuring immunity without the risk of disease. It is sometimes referred to as Injectable Polio Vaccine because it is injected and not orally administered.

† How well a vaccine can trigger the body's immune system to protect against a disease.

polio from the country. Studies from Delhi and Bombay also indicated low immunogenic efficacy.

Warnings about the poor efficacy of OPV in India were evident years before the 1978 launch of the Expanded Programme on Immunization (EPI). This WHO-driven campaign aimed to reduce fatalities from diseases like diphtheria, pertussis, tetanus, poliomyelitis and tuberculosis through effective vaccination. In contrast, during clinical studies, IPV had demonstrated excellent Vaccine Effectiveness (VE). Since 1955, IPV had been successfully employed in the US, Canada, the UK and several northern European countries, resulting in a rapid and substantial reduction of over ninety-five per cent polio cases. Finland successfully interrupted the transmission of Wild Poliovirus (WPV) in 1962 by utilizing IPV campaigns. India confronted a dilemma as to which vaccine would most suit its needs.

Deploying IPV presented yet another challenge, as it had not been licensed for use in the country. In 1985, a manufacturer who attempted producing IPV under a state license in Maharashtra was forced to stop production after a directive from the Government of India. It was not until 2006 that IPV was licensed and its potential to be the vaccine of the future was acknowledged.[4]

OPV had a much longer history in India. Back in 1966, responding to a specific request from India, Albert Sabin generously contributed his vaccine strains to the Pasteur Institute in Coonoor, almost six years before donating the vaccine seeds to WHO. He went a step further by personally training the institute's staff and ensuring the establishment of an OPV manufacturing unit in the world's second most populated country. This initiative led to the successful production of six batches of OPV. However, rather than expanding its manufacturing capacity, the OPV unit was unexpectedly shut down in 1974.[5]

This unfolded at a time when WHO was devising strategies for the widespread use of OPV as part of the EPI in India. The discontinuation of production of OPV in the country meant that it had to be imported for use in EPI.[6] Consequently, the introduction of OPV under EPI experienced delays and when it was rolled out, it was confined to urban areas between 1979–80 and was extended to rural communities only two years later.

Beyond OPV's availability, the country's vast size and mobile population made polio vaccination daunting. With 27 million babies born annually and millions traveling daily on passenger trains, the risk of virus transmission remained high.

During this period, virus outbreaks had been rippling through neighbouring countries of Bangladesh, Nepal, Tajikistan and countries in Africa. The intricate web of poor sanitation, high population density, sub-par health conditions and the relentless onslaught of heat and monsoons – conditions that India too was battling with – were proving to be a breeding ground for the virus. Therefore, when the vaccine was introduced as part of the EPI, the stage was set for an extraordinary battle against a formidable adversary.

Amid these ambitious efforts, a new challenge emerged. In the western reaches of Uttar Pradesh, unverified rumours began circulating that the vaccine was 'haram' for Muslims and would sterilize boys, sowing seeds of distrust.

However, the most critical challenge arose from a short-sighted approach by the health policy makers. Since OPV was not immediately available in the country, the EPI commenced with the administration of DPT and BCG vaccines which were being produced by public sector companies. This strategy had overlooked the well-known fact that DPT vaccination given without a polio shot had the potential to trigger poliomyelitis. In a country with a high prevalence of polio, the introduction of DPT inoculation without prior polio vaccination created a man-made crisis that led to the loss of many million lives.

According to annual EPI reports that tracked vaccination progress against a total of 29 million children receiving DPT injections over the four-year period from 1978, only 4.4 million children received three doses of OPV.[7] This glaring discrepancy set the stage for what seemed to be the world's largest iatrogenic* outbreak of poliomyelitis in India during the early 1980s.[8,9]

Despite including OPV in the EPI, the incidence of polio cases persisted for a decade with two conflicting forces at play – the decrease in cases due to OPV and the increase caused by DPT. Amid these conflicting trends, a nationwide polio epidemic erupted in 1981 in the middle of an already hyper-endemic situation. That year alone saw over 38,000 reported cases, and the final tally was pegged at almost 200,000 cases. John, in a study jointly performed with his colleagues from the CMC, assessed the national productivity loss from this catastrophe at ₹450 billion.[10]

Through the seventies and eighties, new polio cases continued to surface among children who had already received three doses of OPV, indicating poor vaccine efficacy. In a sample study conducted by John in the Vellore region, the incidence of vaccine failure rose steadily – from ten per cent in 1979 to thirty per cent in 1986, and further to fifty per cent by 1989.[11] In response, health authorities implemented various strategies to address the issue, including a prime-boost† approach by administering additional doses.

Based on his trials involving the administration of five doses in infancy, which aligned with the five infant-contacts in the EPI with other vaccines, John proposed a five-dose strategy. However, the Ministry of Health dismissed his suggestion, adhering to the three-dose rule, potentially endangering many young lives.

Undeterred, John explored alternatives, including the use of IPV, which demonstrated predictability and complete protection. Surprisingly, the Ministry of Health did not grant license for IPV in the country.

John then proposed the concept of pulse polio vaccination campaigns‡, a strategy that could potentially control polio. Pulse

---

* A health problem caused by medical treatment itself, rather than by the original illness.

† A vaccination strategy where a person is first given one or more initial vaccine doses (prime) followed by additional doses (boost) to increase protection.

‡ Administering oral polio vaccine as drops into the mouths of children under five years of age.

vaccination, he argued, could disrupt the balance between the vaccinated and the susceptible children at a specific point in time, impeding the ease of transmission of wild polio virus (WPV). However, despite its promising potential, the Ministry of Health, yet again chose not to approve the vaccination campaign.

To circumvent governmental apathy, John drafted a pathbreaking collaboration with the Rotary Club of Vellore and the Vellore Municipality which led to the birth of pulse polio campaigns. The town was strategically divided into sixteen zones, each with a designated station for administering OPV. The campaign was to inoculate children below four years of age with three doses, strategically spaced at monthly intervals, ending towards the end of 1981. The community was mobilized through slide presentations in cinema halls, newspaper announcements and widely distributed handbills.

This was not just a routine vaccination – it was a community-wide endeavour fuelled by a shared vision of a polio-free future. Each campaign spanned four half-days, with four stations operating simultaneously, manned by volunteers from the CMC and municipal health centres. The impact of the campaign was monumental. To assess its reach and effectiveness, a thirty-cluster sample survey* was conducted in February 1982, strictly following WHO-recommended methods. The results were nothing short of a triumph, with a remarkable 62 per cent of children in the catchment area† receiving three doses of the oral polio vaccine.

John's strategic vision and collaborative approach proved that polio could indeed be controlled in small geographical units. Vellore became a beacon of hope and resilience, demonstrating that a community could, on its own, overcome a seemingly insurmountable challenge with hard work and cooperation. The success story echoed far beyond the town boundaries, inspiring other communities to embark on their own journeys toward a polio-free future. John's

* A survey method recommended by WHO, where thirty small groups are randomly selected to measure the reach of health programmes in a population.

† The geographic region or community served by a specific health programme or facility.

Vellore pulse polio campaign set a precedent for effective community-based health initiatives, leaving an indelible mark on the fight against polio in India and in the developing world.

Rotary International carried the message around the world and encouraged its national units to follow the suit. As the organization's efforts began to bear fruit, WHO, caught by surprise, teamed up with UNICEF and Rotary International for its Polio Plus initiative. It passed a resolution in 1988 at the World Health Assembly to 'eradicate polio globally by the year 2000' through mass campaigns.[12]

Meanwhile, the pulse immunization implemented by John's team helped Vellore become India's first polio-free town. Both the concept and the name had come from John, and Vellore, establishing him as a pioneer in polio control measures.[13] The Ministry of Health, albeit reluctantly, took note of this achievement and this marked a turning point in India's polio control efforts.

Building on this momentum, in 1985, the ICMR commissioned a unique project in the larger Vellore region covering a population of 5 million to compare the efficacy of OPV and IPV, a question that had been haunting health administrators. John recounted the Director General of Health Services (DGHS) D. B. Bisht shouting at him that 'IPV will happen only over my dead body'.[14] ICMR refused to fund the project prompting John to secure funding from the European Union to run the study.

As part of the study, half the population received OPV while the other half was given IPV, with two doses at ten and fourteen weeks, followed by a third dose at nine months. The observations made from this project highlighted that though incidence of polio decreased in both groups, the IPV group exhibited a rapid decline.[15] However, John never published the outcome of this study, keeping the word given to ICMR and the DGHS at the time of commissioning the project.[16]

Nevertheless, John's tireless work on polio soon led him to occupy the office of the chairman of the India Expert Advisory Group on polio eradication. With his vision and guidance, India's fight to eradicate polio began.

Soon, WHO's Global Polio Eradication Initiative (GPEI), in collaboration with UNICEF, the Centre for Disease Control (CDC) and Rotary International, devised a strategic plan for India. This led to the inception of the National Polio Surveillance Project (NPSP), a collaborative effort with the Government of India. Up until this point, India had struggled to bring polio under control, but now the goal was set to eliminate the transmission of the disease within the next four to five years.

In 1995, India formally launched the Pulse Polio Programme nationwide. In the following years, the government spent over $2.5 billion deploying armies of vaccinators who campaigned for two days in a year, carrying pulse polio vaccine kits to every nook and corner of the country. Almost 150,000 supervisors coordinated these armies of vaccinators to administer the vaccines to nearly 170 million children below the age of five years.[17]

There were two significant challenges that hindered the ambitious plan – 'failure to vaccinate' and 'failure of the vaccine'. There were challenges within the government machinery too. Despite the existence of an Immunization Division in the Ministry of Health, the NPSP was chosen as the nodal agency for polio eradication. This decision was met with skepticism, as it ran parallel to the Universal Immunization Programme (UIP), operating as yet another vertical national project covering all diseases preventable by vaccines.

In the initial decade of the EPI era, polio continued to persist as an endemic challenge, marked by intermittent outbreaks at intervals of five to seven years. In 1992, the country faced a polio epidemic. A significant decline in cases followed soon after. By 1993 and 1994, the number of cases had dropped to less than half of those recorded in the pre-EPI era. The downward trend continued, with reported cases falling to 3,263 by 1995. The following year saw a further sixty-nine per cent decline with just 1,005 cases.[18] The numbers continued to decrease and would only spike in 2002 due to a surge in cases in Uttar Pradesh and Bihar.

During this period, the EPI primarily focused on vaccine delivery as it was ill-equipped to monitor disease burdens and control trajectories for the target diseases. Without robust public health surveillance and epidemiological intelligence to build comprehensive monitoring capabilities, the programme was limited to merely delivering vaccines.

Therefore, a sentinel monitoring system named the Central Bureau of Health Intelligence was employed. It played a key role in gathering and disseminating summary data to the public domain, although with a notable lag of two to three years. Interestingly, the reported number of cases represented only about ten per cent of the national total, calculated based on the actual incidence of polio. This highlighted the challenges faced during this critical period in public health, where the reported cases provided only a partial glimpse into the broader landscape of polio incidence.[19]

Despite the challenges, by 1999 the wild polio P2 viral strain had been eliminated from India. WHO took note of this success and its director general Margaret Chan advocated for the rest of the world to adopt the lessons learned from India. Meanwhile, India continued its efforts, introducing the effective monovalent OPV in 2005 and bivalent vaccine in 2010 to eliminate the remaining WPV type 1 (P1) and type 3 (P3) strains as well.

The last confirmed case of P3 was reported on 22 October 2010 in Jharkhand, and the last case of P1 was recorded in Howrah, West Bengal on 13 January 2011. India was removed from the list of polio endemic countries after completing a year without any reported case of wild polio.[20] Since the last reported case in January 2011, India has successfully maintained its polio-free status, officially eliminating the wild polio virus. This remarkable transformation is especially significant considering there was a period in the early 1990s when the country faced a hyper-endemic stage, with an average of 500 to 1,000 children being paralyzed daily. Despite this success, one challenge remained: vaccine-associated paralytic poliomyelitis (VAPP), a rare but serious consequence of the polio vaccine.

With the disease under complete control in 2012, WHO moved

into what is called 'the end game strategy'.[21] The strategy was to universally introduce IPV to remove vaccine virus type 2 from trivalent OPV, a switch from tOPV to bOPV, outlining key steps for concluding the polio eradication efforts. This method was adopted as most of the vaccine-related polio cases were originating from P2 strain present in the Sabin OPV. Therefore, the plan was to remove P2 from the vaccine, making it safer for children.[22] Since this strategy would create an immunity gap for P2, the inactivated vaccine (IPV, Salk) needed to be re-introduced.

The GPEI, the Strategic Advisory Group of Experts on Immunization (SAGE) and the World Health Assembly all endorsed the new plan and worked on the universal introduction of IPV in countries relying solely on OPV.[23]

John's guidance, rooted in his findings in Vellore, became a crucial point of reference – and not only in India. As he would describe to *Current Science* in 2018, 'Vellore was the only centre conducting such basic and problem solving research on polio from mid-1960s'.[24] Many of his recommendations and strategies were replicated on a national and global level to eradicate the crippling disease.

21

BATTLING MEASLES – THE INDIAN DEBATE

DURING THE LATE 1970S, A CONTROVERSY ERUPTED ACROSS the Indian healthcare landscape. The raging debate was whether to include the measles vaccine in the national immunization programme, which had just been launched.

In 1978, when India adopted the EPI promoted by WHO, the measles vaccine was excluded because health planners did not consider measles as a cause of concern in the country.[1] Until the time it was included, an estimated 21 million pre-school children contracted measles annually. Of these, 16 million suffered severe symptoms. The tragedy worsened as nearly ten per cent of patients – amounting to around 200,000 young lives each year – were claimed by this relentless disease.

Amidst this crisis, the Indian Academy of Paediatricians (IAP) rose as a beacon of hope. Through relentless workshops and seminars, IAP championed the inclusion of measles in the EPI. At the forefront of this valiant effort was John and his team from CMC, Vellore. Their epidemiological studies across six villages revealed the impact of measles on childhood morbidity and mortality. Driven by their findings, they advocated for widespread vaccination, a crucial step in the battle to protect the nation's children from this devastating scourge.[2]

Despite the high decibel criticisms and strong arguments, the Ministry of Health and Family Welfare wasn't convinced to change the mandate. The Immunization Division of the Ministry stuck to its gun. They argued, refused and dismissed the demand, pointing to the 'less prevalence' and contraindications* report they had received from some of the regions.

John, a paediatrician himself, wrote a powerful editorial in the *Indian Journal of Pediatrics*, arguing that the measles vaccine was effective, safe and urgently needed in India. He also voiced that there was no justification for not including measles in the EPI in India.[3] The Tamil Nadu government chose not to wait for the nod of the Ministry of Health, and initiated measles vaccination in 1980, using a yet-to-be-licensed vaccine on a special government permission and deploying a few million doses donated by Rotary International. With widespread community acceptance and success, the Ministry of Health was compelled to closely examine the outcomes of this significant case study.[4]

In 1985, after much pressure and persuasion, when the EPI was restructured into the Universal Immunization Programme (UIP), the measles vaccine was included.[5] By then, WHO had already made the measles vaccine part of its first standardized vaccination schedule. This was nearly fifteen years after the vaccine's introduction in the West, following its invention by American microbiologist Maurice Ralph Hilleman, often referred to as the 'father of modern vaccines.' Hilleman and his team are celebrated for developing more than forty experimental vaccines and over a dozen licensed vaccines – chief among which protect against diseases such as measles, mumps, chickenpox, rubella, hepatitis A, hepatitis B, pneumococcal pneumonia, meningitis, pandemic influenza and chlamydia.

A notable distinction between Hilleman's contributions and those of his contemporaries like Salk and Sabin lies in his extensive work with the pharmaceutical industry. While his peers focused largely on

* Medical reasons or conditions that make a certain treatment or vaccine unsafe for a patient.

academic or government-funded research, Hilleman's efforts were directed towards advancing vaccine development through collaboration with transnational corporations. His contributions highlight the shift from state-funded vaccine research to the growing dominance of private industry, where profit generation increasingly shaped vaccine development and often took precedence over public welfare.

In 1957, Merck & Co.* recruited Hilleman to spearhead virus and vaccination research programmes at its West Point, Pennsylvania research centre. His recruitment coincided with the global spread of Asian Influenza in early 1957, highlighting the urgent need for enhanced vaccine research.

'Son of a bitch, this is pandemic flu,' Hilleman is reported to have shouted when he came across a news report about the flu outbreak in Hong Kong that affected 250,000 people in 1957.[6] Still a microbiologist at Walter Reed Army Medical Centre, he swiftly procured a virus sample from an infected serviceman returning from Asia. Recognizing the lack of antibody protection against this new influenza strain, he and his team embarked on a relentless nine-day journey, working fourteen-hour shifts to isolate the virus.

Hilleman wasted no time in initiating vaccine production as well as in distributing samples to manufacturers with an urgent plea for mass production. Within four months, US companies had churned out over 40 million vaccine doses, effectively quelling an epidemic that threatened 70,000 lives in the US alone. India too developed its own vaccine in record time in this epidemic. Globally, the 1957–58 pandemic claimed over 2 million lives and continued to spawn new virus strains thereafter.[7]

Hilleman's major contribution to flu research was the idea that influenza A viruses gradually change their antigenic† characteristics. This idea, known as 'drift and shift', became the foundation of modern flu vaccine strategies.‡

* Merck & Co. is known as MSD (Merck Sharp & Dohme) outside of the US.

† Relating to substances (antigens) that trigger an immune response in the body.

‡ 'Drift' refers to small, gradual changes in a virus that happen over time, while a 'shift' is a sudden, major change that creates a new virus type.

He set off the invention of the mumps and measles vaccines with remarkable scientific ingenuity. One fateful night, while researching the measles vaccine, Hilleman was packing his bags for an overseas trip when his five-year-old daughter Jeryl Lynn complained of a sore throat. Suspecting it to be a symptom of mumps, Hilleman rushed to take a swab from her throat and took it to the lab in the middle of the night.[8]

Utilizing his expertise in virology and tissue culture techniques,* he isolated the mumps virus from Lynn's throat swab and successfully adapted it to grow in chicken embryos. This strain, derived from his daughter's swab, has since been known as the Jeryl Lynn strain.[9] Using this strain, through a series of meticulous experiments, Hilleman and his team developed a live attenuated mumps vaccine which showed promising results in early clinical trials. By 1967, the vaccine was licensed for public use in the United States, marking a major milestone in the global prevention of mumps.[10]

By then, John F. Enders, who won the 1954 Nobel Prize for culturing the polio virus, had returned to his initial interest – isolating the measles virus. In 1954, when an outbreak of measles was reported from a suburban boarding school in Boston, Massachusetts, he rushed his colleague Thomas Peebles to collect throat swabs and blood specimens from the affected children.[11] The culture obtained by Peebles from eleven-year-old schoolboy David Edmonston was cultivated to identify the key measles virus, laying the groundwork for the development of the first measles vaccine and most live-attenuated measles vaccines today.

Between 1958 and 1960, Enders and his team carried out trials of the measles vaccine on small groups of children. Initial success led to larger-scale trials involving thousands of children in New York City and Nigeria. By 1961, the vaccine demonstrated 100 per cent effectiveness, leading to regulatory clearances for public use in 1963.[12]

---

* A lab method used to grow cells (from animals or humans) in a controlled environment to study viruses or test vaccines.

In 1968, Hilleman and his team improved the 'Edmonston-Enders' strain to develop a new version, which remains the primary measles vaccine used in most parts of the world.

The success of the measles vaccine paved the way for advancements in combating other viral diseases. Stanley Plotkin led efforts at the Wistar Institute in Philadelphia to develop a rubella vaccine after an epidemic spread in 1963 spanning Europe and the US, causing millions of rubella cases and thousands of cases of congenital rubella syndrome,* which led to various foetal abnormalities and deaths. Two years before the US outbreak, researchers at the Walter Reed Army Institute of Research, led by Hilleman, had identified the rubella virus.

Plotkin's team isolated the RA 27/3 rubella virus strain and created a vaccine candidate with the weakened virus strain.[13] Early clinical trials in children showed high antibody levels and minimal side effects, confirming the vaccine's effectiveness in inducing immunity without spreading the infection.[14]

However, Plotkin's method of using human cell lines† in vaccines faced severe criticism, including from Sabin. But he was confident that the method was safe for creating vaccines based on findings by another researcher, Leonard Hayflick, who had concluded that there were no cancer-causing properties in human cell strains.[15] Despite controversy, Plotkin's RA 27/3 vaccine became widely used, alongside other rubella vaccines in the 1960s and 1970s, eventually being incorporated into Hilleman's Measles, Mumps, Rubella (MMR) vaccine in 1971. By 1979, authorities discontinued all other rubella vaccines in the US in favour of RA 27/3 because of its fewer side effects. The US regulator licensed Hilleman's MMR combination vaccine in 1971, and it has since been used globally.[16]

It is significant to note that most contributions to vaccine

---

* A serious condition where a baby is born with birth defects because the mother had rubella (German measles) during pregnancy.

† Cells originally taken from a human (often decades ago) that are grown in labs for scientific research or vaccine development.

inventions during this period originated in the US, with minimal contribution from Europe and other regions. India, in particular, made no significant advancements in developing these three crucial viral vaccines. This lack of innovation in vaccine research in India during the 1950s and 1960s can be attributed to the apathy of Indian policymakers, whose commitment to advancing research failed to match the enthusiasm of the British era.

Hill's 1944 Report, which outlined a blueprint for enhancing biological research in India, was largely ignored, and its key recommendations remained unimplemented post-independence. The Sokhey committee report was similarly neglected. Although the Bhore committee, formed to prepare the country for the post-colonial era, addressed general healthcare and drug research to some extent, it did not prioritize preventive medicine and vaccine research.

These extraneous factors led to the degradation of an agile vaccine research and preventive medicine system created by the medical corps of the British colonial rulers and IMS, starting with Waldemar Haffkine and Ronald Ross. Therefore, no new vaccine came out of Indian laboratories for a very long time.

India's contribution to vaccine science was limited to producing the age-old vaccines for smallpox, plague, cholera, rabies, typhoid and BCG in state-run laboratories and public sector units, and administering these vaccines to the needy. Even the production of new vaccines like polio and DPT happened only in the 1970s, despite support from some good Samaritan foreigners and multilateral agencies. A broad-based immunization programme would start only in 1978 when WHO kicked off its EPI globally.

In 1985, India introduced a single dose measles vaccine into its UIP amid public debate and controversy. Despite global evidence supporting the effectiveness of two doses in reducing measles-related mortality, India was slow to adopt this approach.[17] WHO's Strategic Advisory Group of Experts (SAGE) recommended administering two doses as early as November 2008, but India still did not implement it.[18] It wasn't until 2010 that the second dose was introduced in twenty-two states and union territories, with the remaining fourteen states and UTs following in 2012, marking twenty-five years since the first dose's introduction.

Initially, India's immunization efforts focused solely on measles, neglecting the associated mumps and rubella vaccines. It took twenty-five years for an Indian manufacturer to develop an MMR vaccine after the US had licensed it in 1967. Until then, the MMR vaccine was imported and marketed by companies like Merck, GlaxoSmithKline Biologicals and Sanofi Pasteur. The Serum Institute of India launched its version, Tresivac in 1993. However, this vaccine was considered premium and recommended by the IAP only for children from families who could afford it.

The Indian Health Ministry was further encouraged by the reports that some countries had restricted their vaccination programme to only measles or the measles and rubella combination. They also took shelter behind reports questioning the effectiveness of the mumps component in the MMR vaccine.

Eventually in 2019, the Indian Health Ministry launched a mandatory measles-rubella vaccination campaign in schools, after the rubella vaccine was introduced in UIP.[19] This campaign also brought to the fore an important discussion that would not have been debated a few decades earlier on a topic like vaccination – informed consent.

22

MISSION INDRADHANUSH

TOWARDS THE END OF THE NINETEENTH CENTURY, REV. Charles Swynnerton served as a chaplain in the British Indian Government. Despite his demanding ministerial duties, he made remarkable contributions to India, particularly in a field that few others had explored.

Whenever he found respite from his official responsibilities, Swynnerton ventured into Indian villages in search of folklore. In the evenings, he would gather villagers around a bonfire set up outside their homes and listen intensely to their stories. Over time, he collected and compiled these tales, eventually publishing them in compendiums primarily intended for children.

In one of his collections, *Indian Night's Entertainment, or Folktales from the Upper Indus,* Rev. Swynnerton recounted the tale of a Brahmin man and a Muslim merchant named Ali. The Brahmin had two sons, both uneducated and ignorant. Concerned about their future, the man acquiesced when Ali offered to tutor the boys for a year. However, the merchant had a condition – at the end of the year, one of the boys would belong to him. The younger son, who displayed remarkable intelligence, received advanced instruction from Ali, while the elder son was taught only the basics. When the year concluded, Ali returned to the Brahmin to claim one of the boys. Over time, the place where this story is set came to be known as AliBrahmin, immortalizing the tale.[1]

AliBrahmin, located in the Palwal district of Haryana ninety kilometres south of New Delhi, is a satellite village of a larger village named Uttawar. Since the 1970s, Uttawar and AliBrahmin have found a place in the history of India due to the forced sterilization drive spearheaded by Prime Minister Indira Gandhi's son Sanjay Gandhi, who believed that India could only progress through his five-point programme. Promoting literacy, family planning, tree planting and abolition of casteism and dowry, the programme was implemented with iron hands.[2]

During the peak of Indira Gandhi's Emergency era, the quaint hamlet of AliBrahman – housing largely Muslim residents – was rudely awakened one early morning by police loudspeakers. The loud cry instructed all men above the age of fifteen to gather at the Uttawar bus stop to be volunteers for a government programme. Upon reaching the bus stop, the men were informed that they had been gathered at the location for compulsory sterilization on the orders of the Gandhi Prince.

Approximately, 400 men had gathered at the bus stop. The authorities did a head count and found that some eligible villagers were missing. In order to trace the missing and collect more 'volunteers' for sterilization, the police engaged in pillaging, vandalism and looting over the next few days. The search and sterilization continued for three weeks, resulting in a total of 800 vasectomies* across Uttawar and AliBrahmin.[3] Of the 175 men in AliBrahmin, more than 100 had been forcibly sterilized.[4]

There was a massive fallout from this mindless initiative, which rendered over 8 million men impotent in just a year. Family planning, sterilization and contraception became dirty words in post-Emergency India.[5] The Ministry of Health and Family Planning was condemned by people for implementing the initiative. The new government that assumed power after the 1977 parliament elections changed the ministry's name to the Ministry of Health and Family Welfare to

* A surgery performed on men to prevent them from fathering children.

fix its public perception and the bête noire of Indira Gandhi, Raj Narain, was charged with damage control.

However, people's lack of trust in the ministry and its programmes continued for a very long time, the effect of which was felt on India's brand new vaccination programme aimed at reducing the soaring infant mortality* and child mortality rates.

Childhood vaccinations on a national scale started in the 1960s with the introduction of the BCG vaccine for tuberculosis and were later expanded to include polio vaccines. Since the early 1970s, diphtheria, polio and tetanus (DPT), diphtheria and tetanus (DT) and tetanus toxoid (TT) vaccines were being provided under maternal and child-health services. Many states and large city corporations like Bombay implemented such initiatives on their own. Nevertheless, it wasn't until the late 1970s that a national programme was launched after the formation of a non-Congress government.

There were intense debates within the healthcare community regarding the necessity and strategy for a comprehensive immunization programme. Critics argued that the entire immunization initiative was ineffective due to several issues such as limited coverage within the current health system, insufficient testing of vaccines to analyze their efficacy, low compliance rates and inadequate infrastructure such as cold chain maintenance.† The moderates proposed enhancing coverage through health education and motivation. Experts like Jacob John advocated for a scientific approach to prioritize vaccines based on need, efficacy and safety, simplifying vaccination schedules and focusing on mothers to improve compliance.[6]

It was eventually decided that India would adopt WHO's EPI programme. EPI arrived in India almost four years after it was launched globally to reduce morbidity and mortality from diphtheria, pertussis, tetanus, poliomyelitis and childhood tuberculosis. The initial goal set was to immunize all eligible children and pregnant

---

* Number of babies who die before turning one year old.

† A system to keep vaccines at suitably cold temperatures from the factory to the clinic.

women with TT to avoid neonatal tetanus by 1990.[7] India also resolved to achieve self-sufficiency in the production of vaccines required for the programme.

Despite best efforts, the launch of the EPI in 1978 wasn't well received by the masses, especially in areas where forced sterilization had been carried out by the previous government. The same ministry that enforced the sterilization policy during the Emergency era – using the same healthcare personnel, including community health workers and auxiliary midwives* who had coerced and misinformed individuals into undergoing sterilization – was now advising parents to vaccinate their children. This state of indecision and uncertainty about vaccination – known now as 'vaccine hesitancy' – prevailed for quite some time.

The skepticism towards vaccination was rooted in the distrust that lingered from past government policies. However, the value of vaccination in saving lives had been recognized much earlier by visionary leaders. India's first Prime Minister Jawaharlal Nehru was one of the earliest to understand the value of vaccination and good hygiene in saving lives. As noted in his book, *Glimpses of World History*, 'Sanitation and health and the conquest over some diseases depend on science. For the modern world, it is quite impossible to do without applied science.'[8] He ensured that India was not far behind the Western countries in immunization programmes. Back in 1948, the United Kingdom initiated a systematic national immunization programme soon after establishing the National Health Service (NHS) to combat diseases like diphtheria, pertussis, and tetanus. Around the same time, India too commenced its vaccination efforts, individually focusing on tuberculosis, and covering plague, cholera and smallpox.[9]

The US, Canada, the UK and most European countries established their national childhood immunization programmes at various

* Health workers, often in rural areas, who help pregnant women deliver babies and provide basic healthcare.

points in the middle of the twentieth century. The US introduced its programme with the Vaccination Assistance Act in 1962. Canada followed suit, expanding its immunization schedule over the years. European countries also began implementing systematic childhood immunization programmes during this period, focusing on preventing diseases like measles, polio and tuberculosis. These programmes were replicated by many other countries and eventually, WHO created the EPI.[10]

China started its childhood immunization programme as a national initiative under the name National Immunization Programme (NIP), almost at the same time India launched the EPI. The Chinese programme started in the aftermath of a devastating smallpox outbreak during the late 1970s. The nationwide vaccination campaign that followed the outbreak eventually evolved into a comprehensive childhood immunization programme, targeting various vaccine-preventable diseases.[11]

The formal launch of the EPI in India marked a significant milestone. Initially, EPI included BCG, three doses of DPT and typhoid vaccine; OPV was added the following year. In addition, two boosters – one administered at one and a half years and the other at five years – were also included to cover children up to five years of age. By 1981–2, the DPT vaccine was well-integrated into the EPI, prioritizing children under two years of age. The use of the Tetanus Toxoid (TT) vaccine was also extended to school children in the final classes of primary and secondary schools.[12]

After the inclusion of the measles vaccine in the programme, EPI was rechristened and relaunched as the Universal Immunization Programme (UIP) in 1985. UIP was planned as a well-thought-out strategy aimed at systematic expansion across districts, with plans to have universal coverage in all districts by 1989–90. It had an ambitious target to reach at least eighty-five per cent of infants and 100 per cent of pregnant women across the country by 1990.

The UIP maintained the initial DPT booster but modified the second booster at five years to DT, excluding the pertussis component.

Concurrently, the measles vaccine was added at nine months, while the typhoid vaccine was discontinued. Over the next two decades, the UIP underwent administrative changes, transitioning to a National Technology Mission in 1986 and later becoming part of the Child Survival and Safe Motherhood (CSSM) programme in 1992 and the Reproductive and Child Health (RCH) programme in 1997. Despite these shifts, its focus remained on four vaccines – BCG, DPT, OPV and measles, targeting six diseases.

It wasn't until 2006 that new vaccines such as hepatitis B, the second dose of measles and the Japanese Encephalitis vaccine were introduced. Initially, hepatitis B vaccination began in ten states before expanding nationally, while the Japanese encephalitis vaccine was introduced in 111 districts across fifteen states with high disease burdens.[13]

Since 1978, immunization coverage among infants had been steadily increasing. Initially targeting children under five years of age, the programme expanded its focus to children under two years old and later to those under one year old with the launch of the UIP. Immunization coverage of infants and pregnant women showed a positive trend, with coverage for infants increasing more steeply in recent years.

The UIP has been one of India's most extensive public health initiatives, targeting approximately 27 million newborns and 29 million pregnant women annually. It has played a stellar role in reducing the mortality rate attributed to vaccine-preventable diseases among children under the age of five.[14] Even so, more than three and a half decades since the launch of the UIP, 100 per cent coverage of children under the age of five and all pregnant women remained a distant target. Therefore, the Narendra Modi government in 2014 revamped the immunization initiative by rechristening it Indradhanush, meaning 'rainbow'.

Mission Indradhanush, an initiative launched in December 2014 with the active support of WHO and UNICEF, aimed to ensure comprehensive vaccination coverage by 2020 for children who are either unvaccinated or partially vaccinated against seven vaccine-preventable diseases – diphtheria, pertussis, tetanus, polio, tuberculosis, measles and hepatitis B.

The initiative was further strengthened with the launch of Intensified Mission Indradhanush (IMI) in October 2017, which was again updated to IMI 2.0 in December 2019. Since then, the programme has undergone changes every second year. The latest NIP, as of 2025, is IMI 5.0, with a special focus on the elimination of measles and rubella and the use of the digital platform U-WIN for routine immunization in all districts of the country.[15]

With graduating versions of Indradhanush vaccines against rubella, meningitis, pneumonia caused by Haemophilus Influenza B,* rotavirus diarrhoea, pneumococcal pneumonia and Japanese Encephalitis were added. The 2023 version of Indradhanush aims to achieve the Sustainable Development Goal of ending preventable child deaths by 2030 and includes a total of twelve vaccines offered to infants and children free of cost.

Although total childhood immunization is nearing its end goals, many questions remain unanswered about the early governmental efforts to ensure vaccination for disease prevention. One glaring issue is the delayed prioritization of immunization, illustrated by the fact that it took thirty-six years for independent India to formulate a national health policy. Even then, the 1983 National Health Policy placed limited emphasis on immunization, reflecting a broader pattern of successive governments neglecting health amid competing priorities.

After Rajkumari Amrit Kaur's pioneering ten-year tenure as India's first woman health minister, the ministry operated without a cabinet minister for the next decade. It was not until 1977, when the influential Raj Narain took charge as Health Minister, that the ministry began gaining prominence. From then until the end

* A bacteria that can cause serious infections, especially in children, like pneumonia or meningitis.

of Narasimha Rao's government in 1996, the ministry was led by capable ministers or the prime minister himself. The era from 1977 to 1996 marked significant progress in vaccination, as infant mortality fell from 120 per thousand to seventy per thousand. This trend continued, with infant mortality declining to thirty-nine per thousand by 2014 and further to twenty-six per thousand by 2022.

Since 1978, the results of vaccination programmes have been steady, even with the growing numbers of newborns and mothers. The National Family Health Survey (NFHS)-4 for the period 2015–16 indicated a national immunization coverage of sixty-two per cent, while data presented by the Ministry of Health and Family Welfare at the 4th Partners' Forum meeting in New Delhi in December 2018 showed eighty-three per cent coverage against a ninety per cent target.

However, the report of 2018 National Statistical Office (NSO) punched holes in the data of the NFHS-4 and suggested only sixty per cent complete vaccination coverage, that is, only 60 per cent of children below five years were vaccinated with all government-prescribed vaccines. According to the NSO data, only 58.4 per cent of children in rural areas and 61.7 per cent in urban areas were fully immunized. In states with high birth rates like Bihar and Uttar Pradesh, the full immunization coverage stood at 48 per cent and 55 per cent. Conversely, states like Andhra Pradesh and Kerala, which perform well, exhibited an average full immunization rate of 74 per cent and 73 per cent respectively.[16]

In the 2022 UNICEF South Asia Immunization Report, India stood at 90–94 per cent coverage for DTP3,[17] a WHO indicator that shows the percentage of one-year-olds who have received three doses of the combined diphtheria, tetanus toxoid and pertussis (DTP3) vaccine in a given year.[18] Though India is behind Bangladesh, Bhutan and Sri Lanka in this yardstick, it is still ahead of Pakistan and Afghanistan in the region.

India faces several challenges in achieving its high vaccination goals compared to its neighbours like Bangladesh, where over 90 per cent of children are fully vaccinated by the age of two. One major obstacle is India's large population, coupled with a relatively high growth rate, with approximately 27 million children born in India each year.[19]

Over the past half a century, vaccines have become a critical tool in healthcare in aiding the prevention of epidemics. WHO estimates that today vaccination prevents approximately 3.5–5 million deaths annually, of which at least half a million are from India.[20] It is a commendable effort, considering the state of affairs in 1880 when more than 50 per cent of all children born globally did not see their sixth birthday. Undoubtedly, vaccination has been one of the biggest catalysts in preventing childhood diseases and reducing their burden over time.[21]

Many deadly pathogens like smallpox virus and wild poliovirus have since been eradicated from the face of the planet with the help of effective vaccinations. With vaccines and better hygiene in practice, child mortality began declining at the beginning of the twentieth century. In India, the under-five child mortality rate has fallen from 53 per cent in 1900 to under 4 per cent in 2020.[22] The UN Inter-agency Group for Child Mortality Estimation reported twenty-eight deaths per thousand children under five years of age, 2.8 per cent, at the end of 2023.

The gradual decline in vaccine-preventable diseases as well as in child mortality is no less a feat. India has achieved it by battling with several challenges in vaccine delivery due to its diverse geography, including snowbound/hilly areas, deserts, tropical forests and remote islands. It has also confronted myriad challenges of cultural diversity, encompassing varying religions, languages, traditions, beliefs and customs that further complicated the efforts to provide vaccination to all. Political instability, including coalition governments and areas affected by naxal or terrorist activities, added to this complexity. Additionally, reaching out to a big and constantly moving migrant population has posed yet another challenge.[23]

Vaccine hesitancy, initially driven by the fears of sterilization, continued with some sections of the society who believed that vaccines are manipulative tools to sterilize people without consent. However, the biggest challenge has been vaccine equity where certain groups of people in need of certain vaccines do not have access to them, but affluent sections have unlimited access to vaccines which are not required by them.

23

THE EARLY PLAYERS

DURING THE EARLY DAYS OF THE COVID-19 PANDEMIC IN 2020, as the entire country looked to vaccine makers for a breakthrough, many laboratories and drug companies jumped into the fray of vaccine development. However, one prominent player remained conspicuously absent – Biological E., a Hyderabad-based pharmaceutical company with nearly six decades of experience in vaccine manufacturing in India.

Around this time, Biological E. was embroiled in a family feud over control of the organization, a conflict that had escalated from the Company Law Board (CLB) in Chennai to the High Court of Hyderabad and eventually to the Supreme Court of India.

In 2017, the High Court in Hyderabad superseded the board of directors of the company, pointing out that the three daughters who owned the company had indulged in acts of oppression against their mother. The Court allowed an appeal by the mother Renuka Datla, who challenged a 2016 order of the CLB and removed her three daughters – Purnima, Indira and Mahima – and their husbands from directorships of the company.[1]

Biological E. was founded by Renuka's father GAN Raju in 1953 along with his friend DVK Raju in Vijayawada. The two distant relatives joined hands upon the return of DVK Raju from the UK after completing his PhD in chemistry at the University of

Edinburgh. He had worked briefly with the pharmaceutical company Sarabhai Merck when he started Biological Products Private Limited with his farmer friend and relative GAN Raju.[2]

As the wheels of time turned, the friends-turned-business partners became family when GAN Raju arranged the marriage between his daughter Renuka and GVK Raju's son Vijay Kumar Datla. Not long after, Vijay Kumar Datla was inducted into the company and appointed the Chairman and Managing Director in May 1972.

In the 1950s, Biological Products Private Ltd. began its operations by manufacturing Heparin* injections. It ventured into vaccine making in 1962 by producing the much-needed DPT (diphtheria, pertussis and tetanus) vaccines, thus becoming India's first private sector vaccine maker. However, it wasn't until 1964 that the company changed its name to Biological E. – 'E' to denote the UK-based Evans Medicals which bought a 40 per cent stake in the company.

Over the years, Evans changed hands and became Medeva, and the stake held by Evans was acquired by GSK. Despite these changes, the company retained the 'E' in its name because by then 'Biological E.' had established itself as a pharmaceutical major in the global market.

Until around 1995, many of Biological E.'s decisions on strategies, products and markets were influenced by GSK, owing to the latter's 25 per cent stake in the company. In 1995, GSK sold the stake back to the Datla family after a friendly takeover bid failed. This decision was primarily driven by GSK's realization that maintaining a minority stake in a pharmaceutical company offered little value when it already operated its own subsidiary in India.

Though Biological E. began producing vaccines ahead of all other private companies in India, it wasn't established as a vaccine company for a very long time. This was because it dabbled in many other product categories – drug formulations including tuberculosis

* A type of medication used to prevent blood clots, often given to patients undergoing surgery or those with conditions that increase the risk of clots.

drugs, cough syrups, digestive enzymes, beauty and skincare products, veterinary products and so on.

Despite the company having a strong foot in the vaccine business, Biological E. kept away from the EPI in 1978 and the remodeled UIP in 1985. However, at the turn of the century, when the government was planning to introduce hepatitis B and H1 influenza B vaccines in its national immunization programme, Biological E. decided to take the plunge and develop the pentavalent formulation* of diphtheria, pertussis, tetanus, hepatitis B and H1 influenza B. The company built a new plant for bacterial, recombinant and viral vaccines and soon, it began establishing itself as a vaccine maker. Mahima Datla, the incumbent Managing Director of the company, explained that 'if we didn't make pentavalent vaccines, we would be dead. It was about whether we wanted to quit the vaccine business or take on the challenge.'[3]

In 2005, Biological E. was roped in by Austrian company Intercell for manufacturing and marketing one of its purified, inactivated† Japanese Encephalitis (JE) vaccines for active immunization of adults, soon after the conclusion of Phase II clinical trials and before starting Phase III trials.‡[4]

However, the unexpected death of Vijay Kumar Datla in March 2013 led to years of turmoil. Not long after, a high-voltage drama erupted at the Hyderabad headquarters for management control. The bitter family feud played out in the open and continued for almost a decade. It was such a high-profile case that when it was first listed in the Supreme Court in December 2017, the three daughters were represented by heavyweight lawyers Mukul Rohatgi, Shyam Diwan and Abhishek Manu Singhvi, while the mother was represented by former finance minister P. Chidambaram.

---

* A vaccine that protects against five diseases. In this case, it includes protection against diphtheria, pertussis, tetanus, hepatitis B and H1 influenza B.

† A type of clean vaccine where the virus or bacteria is killed or inactivated, but still able to stimulate an immune response in the body.

‡ The final big test of a vaccine on large groups of people to check if it works and is safe before it is approved for use.

The key contention was the 80 per cent stake and the position of managing director held by Datla. Perhaps he hadn't expected his life to end so soon, though he was suffering from renal failure. Datla hadn't prepared a clear succession plan or even if he had one, it wasn't shared with anyone in the family or the company.

The Supreme Court made a mediation effort by appointing two former judges of the court. After the failed mediation efforts, Justice Vineet Saran and Justice V K Maheswari, in April 2022, ruled in favour of the daughters while granting a one-time payment of ₹100 million and ₹6.5 million every month to mother Renuka Datla, along with appointing her Emeritus Consultant, granting her a house, security and other benefits.[5]

Despite the turbulence caused by the family feud from March 2013 to April 2022, the company maintained steady revenue and profit growth. From a ₹2.35 billion turnover in 2012 at the time of Datla's death, it crossed ₹10 billion in 2015, ₹11.26 billion in 2017, ₹25.5 billion in 2022 and ₹38 billion in 2023. In the same period, profit moved from a negative territory of ₹140 million to ₹3.5 billion in 2015, ₹3.2 billion in 2017, ₹3.4 billion in 2022 and ₹9.5 billion in 2023.[6] Throughout these years, approximately 80 per cent of the revenue consistently came from vaccines.

By 2020, Biological E. had established itself as a major supplier of vaccines to UNICEF, the Pan American Health Organization and to the vaccination programmes of the Government of India. Additionally, it had pre-qualification status for supplying seven vaccines to WHO, including liquid pentavalent vaccine of DPT plus hepatitis B and H1 influenza B; measles and rubella; and typhoid conjugate vaccines. The company was also recognized as one of the top three global suppliers of pentavalent vaccine, with a backward integration across all the five antigens which enabled the company to maintain antigen quality and cost competitiveness.

Therefore, the absence of Biological E. in the Covid-19 vaccine research was felt acutely when its peers like Serum Institute of India and Bharat Biotech were taking giant strides in working on possible candidates.

However, the company got its act together and by the end of 2020, entered into a co-developing arrangement for a vaccine with global pharma companies, starting with Johnson & Johnson (J&J) in August. In the same month, it also signed a deal with California-based Dynavax Technologies, Houston-based Baylor College of Medicine and the Texas Children's Hospital Centre for Vaccine Development to co-develop a vaccine.

The first vaccine that was planned as a joint QUAD initiative* with J&J was inordinately delayed, despite WHO approving a manufacturing site at Biological E. The second one fructified into Corbevax, as a booster dose for individuals aged eighteen years and older. It was authorized for restricted emergency use and was recommended for use six months after the initial two doses of either Covaxin or Covishield vaccines.[7] Despite being a late starter, Biological E. performed better than many of its peers in terms of producing a non-patent vaccine that would go to the global vaccine alliance COVAX.

While Biological E. was busy developing Corbevax, Ahmedabad-based Zydus LifeSciences was developing a DNA† vaccine with support from the Indian Department of Biotechnology. Zydus too is as old as Biological E. and has been working in the vaccine space since the 1950s. It was founded in 1952 by Ramanbhai B. Patel and Indravadan Modi and was named Cadila Laboratories. The duo got their modest start by producing vitamin supplements in a garage and selling them on the back of their bicycles.

After a long and happy journey together, in 1995 the duo split the company to form two separate entities, both focusing on pharmaceuticals. Of the two new entities, Cadila Pharmaceuticals was

* Quadrilateral Security Dialogue – strategic forum of the US, India, Japan and Australia to promote free and open Indo-Pacific cooperation.

† Deoxyribonucleic acid, the hereditary material in living organisms. Nearly every cell in a person's body has the same DNA.

owned by the Modi family, while Cadila Healthcare was controlled by the Patel family. In the same year, the Patel family began calling their business Zydus, derived from the Greek god Zeus. In 2022, Cadila Healthcare was renamed Zydus Lifesciences Limited.

The first entry of Zydus into the vaccine sector was in 1998, when it formed a joint venture with Korea Green Cross Corporation to manufacture and market a recombinant hepatitis B vaccine. The very next year, the company entered a collaboration with the Swiss Serum and Vaccine Institute to launch a range of vaccines in India, followed by forming a joint venture with the Haffkine Institute, Bombay to undertake research in the field of human vaccines.

In 2013, Zydus and the US-based non-profit Infectious Disease Research Institute (IDRI) joined hands to work on a vaccine for kala azar. Together, the two organizations conducted clinical trials in India to develop, register and market the vaccine. IDRI had been working on the vaccine for more than twenty years, supported by the US National Institutes of Health (NIH) and the Bill & Melinda Gates Foundation.[8]

Cadila Pharmaceuticals, in the meantime, formed a joint venture with Novavax Inc, US, named as CPL Biologicals Pvt Ltd., and developed a vaccine to treat seasonal influenza, calling it the Cadiflu-S.[9] It was touted as the world's first influenza vaccine based on virus-like particle (VLP) technology,* even as the company hoped to get on board with Novavax's vaccine development to work on a pancreatic cancer vaccine, hepatitis E vaccine, varicella zoster virus vaccine and human papilloma vaccine.

At that time, most vaccines in India were still being produced by government-run organizations led by Haffkine Institute, Pasteur Institute and BCG Laboratories. In the private sector, only a few companies were actively involved in vaccine production. Notably, two private sector companies with a long history, dating back to pre-independence days, were Bengal Chemicals and Pharmaceuticals Ltd. and Bengal Immunity Ltd.

* A technology used in vaccines where proteins from a virus are assembled into a particle that mimics the virus but cannot cause disease.

Founded in 1901, Bengal Chemicals and Pharmaceuticals Ltd. initially focused on vaccines/sera, chemicals, synthetics and dyes, but its leadership in technology began declining in the 1960s and the company became unviable in 1970. Despite transitioning into a public sector venture in 1980, the company pulled its shutters in 2000 and had to be revived by the government six years later by infusing a ₹2 billion grant and waiving its debts.

Dating back to 1919, Bengal Immunity Ltd. became a Public Sector Vaccine Institute (PSVI) in 1980. It specialized in producing a wide range of vaccines for the EPI, including cholera, typhoid, anti-rabies vaccines and anti-snake venoms. However, the company could not survive in the twenty-first century.

Despite these setbacks, a few vaccine companies emerged in the public sector in the 1980s. One such company was Bharat Immunologicals and Biologicals Ltd. (BIBCOL), set up in 1989. It was based in Bulandshar near New Delhi and was manufacturing OPV formulations using imported bulk for a long time. Another company that was established in 1983 in Hyderabad was Indian Immunologicals Ltd., a wholly owned subsidiary of the National Dairy Development Board (NDDB), which is an autonomous institution under the Government of India. It initially concentrated on veterinary vaccines but forayed into human vaccines in 1998 with the development of tissue culture rabies vaccine. Subsequently, the company introduced measles and MMR vaccines in 2002, followed by an improved recombinant Hepatitis-B vaccine in 2006.

Yet another public sector vaccine company that came up in the 1980s was the Indian Vaccines Corporation Ltd. (IVCOL) based in Gurgaon. It was founded in 1989 with the intention of producing measles vaccine but faced significant challenges due to the unavailability of the required technology and subsequently ceased operations in 2002.

Top on the list of important private players in the pre-liberalization era is Panacea Biotec, established in 1984 as Panacea Drugs Private Limited. After changing its name to Panacea Biotec in 1993, the company commissioned a state-of-the-art viral vaccine research facility near Chandigarh. By the turn of the millennium, it had formed a joint venture with Cuban company Heber Biotec Ltd. to manufacture hepatitis B vaccines in bulk form.

The company commissioned a recombinant vaccine plant in 2002. In the same year, it formalized a collaboration with the Biotechnology Consortium of India for developing and marketing the anthrax vaccine. Two years later, it entered into an agreement with the National Institute of Immunology, New Delhi, for working on a Japanese Encephalitis vaccine candidate.[10]

A partnership with Chiron, later renamed Novartis, did not go well and was aborted after just six years when Panacea did not benefit from the promised cutting-edge vaccine technologies. But in the year 2004, Panacea's collaboration with Cambridge Bio-stability, UK, for thermostable vaccines* helped improve its vaccine storage and distribution. In 2005, its partnership with the National Research Development Corporation (NRDC) for technology transfer of a foot-and-mouth vaccine and its collaboration with Indonesian PT Bio Farma in 2006 to manufacture and market a measles vaccine helped the company's journey forward. Panacea's association with the Netherlands Vaccine Institute, the same year, for the manufacture and marketing of IPV was a turning point and equally significant was the opening of a vaccine formulation plant in 2007.

In 2005, the company developed a fully liquid pentavalent vaccine against diphtheria, tetanus, whooping cough, hepatitis B and influenza type B known as EasyFive-TT, which was pre-qualified by WHO and used in over seventy-five countries. In 2017, Panacea also introduced the world's first fully liquid hexavalent vaccine, which also protects against wild polio, called EasySix. A collaboration with Serum Institute of India in 2018 to expand market access for EasySix helped further its growth in the global market.

---

* Vaccines that can be stored at higher temperatures, which makes them easier to distribute and store in places with limited refrigeration.

Panacea's vaccine portfolio also includes Enivac-HB, a vaccine to tackle hepatitis B in children and adults; Ecovac-4 against diphtheria, tetanus, whooping cough and hepatitis B; Easyfour against diphtheria, tetanus, whooping cough and influenza type B; and EasyFourPol which includes protection against polio, in addition to the four diseases.

Over the years, Panacea Biotec has become one of the largest vaccine manufacturing companies in India, recognized by UN's health agencies for supplying billions of doses of WHO pre-qualified polio vaccines to over fifty countries worldwide. The company continued to actively develop more vaccines, including recombinant chimeric dengue tetravalent, pneumococcal conjugate and others.

With the addition of Panacea Biotec, the landscape of Indian vaccine makers in the pre-liberalization era became more robust. However, one company, established in the 1960s, would go on to surpass both Panacea and Biological E. in size and impact over the next five decades.

That company is the Serum Institute of India.

24

A STABLE FOR VACCINES

SOLI POONAWALLA'S HORSES HAVE BEEN REGULAR RACERS AT the 2,400-metre Indian Derby held on the first Sunday of every February at the iconic Mahalaxmi Race Course in Bombay since he set up Poona Stud Farm in 1946. Among Soli's two children, young Cyrus, just six years old when the stud farm was established, grew up immersed in this world of racing and breeding.

Born into a family deeply entwined with the racing circuit, Cyrus Poonawalla developed a passion for horses early on. Along with his brother Zavareh, he spent his teenage years involved in equestrian pursuits.

By the time he was twenty, he recognized the limited prospects of horse racing as a business in India. Shifting gears, he briefly delved into automotive ventures along with a schoolmate, to build a prototype sports car modelled on D-type Jaguar. They poured their creativity and enthusiasm into the project, investing a modest $120. Yet, financial constraints soon brought the venture to a halt, leading Cyrus to pivot his focus towards more lucrative endeavours.

The momentous loss of Cyrus's mare had propelled his journey to build the organization that would later become the Serum Institute of India. His decision to sever ties with the Haffkine Institute marked the beginning of a new chapter in India's path towards creating vaccines. Poonawalla was about to transform a personal tragedy into an opportunity that would revolutionize healthcare in India and beyond.

On 12 June 1966, under the scorching summer sun, Soli Poonawalla, sporting a folded fishing hat, laid the foundation stone on a barren stretch of land at Hadapsar, some twelve kilometres from the heart of Pune. By his side were his wife Gool and Cyrus. At just twenty-five years old, Cyrus had kick-started the operations of the Serum Institute of India (SII) from the garage of his father's stud farm. The project began with approximately $12,000 raised by selling a few horses, while Soli contributed the remaining funds needed to launch the venture.[1]

The new facility, located adjacent to the burial ground used for horses at the stud farm, began by hiring expert technicians and scientists from the Haffkine Institute in Bombay. It was an uphill battle in the beginning with challenges of scarce resources and limited revenue.

In 1967, when the facility was fully functional, the SII launched its maiden tetanus anti-toxin production, followed by tetanus toxoid in quick succession, marking the beginning of vaccine production.[2] Soon, Cyrus and his brother launched their first anti-tetanus serum in the market. The duo travelled by train to sell their vaccines and sera to hospitals in Bombay and Ahmedabad, offering rates 40 per cent cheaper than their competitors.

The early days were tough – funding was scarce, equipment was rudimentary and sales numbers were low. But Cyrus and his team persevered. Late nights, failed experiments and dwindling resources were no match to their dedication. In 1969, a breakthrough came in the form of a large order for tetanus antitoxin, earning SII some much-needed recognition.

A few years thereafter, the Serum Institute developed the full three-component DTP vaccine against diphtheria, tetanus and pertussis which heralded its arrival in the arena of vaccine innovation. By 1974, SII began revolutionizing the healthcare landscape with the introduction of the DTP vaccine, safeguarding children against the three diseases.[3] However, it was only in 1981 that they could find the solution to the problem that had haunted the company from its inception – making an anti-serum for snakebites. It was the first time that a company in the private sector in India had developed snakebite anti-serum. The family had another reason to celebrate that year, with the birth of Cyrus and his wife Villoo's baby boy.

Financial challenges continued to plague Serum Institute well into the 1980s. Cyrus sought a $3 million loan from the International Finance Corporation (IFC) but talks collapsed when IFC demanded all current and future assets as collateral. He then considered selling a stake to Institute Mérieux (now part of Aventis), but negotiations failed when Mérieux deemed Serum's $10 million valuation too high given its modest earnings.[4]

Undeterred, Cyrus secured a loan from an Indian bank to develop measles vaccine M-Vac and launched it in 1989. Within a year, SII emerged as one of the nation's leading vaccine manufacturers. Through the 1980s, SII played a key role in helping the country achieve self-sufficiency in critical vaccines against tetanus, diphtheria and pertussis.

However, profitability remained elusive, as sales were primarily confined to government programmes at government-mandated prices, significantly lower than those in export and open markets. By now, the Serum Institute knew it needed more funds to expand and Cyrus began looking at multilateral agencies, while improving quality and upgrading his facilities.

From 1991, things started moving at breakneck speed with the liberalization of the Indian economy. A big breakthrough came in 1994 when WHO accredited the company, enabling it to export vaccines globally. By 1998, the Serum Institute's vaccines were being distributed in more than 100 countries.[5] WHO accreditation* also

---

* A recognition from the World Health Organization, which allows a facility or product to be trusted internationally.

enabled the supply of its vaccines to UN agencies like UNICEF and the Pan American Health Organization (PAHO).

The very same year, the company launched its combined vaccine for measles, mumps and rubella (MMR) under the brand name Tresivac. Tresivac is a mix of three vaccine strains – Edmonston-Zagreb strain of measles, Leningrad-Zagreb strain of mumps and Plotkins RA 27/2 strain of rubella – administered in a two-dose schedule, the first at twelve to fifteen months and the second at four to six years.

Tresivac didn't have a smooth ride. In 1998, reports of meningitis surfaced from two states of Brazil as an adverse reaction to the vaccine. Studies reported that Tresivac caused a high incidence of aseptic meningitis* noted from routine surveillance during two mass immunization campaigns. Cyrus spurred his teams into action and an India-based external scientific team evaluated and picked holes in the Brazilian findings. Similar studies from Brazil also reported that they were unable to isolate the L-Zagreb mumps virus from the cerebrospinal fluid (CSF) of the reported meningitis cases, a necessary step to establish a definitive association between the vaccine and the reported adverse response.

SII also faced significant delays in developing its hepatitis B vaccine compared to its competitors, Shantha Biotechnics and Bharat Biotech. Hepatitis B has been a major global public health problem, with an estimated 300 million chronic carriers of the virus and 820,000 annual deaths due to HBV-related cirrhosis† and liver cancer.[6] In the year 2001, Serum Institute launched GeneVac-B, a purified vaccine based on the surface antigen of hepatitis B. This launch occurred nearly four years after Shantha debuted the first recombinant hepatitis B vaccine in the country.

Unlike that of some of its predecessors, GeneVac-B did not elicit many adverse responses. Early studies reported that it was able to

---

* Inflammation of the protective membranes covering the brain and spinal cord, not caused by bacteria.

† Severe liver damage where healthy tissue is replaced with scar tissue.

generate sufficient immunity comparable to its competitors when administered with the DTP vaccine at six, ten and fourteen weeks of age.[7]

The very next year, Serum Institute launched the Tubervac vaccine, a live attenuated freeze-dried BCG vaccine, despite the company procuring the tested and proven seed virus Danish Strain 1331, from the custody of the sole government manufacturer in India, BCG Vaccine Laboratory. Five years later, it launched ONCO-BCG using BCG strains, a vaccine treatment for bladder cancer, comparable to similar treatments that had surfaced in the West.

Recognizing the importance of strategic growth and diversification, in 2012, the Serum Institute made a significant move by acquiring Bilthoven Biologicals, a vaccine maker owned by the Dutch government that had been operating at a loss. The Serum Institute invested €70 million ($78 million) over three years to expand its production capacity. This acquisition granted the company access to injectable polio vaccine (IPV) technology, which was previously limited to only a few vaccine producers worldwide. With increased production capacity, Serum Institute was able to significantly lower prices in the global market, supplying polio vaccines to UNICEF for its polio eradication initiative.[8]

A decade later in 2022, the Serum Institute would develop a recombinant BCG (rBCG) vaccine, VPM1002 and seek authorization for emergency adult use from the Indian regulator. The Biotechnology Industry Research Assistance Council (BIRAC) of the Department of Biotechnology (DBT) supported the efficacy trial in about 6,000 health workers and high-risk individuals in 2020.[9] By then, some of these initiatives were led by Cyrus's son Adar Poonawalla.

Adar joined Serum Institute in 2001 after graduating from the University of Westminster and assumed the role of CEO in 2011, as his father crossed seventy. His leadership came at a crucial time, guiding the company through a period of transformation as the private sector increasingly took on roles traditionally held by the state, including healthcare.

By the time the Covid-19 pandemic struck, Serum Institute had already become a global powerhouse of vaccine production. Adar's vision positioned the company at the forefront of delivering vaccines, making it a symbol of resilience and innovation. When the dust settled after Covid-19, Serum Institute's annual capacity stood at 2 billion doses – the largest capacity of any vaccine maker globally.

25

FROM VAP TO ROTAVAC

IN THE SUMMER OF 1985, INSIDE THE NEONATAL WARD OF India's premier medical institution – AIIMS, New Delhi – something strange was happening. Newborns were contracting rotavirus, a pathogen notorious for killing hundreds of thousands of children each year through violent diarrhoea. But most of these babies, though testing positive, showed no symptoms. No vomiting, no dehydration, no distress. They were silent hosts to a disease that was, somehow, not behaving as expected.

Halfway across the world, a rotavirus specialist named Dr Roger Glass was preparing for a trip to Calcutta, unaware that a casual evening drink with a young Indian paediatrician from AIIMS named Dr Maharaj Bhan would set in motion a medical revolution. Over drinks, Bhan described the bizarre outbreak, his curiosity piqued by the virus's refusal to follow the rules. That night, two scientists from two nations on opposite sides of Cold War suspicion raised glasses over an enigma – and unknowingly laid the first brick in a bridge of trust.

Just three years earlier, in the shadow of a bruised Indo-US relationship marred by gunboats and geopolitics, Prime Minister Indira Gandhi and President Ronald Reagan had signed a Science and Technology Initiative (STI) that many dismissed as diplomatic nicety. Few imagined it would lead to a joint vaccine venture.

STI kickstarted a series of actions and one of them led to the establishment of the Indo-US Vaccine Action Programme (VAP). VAP emerged out of a consensus that was arrived at after three years of bilateral discussions between the two nations – that vaccines are the most cost-effective health solution to control preventable diseases and India deserves special attention because of its large and growing population.[1] In fact, a well-defined vaccine partnership took almost five years since the signing of the STI by Gandhi and Reagan.

One of the key reasons for the delay in the fructification of the partnership was the deep distrust of India towards the US, given the Nixon administration's support to Pakistan during the Indo-Pakistan War of 1971 that culminated in the deployment of the mighty Seventh Fleet of the US Navy in the Bay of Bengal to intimidate Indian forces at the height of the conflict. Notwithstanding the best efforts by the subsequent governments of Gerald Ford and Jimmy Carter, the hostility continued, and distrust ran deep till the end of the Cold War in 1991 when India opened up for liberalization.

In scientific circles, two projects further sowed the seeds of mistrust – the CIA's yellow fever experiments to use mosquitos as biological warfare in Delhi[2] and the US non-profit aid agency Rockefeller Foundation's apparent attempts to hijack Indian rice germplasm.[*3] However, the US custodian of the VAP, the National Institute of Allergy and Infectious Diseases (NIAID) prevailed and renewed the partnership every five years.

VAP was viewed with suspicion from the beginning by the Indian intelligentsia, who thought it would open up India to US biotechnology corporations and turn it into a laboratory where vaccines and drugs could be tested without regulatory control. Prafull Bidwai, a fiery critic, cited the 1986 US Wistar Institute project wherein bio-engineered rabies vaccine was tested on Argentine cattle without proper permissions from the Latin American nation.[4] In

* The genetic material (like seeds or cells) that carries the traits of a plant or animal and is used to improve or conserve species.

strict contrast, the Wistar project was referred to by the US side as an outstanding example of vaccine collaboration in the fifty-nine-page preparatory material readied as a precursor to the VAP.

The primary goal of the NIAID through VAP was to develop a rotavirus vaccine. Rotavirus, the most common cause of diarrhoea in infants, was one of the prime reasons for higher infant mortality in developing countries. The NIH had previously tried many vaccines to prevent it, including an attenuated bovine vaccine developed at the Wistar Institute. A clear objective of the project was to conduct field trials of the rotavirus vaccine that was being developed using the recombinant method, which involved genetic engineering of the nuclear material obtained from the virus.

However, the biological and environmental consequences of conducting vaccine trials in India, rather than doing it in the US, was a cause for concern for the critics of VAP, like Bidwai. They cautioned about the larger dangers of letting loose the bioengineered monsters which, once released into the environment, would evolve for survival and could have undesirable effects on other organisms, including humans. The frightening part was that there was no recall possible once it was released to the world.[5]

India was struggling to prevent diarrhoea, caused by rotavirus, which was a leading cause of death among children under five years of age globally, with India alone accounting for 22 per cent of these deaths.[6] By the turn of the millennium, rotavirus caused about 111 million gastroenteritis cases a year that necessitated home care, 25 million clinic visits, 2 million hospitalizations and between 352,000 and 592,000 deaths among children under the age of five.[7]

By the age of five, nearly every child would have experienced at least an episode of rotavirus gastroenteritis, with one in five requiring a clinic visit, one in sixty being hospitalized and approximately one in 293 succumbing to the illness. Notably, children in the most impoverished nations account for 82 per cent of all rotavirus-related fatalities.[8] Therefore, a reliable vaccine to prevent rotavirus infection was a top priority of healthcare professionals around the world.

The story of ROTAVAC development started with an outbreak of diarrhoea in the neonatal ward of AIIMS, New Delhi in 1985. VAP hadn't come into existence yet, though negotiations were going on bilaterally under the broader framework of STI. Only in July 1987 would VAP be formalized by the director of NIAID, Anthony S. Fauci, and Secretary of DBT, S. Ramachandran.

Glass, who was attending a WHO meeting on diarrhoea-related diseases in Calcutta, met the young paediatrics professor Bhan who joined the conference from the midst of the AIIMS outbreak. They went out for a drink in the evening and during their casual conversation, Bhan mentioned that he had been following the rotavirus outbreak in the newborn unit of his hospital in Delhi and that he was a bit surprised that despite contracting the viral infection, the neonates were not showing any clinical symptoms.[9]

This interested Glass as he was working on an NIH project to study an unusual group of rotaviruses, collected from newborns from four different continents, that did not cause the disease. This, in turn, marked the beginning of an association that lasted decades, ultimately leading to the development of a vaccine that would protect infants from the deadly scourge.

Bhan, by then, had cultured stool samples of infected neonates and isolated the rotavirus responsible for the infections. His efforts to compare the virus strain with already identified strains failed, leading to the realization that the strain he was looking in the electron microscope had not been documented by anyone.[10] Therefore, Bhan announced the discovery of an India-specific strain of rotavirus, soon to be labelled as the 116E strain that would lead the path to Indian vaccine development.

At around the same time, Durga Rao at the Indian Institute of Science (IISc), Bangalore was documenting cases of rotavirus infections without any accompanying serious symptoms of diarrhoea, like vomiting and dehydration, in a city hospital. He was able to identify a strain which he labelled as I321.[11]

These two incidents led the teams at AIIMS, Delhi and IISc, Bangalore to follow up with the infants to observe whether they continued to be asymptomatic on repeated exposure or not. The teams observed that, upon subsequent exposure, the infants demonstrated a stronger immune response without developing any severe symptoms of diarrhoea, which in turn, led to the idea of developing a vaccine from these strains.

Since both the strains had undergone structural mutations* from the original rotavirus strains through what was described as the 'natural reassortment process',† they worked on the premise that perhaps it could offer immune protection to infants.

AIIMS and IISc continued their informal collaboration by exchanging thoughts and notes on the twin strains. These exchanges led to a more concrete proposal by the time VAP was firmed up as an Indo-US vaccine collaboration in 1988. An airtight proposal to extend the investigation using the two strains to develop an effective vaccine was submitted to the newly formed VAP, the stakeholders of which were the Department of Biotechnology (DBT) from India, the NIAID and the Department of Health and Human Services from the US. Sensing an opportunity, two other entities jumped into the fray – the Government of Norway and the Bill and Melinda Gates Foundation, the latter through an arrangement with PATH, a global healthcare non-profit based out of the US.

The proposal was summarily approved, and work kicked off with funding from DBT, NIH and the United States Agency for International Development (USID). The NIH had contracted a private firm in 1997 to produce clinical-grade pilot lots‡ of the vaccine candidates and evaluate the lots in American adults and children

---

* Changes in the physical structure of a gene in an organism that can affect its properties or behaviour.

† The process where two similar viruses swap genetic material, which can lead to new strains or variants.

‡ Small batches of a product (like a vaccine) that are produced under strict quality control conditions for use in clinical trials.

prior to shipping them to India.[12] During 1997 and 1998, NIAID sponsored clinical trials in healthy adults and active children at the Cincinnati Children's Hospital, one of eight NIAID-funded vaccine and treatment evaluation units.[13] Once the vaccinated individuals in all three segments of trials were found to be asymptomatic the vaccine samples were brought to India for larger trials.

In the meantime, the first ever rotavirus vaccine named RotaShield, produced by Wyeth Laboratories, was licensed in the US in 1998. However, a strange adverse event called 'intussusception', in which part of the intestine slides into an adjacent part, led to its withdrawal within fifteen months.[14] This growing urgency among VAP's US partners to expedite the India project led to the search for a local industry partner.

By 1998, VAP was actively scouting for a local industry partner to manufacture the vaccine in India and conduct larger trials. Just two years earlier, an agriculture researcher named Krishna Ella and his wife Suchitra Ella – an economics graduate from University of Madras – had returned from the US and established a company in Hyderabad that focused on creating innovative healthcare solutions and bio-therapeutics. On account of their work experience in both India and US and with a little push from the Chief Minister of Andhra Pradesh Chandrababu Naidu, VAP found their partner in the couple's newly formed company, Bharat Biotech.

However, immediately after Bharat Biotech had begun work on the vaccines, it faced its first setback when the stock of the virus strain got contaminated with bacteria. It took more than two weeks and the support of the US Centers for Disease Control and Prevention (CDC) to restore the virus strains to their previous levels. Phase 1 and 2 of preclinical trials were carried out collaboratively by Bharat Biotech, AIIMS, DBT and PATH and continued till the safety and immunogenicity of the vaccine candidate were established in 2008.

Thereafter, the protocol development for the phase 3 trials took almost two years. The trials started in March 2011 at three sites: the Society for Applied Studies (SAS) Delhi, KEM Hospital and Research Centre, Pune and Christian Medical College, Vellore. The data of the trial – involving 6,800 infants, monitored over a two-year period and analyzed by the Translational Health Science* and Technology Institute in Delhi – indicated that the 116E-strain based vaccine provided 56 per cent protection in the first year, without any significant loss in efficacy in the second year.[15]

The findings were featured in the June 2014 edition of the *Lancet*.[16] The next year, the vaccine received approval for use from the Indian regulator and in 2017, it was incorporated into the India's UIP. Notably, the total expenditure for the vaccine project amounted to less than $50 million, estimated to be approximately one-tenth of the expense of bringing a similar live attenuated viral vaccine to the market in a developed country.

By 2015, Bharat Biotech had received a license from the Indian regulator under the brand name ROTAVAC and in another three years, WHO prequalified the vaccine for global deployment.[17] By then, two rotavirus vaccines, commercially developed and produced by giant pharma companies, were also prequalified by WHO – RotaTeq of Merck & Co. in 2008, and Rotarix of GlaxoSmithKline Biologicals in 2009.[18]

Glass, by now retired as the director of the John E. Fogarty International Centre had spent his lifetime on the prevention of gastroenteritis from rotaviruses, lauded the vaccine as 'the first ever vaccine entirely developed in India in over 100 years'.[19] He generously praised that ROTAVAC was derived from an Indian strain, identified by an Indian scientist, developed by an Indian company, studied in Indian populations, with support from the Indian government.[20] However, Fauci kept stressing on the US's contributions in the creation of the vaccine and soon after the announcement by the Indian team, he made a statement that said, 'NIAID provided the 116E vaccine strain – the particular strain tested in the ROTAVAC vaccine trial – to Bharat Biotech through a technology transfer agreement in 2000.'[21]

---

* A field that focuses on turning lab research into practical treatments or health solutions.

It is a fact that NIAID cultured and strengthened the 116E strain, but well before that it was identified and isolated by Bhan at the AIIMS paediatrics ward in 1985, which was later given to NIAID for further studies and culturing. Fauci's out of place claim cast a shadow on the critical contributions of the US and the spirit of the collaboration that would nurture future associations.

On the contrary, former principal scientific advisor to the Government of India, K Vijayraghavan, who was also the DBT Secretary for five years till January 2018, summed it up as 'an outstanding example of the new world paradigm in affordable, safe and effective vaccine development' by a unique group of domestic and international partners, committed to social innovation with a clear goal of developing a safe and effective vaccine meant for populations that most needed it at affordable prices.[22] In fact, the unique collaboration made the vaccine available to customers at a price of $1 a dose or lower at the time of its launch in 2013.

Three years after ROTAVAC found its place in the Indian immunization programme UIP,[23] the Serum Institute of India too launched its rotavirus vaccine named ROTASIIL, a heat-stable vaccine that did not require refrigeration for storage and transportation and therefore targeted low-income countries.[24] PATH partnered with SII for the phase 3 trial of this vaccine, with funding from the Bill & Melinda Gates Foundation. The results found the vaccine to be safe, well-tolerated and effective against severe rotavirus gastroenteritis.[25] The company claimed an efficacy of 55 per cent, comparable to the outcome of RotaTeq and Rotarix, based on its studies in Bangladesh and Africa.

Non-profit organizations such as, Médecins Sans Frontières and Epicentre evaluated the efficacy and safety of ROTASIIL studies in Niger. The early results showed that the vaccine was 67 per cent effective against severe and 79 per cent effective against very severe rotavirus diarrhoea.[26] Interestingly, the vaccine for trial in Niger was stored at a temperature of 25°C and transported, thus proving its ability to bypass the cold chain requirements. Soon ROTASIIL was prequalified by WHO and accepted by the Indian government for its immunization programme.

Boosted by the success of the rotavirus venture, VAP formed a Candidate Vaccine Advisory Committee (CVAC) in 2015 as a broader collaboration between NIAID, DBT, ICMR and interested private entities for developing and testing safe and effective vaccines. Under this arrangement, VAP offered scientific oversight and guidance to Indian biopharma* companies to develop vaccines for some alarming health challenges – dengue, chikungunya, respiratory syncytial virus (RSV),† zika, influenza and tuberculosis.[27] In 2019, four projects –TB, RSV, Flavi viruses and foot-and-mouth disease – were selected by VAP under its Adjuvant Collaboration Programme to bring together Indian and US researchers on the lines of ROTAVAC research and development.

In the meantime, yet another big success for VAP was unfolding – the Indian-developed Covid-19 vaccine Covaxin, which used the US-provided Alhydroxiquim-II as the adjuvant.‡ Alhydroxiquim-II developed through NIAID's adjuvant programme was made available by the US-based ViroVax.

Drawing inspiration from the success of the Indo-US vaccine collaboration, the European Union in 2018 initiated discussions on a similar partnership with India to jointly develop effective vaccines against viral influenza. The European Commission (EC), through the EU funding programme for research and innovation named 'Horizon 2020', has committed €15 million with the DBT matching an equal contribution to develop the next generation influenza vaccine. The need to develop better vaccine options was necessitated by reports of 300,000 to 650,000 deaths from seasonal influenza every year globally.[28,29]

* The branch of the pharmaceutical industry that deals with biologic products like vaccines, blood products and gene therapies.

† A common virus that causes lung infections, especially dangerous in babies and older adults.

‡ An ingredient added to vaccines to help boost the body's immune response.

Similar collaborations with Russia and France too had been established well before the Covid-19 pandemic. More partnerships were formed in the wake of Covid-19, and at the G20 meeting in 2023, India asked member countries to join its vaccine research collaborative to help save the world from vaccine inequity.

These collaborative efforts not only strengthened India's position as a global vaccine hub but also paved the way for a more resilient and equitable global healthcare landscape.

26

THE END OF STATE-RUN VACCINE MAKING

ONE MORNING IN 1976, PII, COONOOR ABRUPTLY RECEIVED an order from the Government of India to stop its polio vaccine production. The reason: one batch of its vaccine had failed quality tests at CRI, Kasauli. Instead of finding the root cause and rectifying it, the Health Ministry hastily ordered to halt production of polio vaccines at the facility.[1]

The Pasteur Institute, Coonoor had been meeting the entire polio vaccine requirements of the country since Albert Sabin personally trained the Institute's staff for producing the vaccine, besides donating the vaccine strains from his lab. Theories abound as to why vaccine production at the institute was suddenly stopped.

During those days, the influence of the import lobby – bolstered by alliances with ministers and bureaucrats – was growing stronger by the day. International pharmaceutical companies had formed a group under the banner of Organization of Pharmaceutical Producers of India (OPPI). The American pharma major Pfizer was active in the OPPI lobby, with its India head S.V. Pillai chairing the organization until 1975. Pfizer had been producing polio vaccines since 1963 and was one of the first to receive a strain-by-strain license from the US regulator. They were also exporting vaccine vials to various parts of the globe, including India.

Pfizer's selection as the first provider of oral polio vaccine (OPV) in the US had happened under interesting circumstances. The contract was awarded through a sealed bidding process involving three companies but two abstained, leaving Pfizer to secure the bid at an unusually high price.[2] Therefore, eyebrows were raised when the Indian government suddenly ordered PII, Coonoor to halt OPV production and resorted to import to meet the huge domestic requirement.

Jacob John recalls how the politics of one-upmanship by states led to a prolonged period of disaster during which no Indian manufacturer could produce OPV in the country. The Maharashtra strongman Y. B. Chavan, who was the finance minister in Indira Gandhi's cabinet, pulled strings to shut down the facility and relocate production to the Haffkine Institute, Bombay. Though the vaccine seeds were transferred to the Haffkine Institute on the orders of the Government of India, the Pasteur Institute refused to transfer its equipment, citing its status as an independent society and not a governmental institution. It so turned out that despite years of efforts, Haffkine Institute couldn't produce a single vial of polio vaccine.

Almost eighty scientists and technicians at PII, Coonoor who spent tireless days and nights on vaccine production, including its head Dr G. V. J. A. Harshavardhan, were extremely upset with the government's decision and accused the private vaccine importers of foul play. Many of them left the organization while a few migrated to other fields. Much later in 1978, when the government asked the Pasteur Institute to work on DTP vaccines, the remaining members of the polio team were shifted to the new project. Three years thereon, the same team produced the DTP group of vaccines from scratch.[3]

This vaccine fiasco in a way ended the country's dominance on polio vaccine production. Despite several subsequent endeavours, the country never succeeded in mastering the technology to produce OPV in the public sector. Instead, it ended up depending on imports for a very long time till the private sector came up with its production.[4] Even when the private sector eventually did catch up, the cost of polio vaccine was never the same.

Over a decade later, an honest attempt was made through an Indo-Russian collaboration and a company was established in the public sector specifically to address the polio vaccine shortage under the aegis of the Department of Biotechnology (DBT) – Bharat Immunologicals and Biologicals Corporation Ltd. (BIBCOL), Strategically located in a polio endemic area, Bulandshahar, Uttar Pradesh, the company started off by packaging polio vaccines in vials from the bulk received from its Russian partner, the Institute of Poliomyelitis and Viral Encephalitis (IPVE), Moscow – the same institute from where PII, Coonoor had procured additional seed strains three decades ago. As per the original understanding, the company could start vaccine production in five years upon the successful transfer of technology and seed strains.

The story began changing by 1998, when UNICEF, a major client of BIBCOL, declined to purchase the rebranded vaccine of Russian origin. This was at a time when the polio vaccination initiative in India was supported by UNICEF and the country had been relying on vaccines sourced by companies on behalf of their predominantly Western donors. The US–Russia relationship had become increasingly strained following NATO's eastward expansion and Russia's financial crisis. Institutions like UNICEF, which depend heavily on American financial contributions and are subject to donor-country influence, began adopting stricter procurement policies that mirrored these broader geopolitical undercurrents.

UNICEF informed BIBCOL that its updated procurement standards now required all its vaccine suppliers to have WHO-issued Good Manufacturing Practice (GMP) certification. Since IPVE, lacked this certification, UNICEF halted procurement from BIBCOL, which began impacting supply of OPV to UNICEF and therefore to India's polio eradication programme.[5]

With pressure mounting, India in turn suspended its bulk purchase from IPVE citing its lack of WHO-accredited GMP certification.[6]

BIBCOL struggled to find alternate buyers for its vaccine as it was wholly dependent on India's polio vaccination programme, which hinged on UNICEF's procurement standards. To tide over the crisis, BIBCOL eventually sourced OPV bulk from WHO-approved, GMP-certified suppliers like SmithKline Beecham in Belgium and Biopharma in the US.[7]

Shortly after BIBCOL changed its import source, UNICEF endorsed BIBCOL as a supplier. By packaging from the bulk sourced from its new associates, BIBCOL supplied UNICEF 70 million doses of OPV by early 2000, resulting in a turnover of ₹5.5 billion and turning the company a profitable entity by the turn of the century.[8]

However, the emergence of domestic private companies such as Panacea Biotech in the OPV space intensified competition and threw a spanner in the works. Consequently, BIBCOL was declared financially distressed in the new millennium and the government referred it to the Board of Industrial and Financial Reconstruction (BIFR) for its potential revival. Upon reviewing a revival plan by its bankers, the government endorsed the production of BCG, measles and tetanus toxoid (TT) vaccines to generate additional revenue. However, the company could never venture into producing any of these vaccines and ended up making zinc tablets and diarrhoea management kits for survival.

The story of BIBCOL not only exposes the government's apathy but also showcases the influence of geopolitics and the nexus between global pharma lobbies and multilateral agencies. It is a fact that its foundation was ill-timed, just before the liberalization of the Indian economy in 1991. However, BIBCOL was the result of the long-term Science and Technology Cooperation signed between India and Russia in 1987, in response to the Indo-US STI. Geopolitically, BIBCOL was Russia's response to America's VAP that had kicked off in 1987.

The control of the US and its grant-in-aid agencies over multilateral bodies like UNICEF was so pronounced at the time that the disqualification of bulk polio supplier IPVE on account of GMP compliance was likely nothing more than a planned attempt to stifle Russian collaboration with India. The brazenness with which UNICEF halted vaccine supply to the Indian polio programme on this account was also demonstrative of the agency's arrogance, mainly owing to its Western-driven governance. The US health lobbies were wary of India building closer ties with Russia in biopharma, similar to cooperation in nuclear technology and space science.

Though developing nations wielded significant voting power in UN organizations like WHO and UNICEF, their influence paled in comparison to the leverage held by first world countries who could withhold financial contributions and stall the running of the agencies. Additionally, developing countries are often reluctant to challenge donor nations, as these donors provide crucial technical and financial support to them. Therefore, fingers were pointed to the US in derailing the key Indo-Russian collaboration at a crucial time of a national polio crisis.

Similar to the Indo-Russian collaboration of BIBCOL, another vaccine company was established through an Indo-French agreement. Thanks to its rapidly progressing healthcare, Europe too wanted to collaborate with India in response to the American vaccine project. Named the Indian Vaccine Corporation Ltd. (IVCOL), set up by the DBT in 1989 in Gurgaon, it was to produce vero-cell-based IPV and measles vaccines, using technology from the French public sector unit, Institut Merieux. The cells were derived from the kidney of an African green monkey. This venture did not take off because of management changes at the French institute after the acquisition of Canadian vaccine maker Connaught Biosciences Inc. and subsequently, because of global economic changes and India's liberalization.[9]

It is worth noting that India was almost at par with the developed world in vaccine technology development till the 1920s and the two most important vaccines – against plague and cholera – came from India. This continued to some degree for decades because of the role played by three key institutes, the Haffkine Institute, CRI, Kasauli and PII, Coonoor, and also due to the leadership of Sokhey and Bhatnagar.

A decade after independence, the gap in new vaccine development efforts between the developed world and India widened, so much so that even improvisations on bacterial vaccines such as TT, DT and DPT took a decade or more after they were introduced elsewhere.[10] India was lagging behind in terms of resources in biological research, both in funding and scientific capital. And when the biotechnology revolution set off in the western world, India was left far behind.

Even efforts on tuberculosis and polio – from resource allocation to leadership initiatives of the government through the 1960s and 1970s – were half-hearted. However, a sense of urgency crept in with the launch of the EPI in 1978, partly to meet the objectives of WHO's 'Alma Ata' declaration and thereby be eligible for a grant-in-aid from multilateral agencies, government aid agencies and other donors.

What followed was a governmental decision to redirect many of the age-old organizations, working on various vaccines, and push them to produce the DTP group of vaccines, an essential part of the EPI, for which import dependence was growing. In addition to the usual suspects of PII, Coonoor, CRI, Kasauli and Haffkine, Bombay, many other institutes like the Institute of Preventive Medicine, Hyderabad were also called into service.

Soon after the declaration of smallpox eradication in 1976, several other smaller vaccine-producing units spread across the country, mainly engaged in making smallpox vaccines from the pre-independence era, were transitioned to produce DTP vaccines after shutting down their smallpox vaccine production. This included the King Institute of Preventive Medicine and Research, Chennai; Vaccine Institute, Belgaum and PII, Shillong. The socialist government that replaced the Emergency regime of Indira Gandhi took over many of the private vaccine makers of the time such as Bengal Immunity Limited and Smithstrain Street Pharmaceuticals Ltd, both based in Calcutta, in 1977. Others such as Bengal Chemicals and Pharmaceuticals Ltd., West Bengal Lab and Vaccine Institute, Nagpur were converted to public sector vaccine-making units by 1980.[11]

As a result, there was relief from import dependence in the early 1980s as the country gained momentum in vaccine production, mostly in the public sector and in the government research institutes. A good part of the requirements of EPI was met from public sector supply, with the rest coming from the private sector, domestic and transnational vaccine makers who were importing their vials. By the time EPI was restructured and relaunched as the UIP in 1985, India was in a better position in terms of vaccine supply in most vaccine categories.

However, a gap between the supply and demand existed for at least two vaccines – measles and polio – for which the country was dependent on import.[12] The agency that came forward to resolve this widening gap was a new player in the government, the DBT. It started with setting up the BIBCOL, with Russian collaboration, to fill the polio vaccine gap and IVCOL, with French support, to address the measles vaccine shortage. For a variety of reasons, both turned out to be futile exercises. With the liberalization policies ushered in by Prime Minister Narasimha Rao and his able Finance Minister Manmohan Singh, it was evident to the newly formed Department that it needed to change tracks, leading it to end its public sector efforts with these two entities.

The Department stopped investing in the public sector and began focusing on the private sector instead. It also began encouraging translation of academic research from laboratories to the field, by assisting in building agile industry-academic collaborations. This was followed by encouraging start-ups and small entrepreneurs to step in and find solutions to unresolved health mysteries and combat new health challenges, including inventing and replicating vaccines. These measures set India on a new path.

PART IV

FROM PUBLIC TO PRIVATE SECTOR

(1991–2010)

27

LAHORE TO LABS

HAD THE BCG VACCINE BEEN INVENTED A FEW DECADES EARLIER and introduced by the British in colonial India, could it have spared India from the agony of Partition?

Theoretically, perhaps. Muhammad Ali Jinnah was an eminent politician from the Western part of India and the tallest leader of the All-India Muslim League since 1913. By middle age, he had become addicted to tobacco and alcohol. A heavy smoker, Jinnah worked with a tin of Craven 'A' cigarettes at his desk, smoking fifty or more cigarettes a day for thirty years.

Jinnah had received treatment in Berlin for complications resulting from an episode of pleurisy. Since then, recurrent bronchitis had sapped his strength and weakened his respiratory system to such an extent that delivering a major speech left him breathless for hours. His over-dependence of cigarettes and cigars began taking a toll and his health grew fragile by the early 1930s. In late May 1946, while in Simla, Jinnah fell seriously ill. His devoted sister, Fatima, managed to get him on a train to Bombay, but his condition worsened during the journey.

Alarmed, she urgently contacted his physician in Bombay, Dr Jal Patel, who waited en route and boarded the train outside the city. Upon examining his distinguished patient, Dr Patel found his condition to be 'desperately bad'. Warning Jinnah that he would collapse if he attempted to go through with the reception he had planned at Bombay's Grand Railroad Station, Patel urged him off the train at a suburban station and rushed him to a hospital. It was there that Dr Patel uncovered what would become one of India's most closely guarded secrets.

That secret was frozen onto the grey surface of a piece of film; a film that had the potential to disrupt the Indian political landscape and likely alter the course of history. So valuable was this secret that even the British CID, renowned as one of the most effective investigative agencies in the world, were unaware of it.[1]

The film was an X-ray with black circles indicating pulmonary cavities – gaping holes where vital lung tissue had been destroyed. A chain of white dots revealed areas where pulmonary or pleural tissue was hardening, confirming the diagnosis. Tuberculosis was ravaging Jinnah's lungs. The damage was so severe that he likely had only a few years left to live.

Sealed in an unmarked envelope, these X-rays were secured in the office safe of Dr Patel in Bombay. Jinnah kept the secret within the close confines of his family; only his sister and a few others close to him knew the truth. He believed that the information, if leaked, would hurt his political career.[2] Had Jinnah been an ordinary tuberculosis patient, he would have been confined to a sanatorium for the rest of his life.

Upon being discharged from the hospital, Dr Patel brought him to his office and, with great sadness, informed his friend and patient of the fatal illness he had contracted. Patel told Jinnah that he was nearing the end of his physical endurance. Without significantly easing the overall stress on his system by reducing his workload, resting more frequently and quitting cigarettes and alcohol, he would not live more than a year or two.

Jinnah received the grim news with a stoic calm; his pale face showed no emotion. There was no question of giving up his mission to be confined to a sanatorium, he told Dr Patel. Fortified by biweekly injections from the doctor, Jinnah returned to work, making no real effort to adhere to the medical advice. He was determined not to let his impending death rob him of his place in history. With extraordinary courage and all-consuming zeal, Jinnah pursued his life's goal, his health fading as he made one final, intense push.

'Speed,' Jinnah emphasized during discussions with Louis Mountbatten on India's future, 'is the essence of the contract.'[3] He wanted to ensure two nations would be created through partition – and that he would command one of them before he breathed his last. It is possible that had Mountbatten, Nehru or Gandhi known about this extraordinary secret by April 1947, the partition of India might have been averted. The Indian leadership was so magnanimous that they might have let Jinnah become the prime minister of a united India to avoid a partition, which would cause immense destruction and sow seeds of lasting distrust between Hindus and Muslims.[4]

During the partition, the newly divided nations witnessed horrendous atrocities on the Punjab and Bengal borders as millions fled their homes. Innocent Hindus, Sikhs and Muslims became targets of merciless attacks, facing murder, rape and pillage as they were trying to cross the border on either side of the newly drawn Radcliffe line. Families were torn apart, communities decimated, and centuries-old bonds of camaraderie and co-existence were shattered in a matter of days.

In August 1947, as the dream of India's freedom was turning into a reality, twenty-one-year-old Gursaran Pran Talwar was forced to make an impossible choice. At the stroke of midnight on 15 August, when the tricolour was hoisted in Delhi's Red Fort, Talwar realized his home was no longer in India – it was in newly created Pakistan. With no real-time communication channels, he learnt from the radio and newspapers that Hindus from Lahore were fleeing across the Indus River, while the Muslims were heading in the opposite direction. Determined to save his family, Talwar joined a military convoy put together to rescue Hindus stranded in Pakistan. When

Talwar arrived in Lahore, he found his once-safe home empty, ransacked and damaged. 'I did not know where my family were,' he would recall later.[5]

Talwar's mother had died of tetanus when he was just eight days old. Worried about his father, he was searching through the remains of his ransacked house when he realized that an unruly Muslim mob was approaching. He rushed to the house of his neighbour, the famous poet Hafeez Jalandhary, who would later pen the national anthem of Pakistan. Jalandhary hid Talwar in the secluded women's quarters of his home, risking his life and that of his family.

To search for his missing father without arousing suspicion, Talwar began venturing out in disguise, sporting a beard and skull cap and posing as a Muslim. During his final days in Lahore, he witnessed the travails of fellow Hindus and advised one father-son duo to leave for India as soon as possible. He was shocked to find both father and son shot dead on a street corner just a few days later. Despite the danger, Talwar stayed on, undeterred in his pursuit of his missing father.[6]

Eventually, he did locate his father – not in Pakistan but on the Indian side. His father had crossed the border and safely reached Delhi, where Talwar went on to rebuild his life and that of his family. Alongside this, he laid the foundations for a new branch of science in India – immunology.

At the time of partition, Talwar was completing his master's degree in Chemical Engineering from the University of Punjab in Lahore, after completing his BSc (Hons) in Biochemistry.[7] He would finish his master's degree under very different circumstances, from a refugee camp in Delhi while working two jobs to meet his family's living expenses. In 1950, Talwar earned a scholarship for higher studies in France, where he was admitted into the Pasteur Institute, Paris. After spending six good years at the Pasteur Institute doing his DSc and later conducting research as a Humboldt postdoctoral fellow in Germany, he returned to Delhi to join AIIMS in 1956.

At the newly established institute, Talwar spent the initial years building AIIMS's team, strategy, infrastructure and projects. He played a key role in establishing an independent biochemistry department and elevating its status in medical education and research. He was thus part of a unique team that was building an institution which would go on to become the finest medical institution in the country.

A. V. Hill, who was invited to India to study research gaps in the region, had mooted the establishment of an advanced All India Medical Centre on the lines of John Hopkins in the US, drawing largely from the British Goodenough Committee's report.[8] In 1946, the Health Survey and Development Committee chaired by Sir Joseph Bhore also proposed the establishment of a national medical centre.[9]

After independence, Prime Minister Jawaharlal Nehru and his first Health Minister Rajkumari Amrit Kaur initiated steps to implement the recommendation with support from the government of New Zealand, under the 1950 Colombo Plan for economic development of South Asia.[10] Finally, in 1956, AIIMS was established as an autonomous institution through an Act of Parliament to serve as the nucleus for nurturing excellence in all aspects of healthcare.

At AIIMS, Talwar and his team elucidated the mechanisms underlying the biological effects of hormones like estradiol,[*] laying the foundation for further research in molecular biology[†] and endocrinology,[‡] while also starting his important work on a vaccine against leprosy. Not many had ventured into leprosy vaccines by then.

His resolve deepened when, during a scientific conference, he heard a WHO official respond sharply to a question about leprosy:

---

* A key female sex hormone that plays an important role in the reproductive system and menstrual cycle. It's also important for overall hormonal balance in both women and men.

† A branch of science that studies the structure and function of the molecules (like DNA, RNA, proteins) that make up living organisms.

‡ The branch of medicine and biology that deals with hormones – chemical messengers that control many bodily functions like growth, metabolism and reproduction.

'India has the world's largest number of leprosy patients [3.2 million at that time]. Do we expect Americans to come and work on this disease to find solutions? Scientists in India should take up the problems of India.'[11] Those words struck a chord. They ignited in Talwar a deep sense of responsibility and purpose. Recalling his final days in Lahore and his decision to dig up for a leprosy vaccine, he reflected, 'No one would come to our help, but for ourselves.' That conviction would go on to shape his lifelong commitment to tackling leprosy in India.

Leprosy had long been a scourge in India – not just its physical impact on patients but also the deep social stigma rooted in religious beliefs that surrounded it. It was often seen as a 'divine curse', leading to widespread ostracization of those infected. Religious texts across traditions reinforced this perception: the Hindu scripture *Manusmriti* prohibits matrimonial alliances with families affected by leprosy; the *Book of Leviticus* in the Old Testament considers it as a divine punishment for sins; Islam urges avoidance of those with leprosy, likening it to fleeing from a lion; and Buddhism views leprosy as a karmic disease, the result of past-life sins.[12]

Leprosy is believed to have originated in India around 2000 B.C., spreading to other regions through trade and conflict. During colonial rule, the Lepers Act of 1898 was introduced, mandating the institutionalization and segregation of poor leprosy patients, while exempting the rich and affluent from isolation requirements.[13] A harsh tool of discrimination, the Act was finally repealed by the Parliament in April 2016.[14]

Talwar's field studies and laboratory research at AIIMS suggested that patients with leprosy, caused by multiple types of bacteria (multibacillary), didn't exhibit a generalized immune deficiency. These patients responded normally to most antigens but showed no reaction to the bacteria causing leprosy. Depending on the stage of the disease, the immune system's deficiency can be considered either inherent or acquired due to the leprosy infection.[15]

These findings led Talwar to investigate the factors that made certain immune cells (white blood cells) effective in killing the bacteria in some patients but not in others. Using a radioactive substance to track bacterial growth, he discovered that in patients with severe leprosy, their immune cells and bacteria failed to communicate effectively, allowing the bacteria to multiply unchecked by the immune system.

By the late 1960s, as the research progressed, Talwar accepted an offer from WHO to establish and head the Immunology Research and Training Centre for South Asia in Delhi. The Indian government negotiated with WHO to convert it into a joint ICMR-WHO Research and Training Centre in Immunology. Talwar set up the new centre within AIIMS itself, allowing him to continue the research he was already engaged in. He pursued his work on leprosy in coordination with the AIIMS team working on the subject.

By 1974, under Talwar's leadership, WHO launched a global project called the Immunology of Leprosy Programme (IMMLEP) to develop a vaccine as a preventive remedy and reagents to detect subclinical leprosy.[16]

Many researchers had attempted to develop leprosy vaccines using killed or attenuated bacteria, but those were found to be ineffective in generating immunity. Therefore, when Talwar attempted cross-reactive mycobacteria, the study was looked at with suspicion. Five different mycobacteria were identified and investigated for their ability to cause a delayed hypersensitivity reaction. Eventually, Talwar zeroed in on an atypical, fast-growing mycobacterium, which he designated 'w.' It would later be named after him as *Mycobacterium indices pranii*, 'Prani' being his nickname derived from his middle name.[17]

Pre-clinical toxicology studies* paved the way for Phase I safety trials, demonstrating positive outcomes. Phase II immuno-therapeutic trials in multibacillary patients showed faster bacterial decline and

* Tests done before clinical trials to check if a new vaccine or drug is safe and non-toxic to humans.

clinical improvement with the use of vaccine. Phase III and IV field trials, involving over 400,000 subjects, demonstrated significant protection against leprosy, leading to the approval and marketing of the vaccine under the brand name 'Immuvac' by Ahmedabad-based Cadila Pharmaceuticals.[18]

Talwar's *Mycobacterium w* vaccine is used today as immunotherapy for multibacillary leprosy. It is equally efficient in treating mycobacterial infections such as pulmonary tuberculosis, immunodeficiency and cancers affecting the head, neck, bladder and lungs because of its immuno-modulatory qualities – the ability to modify or regulate the immune system's response.[19] It is also reported to be almost 90 per cent efficient in curing genital warts.[*20]

In addition, when this author met the ninety-six-year-old Talwar at his modest office during the peak of Covid-19, he mentioned the potential of the vaccine in treating SARS-CoV-2 infections. As it turned out, Department of Pulmonary Medicine at the Postgraduate Institute of Medical Education and Research, Chandigarh evaluated this possibility and reported that *Mycobacterium w* vaccine gave promising outcome in patients with severe Covid-19 infections.[21]

For various reasons, Talwar's leprosy vaccine has not been widely adopted in routine immunization programmes. While research in the field of vaccines continues, leprosy remains a concern, with over 200,000 new cases reported annually worldwide, and almost 50 per cent of them coming from India, mostly from the tribal regions of Jharkhand and Chhattisgarh. Despite being curable and vaccine-preventable, it remains the most stigmatized disease[†] even today.

Much has changed since the creation of Talwar's leprosy vaccine and the eventual journey to its licensing and commercialization. By the mid-1980s, Talwar had moved from AIIMS to the ICMR-WHO Centre, but his passion for immunology remained undiminished. In

---

* Non-cancerous skin growths caused by some types of human papillomavirus (HPV), often covered by the same vaccines used for preventing HPV-related cancers.

† Illnesses that cause shame or social judgment, often leading to discrimination against those who have them.

fact, by 1986, he had already embraced on another mission – to set up India's first dedicated centre of Immunology, a vision that found unexpected support at the highest political level.

When Prime Minister Indira Gandhi annually met with Jawaharlal Nehru Fellows as the head of the Jawaharlal Nehru Fund, discussions were centered on the state of India's scientific landscape and often ended with her seeking suggestions for advancing scientific pursuits. On one such occasion, Talwar advocated for immunology, highlighting its significant contributions, particularly in reducing infant mortality through vaccinations. He listed vaccine development as a priority to combat prevalent infections, alongside the importance of diagnostic technology. In no time, Gandhi asked for a proposal.

That hurriedly submitted proposal evolved into the National Institute of Immunology (NII) by June 1981. Talwar was appointed as its first director, while donning other hats, including his professorship at AIIMS. A year later, the ICMR-WHO Research & Training Centre which Talwar was heading out of AIIMS would formally be merged with NII. The NII operated from Talwar's laboratory at AIIMS till a building was constructed on a piece of land carved out of the Jawaharlal Nehru University (JNU) campus in another part of New Delhi.

Almost five years before he met Gandhi and mooted the NII concept, Talwar had already begun exploring a bold new frontier. While researching female hormones during the peak of the Emergency – a time when the government's push for population control had led to widespread controversy over forced vasectomies – he began looking for a more humane and scientifically sound alternative. That's when a radical idea took shape in him: what if there could be a vaccine that acted as a contraceptive for women?

The concept involved targeting a pregnancy-related hormone called human chorionic gonadotropin (hCG), which plays a vital role in helping embryos implant in the uterus.[22] Talwar's approach was to link a segment of hCG with a harmless fragment of the tetanus toxin (TT) so the immune system would treat it like a threat and block the hormone's action, thereby preventing pregnancy.[23] However, its effects were temporary and required booster doses to maintain protection.[24]

Despite criticism and controversy, including allegations of inadequate animal testing and opposition from women's groups about safety and ethics, Talwar's vaccine garnered support from a large global non-profit organization, the Population Council. However, it faced obstacles in securing funding support and regulatory approval. Additionally, the debate over the vaccine's classification as one that induced abortion further complicated its development and funding prospects.[25]

At this critical juncture, the US-based International Committee for Contraceptive Research (ICCR) came forward and converted Talwar's research into a multi-country investigative programme that worked on the safety and effectiveness of the vaccine. The ICCR studies were carried out in fertile women in Finland, Brazil, Chile, the Dominican Republic and Sweden.[26]

During these trials, when the vaccine was tested on women who were sexually active and wanted to avoid pregnancy, researchers found that it did not interfere with menstrual cycles or libido. Most importantly, it significantly reduced the chances of pregnancy, even after years of use.[27] The new version of the vaccine was much better than the initial one, with about three-fourths of the women producing enough protective antibodies.[28] The vaccine's effects were reversible, meaning women could conceive at any time, if they wished to. More importantly, it didn't affect ovulation or menstruation.[29] While these results were promising, further development and testing were needed to ensure its effectiveness in preventing pregnancy in a larger population.

By then, Talwar's research on 'contraceptive vaccines'* had begun to attract significant attention from global public health circles seeking to manage population growth, especially in a world where over a

* A vaccine designed to prevent pregnancy by training the body's immune system to block key reproductive hormones or functions.

million elective abortions took place annually due to unintended pregnancies. Adding to its appeal, the vaccine also showed promising results in treating uterine fibroids* and endometriosis.†

Yet, just as his work was gaining global relevance and momentum, an unexpected roadblock emerged. At the peak of this research in 1994, Talwar was asked to wind up his work at NII. His request for an emeritus position – a customary honor for scientists of his stature – was denied. Even a simple appeal for an office space to coordinate the upcoming 10th International Congress of Immunology, for which he was serving as president, was turned down. To make matters worse, he was asked to discontinue his work on the hCG vaccine immediately upon his departure from the institute.[30]

The treatment meted out to him by some of his senior colleagues befuddled him. It was during this time that he ran into Krishan Tiwari, the director of International Centre for Genetic Engineering and Biotechnology (ICGEB), a prestigious inter-governmental biotech research institute in New Delhi. Tiwari wholeheartedly welcomed Talwar into his institute and offered him the position of Professor of Eminence, along with office space for the secretariat of the International Immunology Congress. It is crucial to note that it was the first time the Congress was being held in a developing country.

Tiwari's offer provided a solution to Talwar's predicament, allowing him to continue his professional journey through ICGEB. Additionally, the Rockefeller Foundation transferred the grant for his work on female reproductive health from the NII to the ICGEB, strongly suggesting that fundings were offered to researchers and projects, and not to institutes.

During 1980–81 when Talwar was a Jawaharlal Nehru Fellow, his research had led to the creation of a technology to mass produce

---

* Non-cancerous growths in the uterus that can cause pain, heavy bleeding or fertility issues.

† A medical condition where tissue similar to the lining of the uterus grows outside it, causing pain and possibly infertility.

antibodies called hybridoma.* Using the new technology, he produced a monoclonal antibody (MoAb)† against hCG, known for its high affinity and specificity. He had licensed the hybridoma technology to two US firms, Carter Wallace and Wampole Laboratories, marking India's first biotech product licensed to US companies, for a royalty payment.

He had used the $780,000 royalty proceeds to establish the Talwar Research Foundation (TRF), a non-profit charitable trust in his name. The Trust began supporting bright women scientists, whose careers had been disrupted by marriage and family, to return to research. It had helped thirty-five women when Talwar decided to channelize the Trust into active research after the conclusion of the Immunology Congress in 1998. He embarked on this new journey with the foundation at the age of seventy-two, beginning a career free from any governmental affiliations – a burden that had troubled him for a while.

By then, a major development was taking place in the field of immunology; new possibilities emerged for monoclonal antibodies against hCG, something Talwar had visualized decades ago. Research reports began pouring in from different parts of the world suggesting the production of hCG outside of the placenta in various advanced-stage carcinomas,‡ including cancers in lung, bladder, colon, pancreas, breast, cervix, vulva, vagina, prostate, mouth and intestine.

Studies also confirmed that antibodies generated against hCG specifically target the tumour secreting hCG, demonstrating selectively binding to these cells while sparing other tissues in the body. Remarkably, these hCG antibodies exhibited significant cytotoxic properties§ on the tumour cells producing hCG outside

---

* A lab technique used to produce large amounts of a specific type of antibody by fusing two different kinds of cells.

† Lab-made molecules that can mimic the immune system's ability to fight off harmful pathogens like viruses.

‡ A type of cancer that starts in the skin or tissues that line internal organs.

§ The ability of a substance (like a drug or antibody) to kill cells – especially harmful or the placenta.[31] In brief, Talwar's hCG work had the potential of a pertinent solution to a wide range of cancers. This development brought new players to his desk, both pharma giants and US non-profits.

When Talwar retired from NII, he was asked to leave the hCG vaccine project he was working on at the time. Since there had been no progress on the project at NII for almost ten years, he revived it under the banner of the TRF. In 2006, the Indo-US VAP came forward and offered him a grant to resume the project, transforming the conventional hCG contraceptive vaccine into a genetically engineered recombinant vaccine with consistent characteristics.[32] In the new vaccine, the β-subunit of hCG* was connected to a protein called heat-labile enterotoxin (LTB)† in bacteria *Escherichia coli,* instead of the previous carrier tetanus toxoid, to avoid suppression of immunity when it is used repeatedly.[33]

Talwar's hCG vaccine has since been developed as a genetically engineered recombinant vaccine and passed on to the Indian vaccine company Bharat Biotech for confirmatory trials and production under GMP. The Drugs Controller General of India and the Institutional Ethics Committees have granted permission to conduct trials at AIIMS and Sir Gangaram Hospital in New Delhi, though its progress was interrupted by the Covid-19 pandemic.[34]

By the time Talwar turns 100 on the Gandhi Jayanti of 2026, he will likely witness the full flowering of his life's work, with the hCG vaccine being used not only as a pioneering contraceptive for women but also as an affordable therapy for a variety of cancers around the world. If so, he may be heralded as the inventor of the first birth control vaccine and of the most cost-effective cancer treatment ever developed.

---

cancerous cells.

* A part of the hCG hormone that is specifically targeted in Talwar's vaccine to block its reproductive function.

† A harmless bacterial protein used to help the body recognize and react to the vaccine more effectively.

Though honoured with the Padma Bhushan by the Government of India and the *Officier de la Legion d'Honneur* by the Government of France, Talwar remains a man of quiet pride and enduring purpose. For him, the true reward lies not in the accolades, but in the impact of his science – in the lives improved, suffering alleviated and knowledge pursued.

28

RECOMBINANT BREAKTHROUGHS

WHEN TALWAR WAS JOINING PUNJAB UNIVERSITY IN LAHORE for his graduate studies, a poor peasant's son from the nearby Raipur village in Multan was completing his Master of Science (MSc) degree with the help of scholarships at the same University. The peasant's son had a journey almost parallel to Talwar's, as he and his family had also endured the hardships of partition, relocating to Delhi and living in refugee camps.

He went to Europe for higher studies, making a mark in biotechnology during the nascent stage of this branch of science. He joined the University of Liverpool on a scholarship from the Indian Government to study insecticides and fungicides, but due to a lack of space in the laboratory, he was forced to pursue organic chemistry. He ended up securing a PhD in 1948 on the chemistry of melanin,* the pigment that gives colour to the eye, hair and skin. Back in Delhi, he struggled to find a job and joined the Swiss Federal Institute of Technology (ETH) in Zurich on a no-payment fellowship. By 1949, he joined the University of Cambridge to work on peptides† and nucleotides‡ under Alexander Todd, who would receive the Nobel

---

* A natural pigment found in organisms, responsible for colour in the skin, eyes and hair.

† Short chains of amino acids, which are the building blocks of proteins.

‡ The basic building blocks of DNA and RNA.

Prize in Physiology seven years later for unravelling the chemistry of bile acids.[*]

The peasant's son would become one of the key scientists who would pave the way for advancements in biotechnology in the 1960s, which in turn would set off a genetic engineering revolution, and launch a brand new industry in the West. As this transformation unravelled, for his work to help understand the genetic code, the peasant's son would be awarded the Nobel Prize in Physiology/Medicine in 1968, at the age of forty-six.

The peasant's son was Har Gobind Khorana.

In the 1950s, while working as a postdoctoral researcher in Stanley Cohen's laboratory at Stanford University, Khorana started his research involving nucleic acids, and their purpose in understanding the genetic code. Cohen was the tallest figure in this emerging field of mixing technology with biology, and would win the Nobel Prize in Physiology/Medicine in 1986, eighteen years after his student Khorana won the same prize. In time to come, Cohen would be known as the founder of biotechnology, along with Herbert Boyer, the first scientist to produce synthetic insulin and growth hormones in a lab.

It was in 1973, during a conference in Hawaii, that Cohen's path crossed with Boyer's. Though they had been working independently on different aspects of DNA manipulation – a field still in its infancy – their conversations during conference breaks revealed a shared vision: introducing foreign DNA into bacterial cells. This intellectual synergy sparked the idea of collaborating by combining Cohen's expertise in plasmids[†‡] with Boyer's pioneering work on restriction enzymes.[§] That serendipitous meeting laid the groundwork for the first successful recombinant DNA experiment – a breakthrough that

---

* Compounds made in the liver that help digest fats.

† A small circular piece of DNA used in labs to carry genes into cells – like a USB stick for transferring genetic instructions.

‡ Small, circular pieces of DNA that exist independently in bacteria.

§ Special proteins that cut DNA at specific spots.

would revolutionize biotechnology and give birth to what we now know as recombinant DNA technology.

For the uninitiated, recombinant DNA technology is the method of joining two or more different DNA strands after slicing and splicing them to create a new combined hybrid, one with altogether different qualities. The tools that slice and splice the DNA are nothing but different types of enzymes.

In recombinant DNA technology, the first step is to isolate a specific DNA sequence which contains the gene with desired traits or the gene of interest. Once the donor is identified and isolated, this DNA is cut using enzymes called restriction endonuclease, creating fragments with sticky ends. Another DNA molecule, called a vector, is isolated to carry the gene into host cells.* Both donor and vector DNA are cut and mixed, allowing their sticky ends to bind and fuse. The fragments are sealed together using another enzyme to form a recombinant DNA. Thereafter, it is introduced into host cells, and the cells with the inserted DNA are marked. These cells multiply, propagating the recombinant DNA and expressing the desired traits from within the host.

Genetic engineering, and therefore new age biotechnology, has significantly been driven by recombinant DNA technology. This technology allows scientists to manipulate and modify DNA molecules, leading to the creation of genetically engineered organisms with desired traits. Recombinant DNA technology has revolutionized genetic engineering by enabling the transfer of genes between different species, thereby opening new avenues for applications in medicine, agriculture and biology.

Many pathbreaking inventions emerged from recombinant technology in the 1960s and 1970s. However, the story of the hepatitis B vaccine has been somewhat overlooked compared to that of insulin and cancer-fighting interferon,† both of which were

---

* Cells into which recombinant DNA is introduced so they can produce the desired product.

† A protein produced by cells in response to viruses; used in cancer treatment.

prominent examples of the technical and commercial prowess of the new technology.

However, the recombinant hepatitis B vaccine turned out to be more consequential than scientists and the industry had originally envisaged. In fact, with recombinant DNA technology in action, the vaccine innovation system itself underwent a paradigm shift from being a publicly funded, public-health-oriented system to an industry-led initiative; and the shift was almost complete by the turn of the millennium.[1]

The recombinant hepatitis B vaccine was initially received poorly, despite the fact that one in every four people was infected with the virus. As of 2019, WHO estimated that 296 million people were living with chronic hepatitis B infection, adding 1.5 million new infections and resulting in an estimated 820,000 deaths a year, mostly from cirrhosis and hepato-cellular carcinoma.* The infection spreads through bodily fluids of blood, saliva, vaginal secretion and semen, and is also passed on from mothers to their babies.[2]

Strangely though, the story of the recombinant hepatitis B vaccine began from a man and his childhood fantasy. Growing up in Brooklyn, Baruch Blumberg dreamt of being like Ernest Shackleton, who led an expedition to the South Pole or Charles Darwin, who voyaged around the world. His heroes were Lewis and Clark, the intrepid explorers of the American continent.[3]

Blumberg originally enrolled in a graduate programme in mathematics at Columbia University and then switched over to medicine at Columbia's College of Physicians and Surgeons. He could never have imagined that this decision would take him around the world, much like his childhood heroes. All these efforts were rooted in one daunting question – why did some people contract certain diseases and not others, despite living in the same environment and being exposed to the same types of microbes?

Through the 1950s, Blumberg embarked on a global search for

---

* A common type of liver cancer.

answers, collecting human blood samples from various regions and racial groups along the way. Upon returning from his field trips, he continued investigating the blood samples for any genetic variations. While examining samples from Australian aboriginals infected with 'yellow jaundice', he identified a surface antigen that had never been recorded before and he called it the Australia antigen. Further studies demonstrated the antigen's potential to cause liver cancer as well.[4]

Using the Australian antigen, Blumberg, along with microbiologist Irving Millman, developed a screening test to diagnose viruses and used it on hepatitis B patients. This revealed that it could, in fact, help diagnose hepatitis B infections. Blumberg and his team went on to prove that this antigen was associated with hepatitis B infection and was part of the virus itself – a small protein that eventually came to be known as the Hepatitis B Surface Antigen (HBsAg) because it was found on the surface of the hepatitis-causing virus.[5] In 1965, while working at the Institute for Cancer Research in Fox Chase, Philadelphia, Blumberg published a paper detailing the new antigen and its relation to hepatitis B.[6,7]

In the late 1960s, Blumberg and Millman postulated that the non-infectious HBsAg particle could be separated from the virus and used to develop a vaccine. Subsequently, Millman developed a hepatitis B vaccine from the plasma of infected individuals for the US drug company Merck & Co. It was also touted as the first ever cancer vaccine as the hepatitis B virus was a leading cause of liver cancer. For his discoveries, Blumberg received the Nobel Prize in Physiology or Medicine in 1976.[8]

Blumberg generously shared his patent for antigen separation with everyone in order to aid its widespread distribution and use. Many pharma companies began using this technology and strains from Blumberg to commercially develop the vaccine.

In the meantime, in 1981, the US Food and Drug Administration (FDA) approved a plasma-derived hepatitis B vaccine. It was an attenuated vaccine derived from blood plasma containing HBsAg collected from the infected, then treated with formaldehyde and subjected to heat treatment. Merck manufactured and marketed the vaccine under the brand name 'Heptavax', the first ever commercial hepatitis B virus vaccine. It would be discontinued in 1990 when more sophisticated vaccines arrived in the market.[9]

By 1986, second-generation genetically engineered, DNA-recombinant hepatitis B vaccines, without any blood materials, were developed by various companies. It was a goldmine for vaccine companies, given the fact that one in four persons worldwide was carrying the virus.

Since the late 1980s, the Indian market too had been flooded with hepatitis B vaccines produced by multinational giants MSD, SmithKline-RIT and its successor SmithKline Beecham. The reason was that over 40 million Indians were hepatitis B virus carriers and over 115,000 deaths were reported every year in India from hepatitis B related complications. Viral hepatitis and its complications such as liver fibrosis,* cirrhosis or liver cancer caused by various hepatitis viruses A, B, C, D and E were also widespread in India.

Therefore, when the second-generation vaccine arrived on the scene, it became imperative for India to develop its own version of HBsAg recombinant vaccine. This urgency was heightened by the reluctance of the western vaccine makers to share the strains or underlying technology, driven by the vaccine's enormous market potential. In response, a few Indian companies began independently exploring avenues to develop an indigenous version since the technology was not patented.

The first firm to get into the space was Shantha Biotechnics, a Hyderabad-based biotech start-up set up by K. I. Varaprasad (a.k.a. Varaprasad Reddy). Many swung into action and approached the Indian Institute of Science (IISc) for support and collaboration. IISc was then headed by Dr G Padmanaban who discovered that *Plasmodium falciparum* synthesizes heme *de novo*† for its survival,

* The build-up of scar tissue in the liver due to damage.

† Making a compound from scratch, not using what's already available.

contrary to the earlier belief that *Plasmodium* entirely depends on the host. This opened up new biochemical targets for the development of novel antimalarial drugs, since heme biosynthesis is crucial to the survival of the parasite but different enough from human pathways to be selectively targeted.

In the 1980s, Padmanaban also opened the doors of his laboratory to the Swedish pharmaceutical giant Astra, bringing on board a team of half a dozen young scientists to pursue research on malaria, tuberculosis and diarrhoea. Two years later, when Astra established its own dedicated research centre – the Astra Research Centre – the collaboration took on a more formal shape.[10] One of his students during this period was an aspiring biochemist P. N. Rangarajan. After completing his PhD in 1989, Rangarajan moved to Salk Institute for Biological Studies, US to do his postdoctoral work. There he came across a novel yeast *Pichia pastoris* which could control the expression of foreign genes.

When Rangarajan returned to IISc in 1993 after completing his post-doctoral work under Prof. Ron Evans, hepatitis B was still a major killer disease in India. Almost 117,000 people were dying every year and the country had a prevalence of 3.7 per cent of the virus.[11]

The market was flooded with hepatitis B vaccines named ENGERIX-B from SmithKline Beecham and RECOMBIVAX HB from MSD. Both RECOMBIVAX HB and ENGERIX-B were available for paediatric and adult use, though Indian customers largely depended on ENGERIX-B.

ENGERIX-B used the common baker's yeast *Saccharomyces cerevisiae* for making the vaccine. Rangarajan wanted to use *P. pastoris* instead. He saw that *P. pastoris* combined the advantages of bacterial and mammalian expression systems. As a single-celled organism, it is easy to grow and can be used to perform complex manipulations on proteins. It can also be made to grow to higher cell densities compared to baker's yeast and produce greater amounts of the recombinant protein with the same effort.

Rangarajan cloned the gene encoding* of the HBsAg and expressed it in *P. pastoris*. A recombinant *P. pastoris* strain expressing high levels of HBsAg was selected and standardized in a four-step process to purify HBsAg from the yeast cell extracts. The purified HBsAg was then made to adsorb aluminium hydroxide, which generates antibodies against HBsAg when introduced in humans.[12]

By the mid-1990s, the Ministry of Human Resource Development had come up with a Technology Development Mission to encourage collaborations between scientists and industries to design and develop solutions that are useful for the country. Rangarajan decided to explore it. He was inspired by the exposure at the Salk Institute, which had a tie-up with the drug company Ligand Pharmaceuticals, allowing his mentor Evans to translate his research to developing drugs.[13]

It so happened that in 1998, two years into its operations and armed with the institutional tie-ups for the Rotavirus vaccine project, Hyderabad-based Bharat Biotech approached Rangarajan to explore the development of the indigenous recombinant hepatitis B vaccine. This was within months of the launch of India's first indigenously developed hepatitis B vaccine by Shantha Biotechnics.

* Copied a specific gene from the virus and inserted it into yeast to make it produce part of the virus used in vaccines.

29

SHANVAC-B – THE *SHAANDAAR* STORY

IN THE GREAT INDIAN VACCINE STORY, FEW HEROES EMERGE from outside the world of science. Even fewer walk into the biotech battlefield armed with nothing but moral fire, a resurrected idea and fondness for a mother whose quiet strength lit their way.

K. I. Varaprasad (a.k.a. Varaprasad Reddy) wasn't a scientist, nor was he a businessman groomed in the corridors of capital. He was, in every sense, an outsider – a man shaped by despair, rebellion and an almost irrational belief that even a lone individual could challenge the monopoly of multinational giants and win.

His story didn't begin in a laboratory. It began with exile – a young boy sent off to live with a communist uncle fighting for justice, to learn discipline and values in life. Reading communist pamphlets and the popular *Soviet Land* magazine, the boy learned early that justice didn't come on a platter; it had to be fought for. And decades later, at a WHO conference in Geneva, Varaprasad would find his war. Not one of ideology, but biology.

The enemy: Hepatitis B.

The weapon: A vaccine India didn't yet have.

The battlefield: The global pharmaceutical market, ruled by Western corporations.

Born as a single child in an agricultural family in the Nellore district of Andhra Pradesh, young Varaprasad had lofty dreams. After completing his engineering studies from Andhra University in 1970, he found a job with India's Defence Research and Development Organization (DRDO).

When he was confronted with having to compromise the very values he stood for, Varaprasad left the defence establishment and joined the Andhra Pradesh Industrial Development Corporation, a government entity promoting industry. For a similar reason, he would leave this government job in 1985 and join a struggling firm manufacturing high-end batteries, picking up orders to supply his erstwhile employer DRDO.

Despite bringing in capital to infuse as equity and reviving the company, Varaprasad did not last there long. He was unceremoniously sacked by his partner due to differences in business approach. Here again, his values were a stumbling block to running the business the way his partner wanted. In his pursuit of a purpose, Varaprasad travelled to see some of his friends and relatives, both in India and abroad. On one such trip in 1992 he ended up attending a WHO conference in Geneva, he found exactly that.

It was a turning point. The Geneva conference exposed him not only to the grim toll of hepatitis B, especially in developing countries like India, but also to the stranglehold Western firms maintained over the life-saving recombinant vaccine. This encounter planted the seed of an idea – one that would soon take root in a small Hyderabad lab.

Varaprasad then decided to explore ways to access the technology needed to make a recombinant vaccine to address the hepatitis B menace in India. He approached a Western firm and was bluntly told that India wouldn't be able to afford such sophisticated technologies and even if he could pay for it, Indian technicians wouldn't be able to understand or replicate it.[1]

There may have been some truth to the statement. Almost at the same time, another Hyderabad-based start-up Transgene Biotech Limited (TBL) claimed to have acquired the technology, and that it was struggling to translate it into a vaccine, running trials and setting up a manufacturing facility. TBL had since claimed to have resold its recombinant hepatitis B vaccine technology to another firm and invested the proceeds in non-vaccine projects.[2] However, no details were available as to from whom it acquired the technology or to whom it resold the technology.

Despite the ominous possibility of failure, Varaprasad was determined to keep going, convinced that there were enough capable Indians who could learn, modify and replicate the process. Without much deliberation, he set up Shantha Biotechnics in Hyderabad and began functioning from the campus of Osmania University, on a special arrangement.

But building a genetically engineered vaccine from scratch was a race against time, and the pressure often pushed people to the edge. When a key member of his team tried to fudge the test data in a desperate attempt to meet accelerated timelines, Varaprasad acted decisively. Around that time he also cemented his relationship with Dr Guntaka Rami Reddy, a microbiologist at Columbia University, and sought his mentorship for the project.

By 1994, Rami Reddy suggested a better place where Shantha's innovations and talents could be better nurtured – the Centre for Cellular and Molecular Biology (CCMB). It was a modern biology cell research centre, spun off by CSIR in 1977 from the then Regional Research Laboratory, Hyderabad, which itself would later become the Indian Institute of Chemical Technology (IICT).

Even with access to a cutting-edge research environment, building a capable team remained a challenge. Varaprasad reached out to almost 100 Indian scientists working abroad, hoping to lure them back with the promise of purpose and nation-building, but only two opted to join the audacious venture. In the meantime, Rami Reddy helped in the crucial part of the puzzle – recombining the DNA. He also trained key members of the team for which Varaprasad would pay him almost ₹7 million.

Soon Varaprasad realized that just as technology and skilled human resources, capital too was a scarce resource. He approached every bank in Hyderabad seeking a loan to fund his venture with a clear business plan and roadmap, but none of them entertained a firm with no revenue, no assets and no balance sheet. Desperate, Varaprasad sold the family silver – disposed of some of his ancestral property – and raised funds from close family and friends. In the end, he succeeded in raising a reasonable capital of ₹19 million.

Unfortunately, this funding wasn't sufficient to sustain the firm beyond a few years. By 1995, the funds had dried up, and Varaprasad was desperately seeking to replenish his coffers. Just as it seemed like the end of the road for his venture, a surprising opportunity emerged. The foreign minister of the Sultanate of Oman, Yusuf Bin Alawi Abdullah was brought on board. An acquaintance introduced Varaprasad to the Omani foreign minister's representative Khalil Ahmed, who would later become the executive director of the company, representing Omani interests and steering the company through troubled times. Motivated by the need for an affordable hepatitis B vaccine for his country, Abdullah invested ₹19 million in his personal capacity in exchange for a 50 per cent stake in the company. He also arranged long-term loans from Oman International Bank at low interest rates, providing Shantha Biotechnics with a much-needed financial lifeline.

The newly infused funds helped the company begin setting up a manufacturing facility at Medchal on the outskirts of Hyderabad even as work was progressing rapidly at the rented CCMB lab. Varaprasad was hoping the company would turn around with the much needed success of a recombinant vaccine.

At the CCMB lab, Varaprasad's team had been exploring many ways to tackle the issue. At the time, most of the researchers globally were using the common baker's yeast *Saccharomyces cerevisiae* for recombining DNA fragments. In the West, scientists were using this yeast for making the hepatitis vaccine as well. The companies that had developed the recombinant technology for slicing and splicing DNA kept it close to their chest.

However, following the advice of Osmania University microbiologist Gita Sharma, the new Shantha team, led by KSN Prasad, decided to explore a different yeast – *Pichia pastoris*. Eventually, the team began making progress in using *Pichia pastoris* yeast instead of the common baker's yeast for recombining DNA fragments.

Since the early 1980s, *Pichia* had been on the radar of researchers, after scientists at the Salk Institute Biotechnology/Industrial Associate Inc. (SIBIA) in La Jolla, CA isolated the key gene responsible for the yeast's alcohol oxidase promoter, known for its ability to control the expression of foreign genes. They had further developed vectors, strains and tools for manipulating the organism's genetics. Among their early successes was the cloning of the surface antigen of the hepatitis B virus (HBsAg).[3]

Pichia pastoris used for single-cell protein production gained importance in the 1980s when Phillips and SIBIA repurposed it as a system for heterologous protein expression.[4] A cost-effective eukaryotic platform widely used for large-scale protein production, Arizona-based RCT acquired the Pichia Classic Expression System from Phillips Petroleum in 1993, and resold its licenses to over 300 companies worldwide. It was now being distributed and supported by a firm named Life Technologies under license from RCT.[5] Varaprasad was one of the earliest buyers of the expression systems from RCT, and the first from India.

Fueled by sparse yet promising conversations with scientists who had dabbled in *Pichia* work, the Shantha team led by Prasad plunged into dense scientific literature, mining fragments of knowledge from scattered papers authored by Western researchers. With no roadmap, they embarked on a high-stakes scientific odyssey.

By October 1995, Shantha had moved into its newly constructed manufacturing facility, and within an impressive span of six months, the first batch of its hepatitis B vaccine was ready. Phase I clinical trials – aimed at assessing safety and tolerability – were conducted at the Nizam's Institute of Medical Sciences in Hyderabad. In a remarkable gesture reminiscent of Louis Pasteur, who once tested a rabies vaccine on himself, Varaprasad offered himself and his family as the first human volunteers. Soon, many of Shantha's staff members followed his lead, standing as proof of their collective belief in the mission. Phase II trials began in December 1996 at Nizam's Institute and KEM Hospital in Mumbai. When the trial results were released in April 1997, they marked a moment of celebration – the vaccine had cleared every benchmark with resounding success.[6]

As the first glimmers of success emerged with the recombinant vaccine molecule finally taking shape, it was only the beginning of a much tougher battle. Translating the fragile success of the lab into industrial-scale production was like turning a paper boat into a warship. Disappointingly, most of the published work had only dealt with making large colonies of yeast by shaking it in flasks, which was the normal method deployed in laboratories. However, scaling the system to industrial-sized fermenters was a challenge. This was overcome by gradually increasing the size of the fermenters – an incredible leap from millilitres to thousands of litres.

But the Shantha team pressed on. Working without a safety net, the team scaled up the fermenters in carefully calibrated steps; testing, failing and adjusting their process with every batch. Each additional litre brought new risks – of contamination, instability* or loss of potency. And yet, against all odds, they succeeded. The fragile yeast held up. The process stabilized. The vaccine endured. The factory could now breathe life into the dream of an affordable hepatitis B vaccine at scale.

In August 1997, as part of the silver jubilee celebrations of India's independence, Shantha launched India's first recombinant hepatitis B vaccine, Shanvac-B, heralding the country's entry into the global biopharma club. Chief Minister of Andhra Pradesh Nara Chandrababu Naidu kept away from the launch, despite Varprasad's personal invitation. Renuka Chowdhary, who was the health minister

* The vaccine breaks down or stops working over time.

in the cabinet of Prime Minister I. K. Gujral, and the Science and Technology Minister Y. K. Alagh attended the event and lauded the efforts of the team.

But a bigger surprise was in store. Taking the global bulls by its horns, Shantha launched Shanvac-B at about $1(₹50) per unit, significantly lower than the $23 to $30 price range set by its foreign competitor SmithKline Beecham.

Analysts scoffed at Shantha's audacity, projecting modest first-year sales of just $100,000, convinced that a one-dollar vaccine could never turn a profit, let alone penetrate a market dominated by Western giants. But Varaprasad had bet not on price, but on scale and impact – and his instincts were spot on. By March 1998, Shanvac-B shattered expectations, raking in over $1.6 million in sales that year. 'Unless it is made for one dollar, nobody can afford this,' Varaprasad had said. Despite the low pricing, Shanvac-B achieved healthy net profit margins of around 20 per cent, proving that affordable healthcare and commercial viability didn't have to be at odds.[7]

Over the next decade, hepatitis B vaccine consumption in India soared – from a few hundred thousand doses in the early 1990s to over 30 million doses by 2008 – driven by growing support from donor agencies and public health programmes. In tandem with this surge, market prices plummeted dramatically, falling from around $23 per dose to as little as $0.23, one of the most dramatic drops in vaccine pricing anywhere in the world.

The greed of transnational pharma companies was an immediate casualty of Shantha's success with Shanvac-B, crashing the price of hepatitis B vaccines in the market. Foreign companies who were having a free run in the Indian market received the biggest setback as the results of a comparative study of the vaccine with its foreign competitor's vaccine came out. Eventually, the market leader SmithKline too slashed the price from $23 to close to $0.23 and later to $0.15 cents per unit.

Shantha had held a mirror to the true face of foreign vaccine companies operating in India. Indian health administers and regulators were stunned to discover that a company claiming to 'exist to save lives' had been selling a life-saving vaccine at 150 times its cost!

By now there was no dearth of funds for Shantha Biotechnics. A few months before the Shanvac-B launch, Varaprasad had signed an agreement with the newly set up Technology Development Board (TDB) of the Department of Science and Technology (DST) for loan assistance to commercialize the vaccine. This was to enable the mass production of the vaccine so that average Indians could afford the vaccine.[8]

Recognizing Shantha's potential, both Morgan Stanley and the State Bank of India Mutual Fund stepped in with a combined investment of $10 million in 2000. Two years later, further validation came when Pfizer partnered with Shantha to co-market its hepatitis B vaccine in India under the brand name HepaShield, impressed by its quality and efficacy. Later, Pfizer obtained first refusal rights from Shantha to exclusively market all its vaccines under development outside of India.[9]

Then came knocking a visitor – Cyrus Poonawalla. He had been watching the Shanvac-B developments, even as his own teams were grappling with the challenges of developing a hepatitis B vaccine. He reached out to Varaprasad suggesting he wanted to visit the Shantha facility. After the visit, Poonawalla turned to Varaprasad and asked, 'How much for the company?' Varaprasad politely responded, 'Not for sale.' Poonawalla once again approached Varaprasad a while later, this time through Ms Poonawalla at a private function. Again, the offer was politely declined by Varaprasad.[10]

Ten years into operations, Shantha was making 100 million units of the vaccine a year and selling in more than fifty countries, in addition to picking up 40 per cent of UNICEF's global supply. This was made possible with the help of WHO certification, which came its way by 2002.

Buoyed by this global validation and early success, Shantha began setting its sights on other public health challenges. After a brief foray into Japanese encephalitis (JE) vaccines and interferon therapy* for cancer, Varaprasad turned his attention to cholera – one of India's most persistent water-borne diseases. In fact, even as Shanvac-B was taking off, cholera had already caught his eye as the next battleground.

He realized that over a billion people globally are at risk of the rapidly dehydrating diarrhoeal disease, caused by different serogroups of the bacterium *Vibrio cholerae*. He also noticed that the disease had always been associated with poverty, poor sanitation and lack of potable water. He had seen devastating cholera outbreaks in different parts of the world that had resulted in hundreds of thousands of deaths. He was shocked to see a WHO report that highlighted the fact that half of the cholera cases and deaths were reported in children below five years of age.[11]

Cholera remained a worrying public health challenge in the world, endemic in many countries and causing epidemics in some of the low and middle-income countries. An estimated 2.86 million cholera cases a year presented in endemic countries, and of that, an estimated 95,000 died.[12] No one had seriously worked on a vaccine against cholera since Haffkine in India, though the challenge has been growing in leaps and bounds.

An effective vaccine to prevent cholera had always been a priority of Indian health administers. Varaprasad knew this well, and as early as 2004, he directed the company's resources in addressing the problem of cholera. To save time on production, he reached out to WHO using his good relations with the world body. WHO facilitated the transfer of a version from Vietnam where the original Whole Cell bacteria (WC) vaccine was licensed in 1997 and was used for endemic situations. It was reformulated to meet WHO and GMP requirements.[13] By April 2009, Shantha succeeded with the first indigenized bivalent oral cholera vaccine named 'Shanchol', offering protection against two serotypes (O1 and O139) of *V. cholerae*.

---

* A treatment using proteins (called interferons) that boost the immune system to fight diseases like cancer or viral infections.

Shantha has been producing the vaccine since 2009 as Shanchol for the South Asian market, while EuBiologics has produced it by name Euvichol since 2015.[14] In addition to Shanchol, there were just two more vaccines for cholera in the market, approved by WHO – a killed whole-cell monovalent (O1) vaccine sold under the brand name Dukoral and a single-dose, FDA-approved oral vaccine called Vaxchora, used in the US for people travelling to an area of active cholera transmission.[15]

By 2017, Shantha delivered 10 million doses of Shanchol to twenty-five countries across the world, the highest ever distribution since receiving WHO pre-qualification in 2011. Meanwhile, Shantha also worked on vaccines for rotavirus, HPV,* pneumococcal infections† and started producing alpha 2-b interferon‡ as a cancer therapy. It also established a US subsidiary to focus on various monoclonal antibody therapies for cancer.

In the meantime, Shantha changed hands and went out of Varaprasad's control by 2006. French Mérieux Alliance, which changed its name to Institut Mérieux in 2009, acquired the 50 per cent stake of Omani investor Yusuf Bin Alawi Abdullah. Mérieux Alliance gradually picked up another 10 per cent stake from a team of employees and some non-resident Indian investors, taking its total stake in Shantha Biotechnics to 60 per cent.[16]

The deal that valued the company at $175 million by Morgan Stanley left Varaprasad with a 16.7 per cent minority stake. He had already parted with 1.3 per cent stake to his employees. Another 22 per cent stake was held by Varaprasad's friends, family and associates.

Institut Mérieux formed a subsidiary 'ShanH' to manage Shantha, bought the available shares from Varaprasad's friends, relatives and employees and kept increasing its stake. The stake went up to 80 per

---

* A virus that can cause cervical and other types of cancers, especially in women.

† Infections caused by *Streptococcus pneumoniae* bacteria, leading to illnesses like pneumonia, meningitis and ear infections.

‡ A lab-made version of a natural protein that helps the immune system fight diseases like cancer and hepatitis.

cent by July 2009. In a final move, they took over most of Varaprasad's 16.7 per cent stake and breached the 97 per cent mark.

In 2013, this entire accumulated stake was bought by the French vaccine maker Sanofi Pasteur, a division of the European drug company Sanofi-aventis for a valuation of 550 million euros (₹37.7 billion) in an offshore deal.[17] One of the serious Indian contenders to take over the stake from Institut Mérieux was the Serum Institute, which tried bidding ₹30 billion through Khalil Ahmed using the first right of refusal given to the Omani investors, but Varaprasad thwarted the move cleverly. After the deal, Sanofi-aventis offered to buy the remaining 3 per cent stake from Shantha employees and Varaprasad's relatives after getting the clearance from India's regulator Foreign Investment Promotion Board (FIPB).[18]

This acquisition was the culmination of a remarkable transformation – from a modest Indian start-up born out of moral conviction into a formidable player in the global vaccine market. For two decades, Shantha had defied odds, battled multinationals on pricing and access, and carved a space for Indian innovation on the world stage.

Yet, the story didn't end there. In a twist worthy of its unpredictable journey, as this book goes to print, Shantha has once again changed hands – returning to an Indian promoter with the blessings of Varaprasad himself.

Shantha's legacy goes far beyond corporate transactions. It ignited a broader biotech revolution in India, inspiring a wave of innovation and enterprise.

30

IMMUNIZED AMBITIONS

IF THE LAUNCH OF INDIA'S FIRST INDIGENOUS HEPATITIS B vaccine in August 1997 shook global pharma giants, it stirred something deeper in another ambitious biotech startup just across the city – Bharat Biotech.

At the helm was Krishna Ella, a quiet but determined agricultural researcher who had returned from the United States and started a vaccine company. He began collaborating with VAP to develop a rotavirus vaccine with the blessings of the Chief Minister of Andhra Pradesh, Chandrababu Naidu. Bharat Biotech built its foundation with far more institutional support and financial backing than most startups of its time – ₹55 million from IDBI Venture Capital, a ₹32.5 million loan from the Technology Development Board of the DST and a ₹5 million loan from the Centre for Technology Development of the USID. Yet, the crucial vaccine breakthrough had happened elsewhere. Ella found himself playing catch-up in a game he thought he would lead.

Concerned not just by the scientific developments but also the disruptive pricing that had now redefined the playing field, Ella moved quickly. He reached out to IISc, and was soon introduced to biochemist Rangarajan, who agreed to take up the challenge. Thus, in 1998, under the Technology Development Mission (TDM), IISc began to develop a Hepatitis B vaccine for Bharat Biotech.

The path was smoother for IISc, especially when compared to the five-year struggle faced by Varaprasad. It had access to an indigenously designed vaccine sample and more importantly, years of studies and trials conducted by another firm. When Rangarajan learned that Shantha Biotechnics had used *Pichia pastoris*, he decided to adopt the same approach.

Rangarajan cloned the gene responsible for producing HBsAg and successfully expressed it in *Pichia pastoris*. He then selected high-yielding strains and developed a four-step purification process to extract the antigen from the yeast cells. The purified HBsAg was combined with aluminium hydroxide and tested as a vaccine. The results were promising; it triggered the body to produce protective antibodies that could neutralize the hepatitis B virus and prevent it from infecting liver cells.[1]

Though Rangarajan was able to replicate Shantha's vaccine Shanvac-B in record time thanks to his deep laboratory experience, there was yet another hurdle – conducting clinical trials. That job was left to Bharat Biotech, which was in a hurry to launch the vaccine, seeing the rapid sales and growing valuation of Shantha Biotechnics. Consequently, without toiling and moiling for any comprehensive clinical trials, regulatory review or formal approvals, Bharat Biotech moved ahead with manufacturing the vaccine soon after receiving the technology from Rangarajan's team.

Thus, just fourteen months after the launch of Shanvac-B and within ten months of forging a partnership with IISc, in a bold and audacious move, Bharat Biotech unveiled a hepatitis B vaccine named Revac-B in October 1998. The launch was a high-profile event graced by Dr A. P. J. Abdul Kalam, then Scientific Advisor to the Defence Minister, who was at the height of national admiration following the successful Pokhran-II nuclear tests that May. Padmanaban, who played a guiding role in the vaccine development too blessed the launch, not knowing that the company would announce that Revac-B had been developed entirely in-house at Bharat Biotech's R&D facility over two years, using *Saccharomyces cerevisiaex* – not *P. pastoris*. No mention was made of Rangarajan's role or IISc's contribution.[2]

Ella told the media present that he chose *S. cerevisiaex* because it was the only strain licensed for use by the US FDA, WHO and the EU regulators.[3] This was despite the fact that the US FDA, WHO and EU regulator EMA do not license virus strains individually; instead, they approve the final vaccine product as a whole, which includes the virus strain (if applicable), production process and comprehensive data on formulation, safety, efficacy and quality. The Revac-B controversy hung in the air for quite some time as the local media caught hold of it, suggesting that Bharat Biotech did not have the license to use the *P. pastoris* in the vaccine, that the vaccine had been released without clinical trials and so on.[4] In an interview to *Business World* in 2001, Ella conceded that he had received a call from RCT informing him of its global patent for the yeast.[5]

The media frenzy eventually died down but in 2001, Pushpa Mittra Bhargava, the founder of CCMB and a respected figure in the Indian scientific establishment, filed a writ petition before the Andhra Pradesh High Court. The petition questioned the scientific veracity and public health implications of Revac-B and sought an independent test of the vaccine's composition and quality.

In his petition, Bhargava alleged that Bharat Biotech was manufacturing Revac-B using *P. pastoris* as the expression system, despite being licensed to use only *Saccharomyces cerevisiae*. He used Shantha's claim, which was based on its internal investigations, including DNA sequencing and PCR analyses, purportedly indicating the presence of *Pichia* DNA in Revac-B samples. Based on these findings Bhargava sought the court to prohibit Bharat Biotech from manufacturing or marketing the vaccine using *P. pastoris*.

On 7 August, Chandrababu Naidu, the Chief Minister of Andhra Pradesh, intervened after the matter reached the Drug Controller General of India. He wrote a letter to Union Health Minister C. P. Thakur, suggesting that the controversy was rooted in business rivalry, and asked the minister to instruct the DCGI not to give undue importance to the complaint filed by certain parties.[6]

Notwithstanding this, the DCGI decided to form an expert committee comprising representatives from the ICMR, the National Institute of Biologicals and officers from the Central Drugs Standard Control Organization (CDSCO). They were asked to suggest experts in DNA sequencing to inspect Bharat Biotech's facility and ascertain the status of its hepatitis vaccine production and the yeast used in the vaccine. However, it could not proceed further as the matter was being heard by the High Court. On 4 October 2001, a single-judge bench of the Andhra Pradesh High Court passed an interim order directing the director of CCMB to collect three vials of Revac-B from the open market, three vials from the petitioner (Bhargava) and three vials from Bharat Biotech itself, and conduct tests to ascertain the contents. The court asked for a report to be filed within five days.

Bharat Biotech immediately challenged the order. In a writ appeal, the company contended that Bhargava was not a disinterested party, as he had professional ties with Shantha Biotechnics. Nor could CCMB be considered an impartial testing authority.[7] The division bench on 21 November 2001 vacated the single-judge's interim order, noting the potential for bias of the petitioner and recommending that any such testing, if warranted, should be undertaken by a truly neutral and recognized laboratory.[8] Neither did the testing take place, nor did the case proceed further. But the episode left behind a trail of unanswered questions.

Around the same time, a serving IPS officer from Andhra Pradesh, M. L. Kumawat approached the National Consumer Disputes Redressal Commission (NCDRC) demanding ₹120 million in compensation from Bharat Biotech, alleging that he suffered serious side effects after taking the second dose of its hepatitis-B vaccine, Revac-B. In its defence, Bharat Biotech accused the complainant of attempting to malign the company's reputation by misusing his official position and manipulating media coverage, allegedly in collusion with Bhargava.

After a prolonged years-long legal battle, the forum noted that the adverse effects could have resulted from improper administration or storage, and that Kumawat's doctor's decision to switch brands between doses was questionable. Crucially, the forum found the use of *P. pastoris* as an expression system was neither illegal nor in violation of any patent, as no infringement case had been filed by the original patent holder, RCT, US. The national forum dismissed the complaint, finding it to be frivolous and lacking in evidence.[9] The matter was pursued by the complainant for two decades and finally reached the Supreme Court, which dismissed the case in 2020.[10]

Notwithstanding these legal challenges, the manual distributed to doctors and labs later on contradicted Bharat Biotech's public position – it said Revac-B is produced in genetically engineered yeast cells of *P. pastoris* which carry the gene that codes for the major surface antigen protein of the hepatitis-B virus.[11]

IISc was extremely miffed that Bharat Biotech did not acknowledge Rangarajan or its contribution, as Rangarajan revealed in an IISc publication many years later: 'Bharat Biotech, the first company to get the technology from us, did not acknowledge our contribution.' Since the understanding with the Ellas was not exclusive, IISc decided to transfer the technology to two other Hyderabad-based vaccine companies – Biological E. Ltd. and Indian Immunologicals Ltd. (IIL).[12] The decision was taken with the intention of bringing the price of the vaccine down, to make it accessible.

What was alleged by rival camps was that Bharat Biotech launched the vaccine without conducting any clinical trials – not even the critical phase III trial. According to Rangarajan, Bharat Biotech first approached him in 1998 for developing a recombinant vaccine against hepatitis B. Even assuming the earliest contact was in January that year, launching the vaccine by October left no realistic window for a proper clinical trial. Typically, phase III trials alone take at least two years, often longer depending on sample size, endpoints and complexity. For Varaprasad, this was deeply unsettling. He believed Bharat Biotech had rushed to market with a stripped-down version of Shanvac-B, sidestepping critical safety and efficacy evaluations. However, later, the doctor manual of Revac-B stated it had successfully conducted phase III trials with a sample of 196 adults.[13]

Despite a long and spirited fight that laid bare the lapses behind Bharat Biotech's vaccine launch, Varaprasad eventually had to relent. Politically, Ella held the upper hand. With Chandrababu Naidu playing kingmaker in the newly formed BJP-led government under Atal Bihari Vajpayee, Ella had powerful backing in Delhi, recalls Shaukat Hussain Muhammed, long time Business Editor of Hyderabad-based *Deccan Chronicle*.[14]

But Varaprasad never truly let it go. In every forum he had access to, he accused Bharat Biotech of what he described as a 'blatant violation' – compromising public health. Long-time *Hindu Business Line* Chief of Bureau in Hyderabad Somasekhar Mulugu recalls the frequent spats between the two and how Ella used to respond to Varaprasad in a defiant tone.[15]

Upon receiving the technology from IISc, Biological E. and IIL launched their vaccines in the market in quick succession after conducting clinical trials. The former launched the vaccine by 2004 as BEVAC and the latter in 2006 as Elovac-B, both as monovalent vaccines at the first instance.

Further, both firms combined the vaccine with DPT and Haemophilus Influenzae B (HiB) and launched it as a pentavalent vaccine – Biological E. introduced COMBE Five in 2011 and IIL launched Vaxtar-5 in 2018. By then Shantha had received WHO prequalification for its pentavalent vaccine. By the end of 2023, since its launch in 2004, Biological E. had sold 225 million doses of BEVAC and 850 million COMBE Five. IIL had sold 145 million and 169 million vials of Elovac-B and Vaxtar-5 respectively.[16]

Unlike Bharat Biotech, both companies openly acknowledged IISc's vital role in the technology and the vaccine development process. They even made a payment of 1 per cent royalty on total sales to IISc for some years. Following the success of this collaboration, IIL signed a new contract with IISc's Society for Innovation and Development

(SID) to develop a DNA-based rabies vaccine and offered a grant of ₹5 million to IISc for five years. This collaboration eventually led to IISc helping the company set up its recombinant DNA laboratory.[17]

More trouble was in store for Bharat Biotech. By 2011, WHO suspended procurement of Revac-B from Bharat Biotech after a site audit found deficiencies in the company's good manufacturing practices. Additionally, WHO terminated the pre-qualification process for all other Bharat Biotech vaccines and kept it under watch for any UN procurement.[18]

Since then, controversy has frequently trailed Bharat Biotech. Its long awaited rotavirus vaccine too has sparked debate because it demonstrated only 56 per cent efficacy in a phase III clinical trial. Experts raised concerns over inadequate safety data and questioned the justification for its inclusion in routine immunization.[19] 'Can you name any other vaccine with just 50 per cent efficacy that's part of a public health programme?,' asked Dr Jacob Puliyel, former head of Pediatrics at St. Stephen's Hospital in Delhi. He said it would be a coin toss whether the vaccine would work for an individual and even if the entire population were vaccinated, it would only reduce rotavirus deaths by half.[20]

Despite years of debate and pushback, the hepatitis B vaccine was officially included in India's UIP in 2018, with the mandate to administer the first vaccine dose within twenty-four hours of birth to prevent perinatal transmission.[*21] However, this was done once the National Viral Hepatitis Control Programme launched that year under the National Health Mission, and the government began offering free diagnosis and treatment for chronic hepatitis B cases.

The battle for scientific integrity, equitable access and regulatory accountability in India's vaccine story had a defining moment in the hepatitis B vaccine saga. What began as a race between innovation and ambition eventually exposed the fault lines in the country's

* Passing of an infection (like hepatitis B) from mother to baby during childbirth.

emerging biopharma ecosystem,* where ethical shortcuts, political patronage and institutional opacity could overshadow public health priorities.

In this turbulent journey, it was the persistence of a few idealists, the strength of public research institutions and the eventual awakening of policy systems that had ensured quality vaccines. The challenger had not only disrupted global pricing norms but also forced the country to confront deeper questions about how science should serve society.

After all, in the race to save lives, how you win matters as much as the victory itself.

* The network of companies, research labs, regulators and hospitals involved in developing and delivering medicines and vaccines.

31

THREE RAMS, ONE REVOLUTION

IN 1942, G. N. RAMACHANDRAN ENROLLED FOR A MASTER'S programme at the Indian Institute of Science's (IISc) Electrical Engineering Department, after earning a BSc (Honours) in Physics from the University of Madras. There, he soon encountered Chandrasekhara Venkata Raman, better known as C. V. Raman.

For Ramachandran, who hailed from Gopalasamudram, a small village on the banks of the Thamirabarani River in Tirunelveli, Tamil Nadu, meeting Raman in the fall of 1942 was a defining moment. Though initially set on pursuing a career in electrical engineering, this encounter would significantly shape his scientific journey.

C. V. Raman, a towering figure in Indian science, had been associated with IISc since 1933, three years after receiving the Nobel Prize in Physics for his groundbreaking discovery of the Raman Effect – a phenomenon describing the scattering of light when it passes through matter.* Raman's contributions and the Nobel Prize played a crucial role in advancing scientific research in India. As the first Indian director of IISc, Raman's leadership left a lasting impact on the institute, which had been established through the vision of industrialist Jamshedji Tata and built on a 371-acre land grant

* A phenomenon where light changes its course slightly when it passes through a material, revealing information about the material's structure.

from Mysore's King Krishnaraja Wadiyar IV in the early twentieth century.[1]

Raman was immediately drawn to Ramachandran, recognizing him as a promising scientist. He advised Ramachandran to redirect his focus from electrical engineering, which he viewed as too application-driven, towards his strengths in fundamental research and theoretical approaches. Consequently, Ramachandran chose to leave the Electrical Engineering Department and joined Raman's team in the Physics Department instead.[2] Raman drew Ramachandran into his own area of research, light and X-ray studies. Under his mentorship, Ramachandran pursued research in optics and X-ray topography* of diamonds, eventually earning a Doctor of Science (DSc) by 1947.

After his DSc, Ramachandran continued his research at the Cavendish Laboratory in Cambridge University. Raman reportedly sent a letter of reference to Lawrence Bragg, who had become the youngest Nobel laureate at twenty-five, jointly with his father William Henry Bragg, for their analysis of crystal structure using X-rays.

By the time Ramachandran completed his doctorate at Cambridge University in 1949, he found his interests drifting from Physics to Biology. He was influenced by the lectures of Linus Pauling, the only person to have ever been awarded two unshared Nobel Prizes, for Chemistry and Peace.

Ramachandran returned to IISc as an Assistant Professor in the Physics Department under Raman. However, this tenure was short and in 1952, Raman sent him to establish an Experimental Physics Department at the University of Madras. There, he began undertaking work that soon earned him recognition as the Father of Biotechnology in India.

Along with a trustworthy research partner, Ramachandran unravelled the triple helical structure† of collagen, a protein abundant

---

* A method of using X-rays to capture images of the internal structure of crystals or materials.

† A specific shape (like three intertwined ropes) that collagen protein takes in the body to

in human connective tissues like tendons, ligaments, skin and bones, providing structural support, strength and elasticity to tissues and organs. When his research was published, Ramachandran received acclaim from eminent structural biologists worldwide, including DNA structure pioneer Francis Crick, who later proposed a modified version to Ramachandran's collagen structure. Ramachandran delved further into understanding the finite structures of proteins, pioneering what is now known as the 'Ramachandran Plot'.*

In 1964, C. V. Raman would nominate his protege for a Nobel Prize in Chemistry for his work on collagen structure – one of only five nominations ever made by Raman and the only time he nominated an Indian.[3] The Nobel Prize Committee did not select Ramachandran because it found his work on collagen incomplete at the time.[4]

In 1970, he returned to IISc, invited by the eminent space scientist Satish Dhawan, who was concurrently serving as the director of the Institute and head of the Indian Space Research Organization (ISRO). By then, Raman had passed away after establishing a new institute in his name for advanced theoretical physics research using his personal wealth – the Raman Research Institute (RRI).

During his second tenure at IISc, Ramachandran founded the Molecular Biophysics Unit (MBU), the first dedicated academic initiative in the country to explore the combined effects of biology and physics. This unparalleled initiative marked a new chapter in India's history – the advent of biotechnology.

As Ramachandran was concluding his active work at IISc, another renowned physicist, Prof. M. G. K. Menon advised Prime Minister Indira Gandhi on the urgent need to support India's journey in biotechnology. Menon was concerned that India might lag behind the advancements being made by the Western nations. This was an era where biological research was gaining global momentum, and the

---

provide strength and flexibility to skin, bones and connective tissue.

* A scientific chart used to understand and predict how proteins fold into shapes.

potential to modify the functions of life forms through recombinant DNA techniques was becoming increasingly feasible.

Menon did not stop there. With eminent scientists like M. S. Swaminathan on board, Menon identified biotechnology as a promising area for India's future in the Sixth Five Year Plan (1980–85). The plan proposed to bolster capabilities in immunology, genetics and communicable diseases.[5]

Pursuing the Sixth Plan proposal, the National Biotechnology Board was established in 1982 to formulate a long-term strategy for promoting biotechnology in the country. It was chaired by Prof. Menon himself, who was also serving as a Member (Science) in the Planning Commission. The task of appointing a suitable candidate with a strong background in biotechnology to head the Board was entrusted to Swaminathan and he turned to another Ram – S. Ramachandran.

At the time, S. Ramachandran was engaged in efforts to revive Bengal Immunity Limited, a public sector vaccine manufacturer in Calcutta. Having moved to the city in 1977 from Hindustan Antibiotics Limited, he had already made a name for himself as a capable institution builder, driven by the larger goal of strengthening India's biotechnology ecosystem. It was in the midst of the Calcutta mission that he received a call from the renowned agricultural scientist.

Once on board, Prime Minister Indira Gandhi granted S. Ramachandran full autonomy to strategize and implement the Board's initiatives. By April 1983, he had formulated a Long-Term Plan in Biotechnology, identifying key priority areas for the nation's biotechnological advancement. He then advocated for elevating the Board into a full-fledged department under the Government of India – a proposal that unsettled the Department of Science and Technology. In 1986, this vision materialized when the Board was transformed into the Department of Biotechnology (DBT), with S. Ramachandran as its first Secretary. The Department began its operations with a modest initial budget of ₹60 million. Decades later, it would be integrated into the Ministry of Science and Technology as part of a broader effort to consolidate all science departments under a single ministry.

Shortly after its establishment, DBT launched an ambitious initiative to make India self-reliant in vaccine production. The plan encompassed deploying new technologies, scaling up the production of polio, measles and DPT vaccines, developing tissue culture-based anti-rabies vaccines and pioneering research on hepatitis B vaccines using advanced biotechnological methods.

This plan led to the creation of the National Technology Mission on Immunization, a collaborative effort between the Ministry of Health and Family Welfare and DBT. DBT's primary role in this mission was to bridge critical R&D gaps in vaccine production and ensuring India's path toward vaccine self-sufficiency.[6] Soon, DBT started expanding its reach, bringing most of the institutes engaged in biotechnology research in the country into its fold while establishing new institutes to focus on emerging areas of biological science research.

Established in 1981, the National Institute of Immunology was the first autonomous institute to be brought under DBT. Shortly thereafter, S. Ramachandran initiated the transformation of the National Facility for Animal Tissue and Cell Culture in Pune into the National Centre for Cell Science. The late 1990s and early 2000s witnessed the establishment of additional institutes such as the National Institute for Plant Genome Research (NIPGR), the National Brain Research Centre (NBRC), the Centre for DNA Fingerprinting & Diagnostics,* the Institute of Bioresources and Sustainable Development and the Institute of Life Sciences.

This momentum continued with the establishment of more notable institutes such as the Translational Health Science and Technology Institute (THSTI), the Institute for Stem Cell

* Techniques used to identify individuals based on their unique genetic code and to diagnose diseases using DNA.

Biology* and Regenerative Medicine† (INstem), the National Agri-Food Biotechnology Institute (NABI) in Mohali and the National Institute of Biomedical Genomics‡ (NIBMG) in Kalyani, West Bengal. Throughout this period, there was a renewed focus on sectors such as healthcare and vaccine development. Later, a total of thirteen institutions were brought under an autonomous body named the Biotechnology Research and Innovation Council (BRIC), aimed at promoting multidisciplinary research and academic innovations.

In 1990, the first significant move towards industry collaboration was taken when DBT initiated the establishment of the Biotech Consortium India Limited (BCIL), with the participation of financial institutions and a venture capital fund. It was envisioned as an agency to expedite the commercialization of innovative biotechnology solutions and pave the way for future collaborations between industry and academia. Over the next decade, significant changes unfolded in the Indian biotechnology sector, particularly with liberalization opening up the Indian economy.

Since then, many global companies established their manufacturing facilities and clinical trial arrangements in India, with DBT facilitating and acting as a regulator on critical biosafety and clinical trial issues. The era of foreign investment and contract manufacturing necessitated increased oversight, which was provided by DBT and other regulators like the CDSCO.

In 2004, Maharaj Bhan, who was instrumental in developing the indigenous rotavirus vaccine, was appointed to lead DBT. With his knowledge of the industry, Bhan enhanced the growth of the biotechnology sector by establishing a formal industry-academia interface. The introduction of domestically developed vaccines and

---

* The study of special cells (stem cells) that can develop into many different cell types in the body and help heal or grow tissues.

† A type of medicine that tries to repair or grow back damaged tissues or organs, often using stem cells.

‡ The study of the complete set of DNA (called the genome) in a person or organism, used to understand genes and how they affect health.

ensuing competition led to a dramatic hundred-fold reduction in vaccine prices. Market dynamics began to shift, liberating Indian citizens from the grip of multinational pharmaceutical corporations.

Gradually, the message of affordable vaccines spread beyond Indian borders to economically weaker countries plagued by high infant and childhood mortality rates. Global pharmaceutical giants began seeking out Indian companies to develop new processes to create vaccines, while global aid agencies lined up to procure vaccines. A new era had begun in the Indian healthcare sector.

This environment gave rise to the formation of Biotechnology Industry Research Assistance Council (BIRAC) in 2012, a not-for-profit entity aimed at promoting innovation and product development through active collaboration between the private sector and academic institutes. BIRAC began supporting small companies to develop innovative solutions to address unresolved health challenges, where larger private players hesitated to venture. An important early success was the launch of ROTAVAC by Bharat Biotech, which DBT had been involved in since the 1990s.

For instance, it aided in the development of JE vaccine SA14-14-2 by Themis Biosyn Ltd with support from Gujarat Industrial Investment Corporation. BIRAC has also been supporting Indian companies in manufacturing the Cervarix vaccine, protecting women against human papillomavirus (HPV) and reducing the risk of cervical cancer.*

In 2017, BIRAC launched the National Biopharma Mission (NBM), branded as 'Innovate in India' (i3), with a project cost of ₹15 billion, supported by a loan from the World Bank. Under this initiative, BIRAC has been facilitating the development of critical biopharma projects, including the recombinant BCG vaccine, the repurposing of Covid vaccine candidates tested by the Serum Institute and the Protein Subunit platform tested by Biological E.

* A type of cancer that occurs in the cells of the cervix (the lower part of the uterus). It is often caused by a virus called HPV.

Additionally, BIRAC has supported the development of vaccines for dengue, chikungunya, flu and cholera, further strengthening India's position as a global vaccine powerhouse. As of 2025, NBM has supported the development of India's first inactivated Chikungunya vaccine (BBV87) by Bharat Biotech, which has progressed through Phase II and III trials; the indigenous Hepatitis E (HEV) vaccine under development by Zydus through a translational research consortium; and Indian Immunologicals Limited's live attenuated tetravalent recombinant dengue vaccine, which has advanced through Phase I and II clinical trials.[7]

BIRAC's initiatives – from the Biotechnology Ignition Grant and Bio-incubation Scheme to the establishment of bio-incubation centres* and catalytic funding initiatives – have played a crucial role in fostering a culture of biological innovation in the country. These strategic interventions have not only seeded a culture of scientific entrepreneurship but have also propelled the biotech start-up boom across the country. As of 2024, Indian bio-economy had surged from $86 billion in 2020 to $165 billion, contributing nearly 4.25 per cent of the country's GDP. Of this, the biopharma sector contributed $58.40 billion, of which vaccines had a share of $16.8 billion. The number of biotech startups in the meantime crossed 10,000 – a 100 per cent jump since 2020.[8]

It has been nothing short of a revolution, one that marked India's emergence as a global powerhouse in vaccine development, manufacturing and export. This enviable feat was made possible by visionary policy support, entrepreneurial grit and BIRAC's unwavering commitment to enabling innovation at scale. This quiet revolution in biotechnology didn't just build companies – it built a nation's confidence in its own scientific and public health systems, and in the possibility of a healthy future.

---

* A special place (often inside a university or research institute) where new startups or scientific ideas are supported with space, mentoring and funding.

32

THE CONJUGATE VACCINE CLASH

THE MOON HAS LONG CAPTIVATED THE HUMAN IMAGINATION. Yet its silvery glow can often eclipse its imperfections. It was Galileo Galilei who first uncovered the Moon's rugged reality. In 1609, using his newly crafted telescope, he turned his gaze skyward and made a startling discovery – contrary to popular belief, the moon was not a perfect sphere. Its surface was scarred by mountains and deep cup-like depressions, later named craters.

Today, researchers have identified over 100,000 craters on the lunar surface. Many of these have been named after pioneering scientists, immortalizing their contributions to human knowledge. Among them is a crater named 'Avery', honouring the legacy of Oswald Avery, a Canadian American medical researcher.

Nearly a century ago, Avery embarked on a study of pneumococcus, the bacteria responsible for pneumonia. Through meticulous research, he identified four distinct types of pneumococcal bacteria – a discovery that would shape the development of conjugate vaccines and prove to be one of the most significant advancements in modern immunology.[1]

In a 1915 paper, Avery posited that people who appeared to be healthy could be carriers of pneumonia, and suggested that it is important to identify the type of bacteria in order to determine treatment options.[2] Not stopping there, Avery mooted the idea of 'conjugate vaccines'.

In his 1927 experiments conducted on rabbits, Avery studied the immune response to the pneumonia-causing bacterium *Streptococcus pneumoniae*. He found that the antibody-generating action of complex sugar molecules in the body known as polysaccharides, which also act as antigens, could be enhanced by combining them with a protein. Vaccines made by combining polysaccharides with protein carriers have since come to be known as conjugate vaccines.

However, Avery's most significant contribution to medical science came over two decades later. In 1944, he isolated DNA from the nucleus of cells and identified it as the material from which genes and chromosomes are made. This groundbreaking discovery laid the foundation for many future inventions and the field of genetic engineering. Avery's paper, published in the *Journal of Experimental Medicine*, inspired James Watson to collaborate with the British biophysicist Francis Crick in deciphering the structure of DNA.[3]

Avery never received a Nobel Prize, despite being nominated through the 1930s, 1940s and 1950s till his death in 1955. This made Nobel laureate Arne Tiselius pronounce Avery as the most deserving scientist not to receive the Nobel Prize.[4] Despite Avery unearthing the possibility of conjugate vaccines, the first such vaccine to be used in humans would take another six decades to be developed.[5] The first conjugate vaccine to be deployed was the Haemophilus influenzae type b (Hib) conjugate against infections such as meningitis caused by the Hib bacteria. Scientists began combining Hib conjugate vaccine with other carrier proteins, like diphtheria toxoid or the tetanus toxoid. When the vaccine was first introduced in the US in the late 1980s, the incidence of Hib dropped over 90 per cent in a short period of time.[6]

Avery's work on *S. pneumoniae* in the 1920s was continued by other researchers, given its ferocity and destructiveness. Popularly known as pneumococcus, the bacteria causes infection in the lungs, namely pneumonia, and also in the thin layer covering the brain, the meninges. The infection on the meninges is widely known as meningitis. It can even infect the blood, known by the name bacteremia.* Infections of the brain and blood cause significant mortality among children below five years of age.

Pneumococcus kills at least a million children every year, more than the combined total of fatalities due to malaria, AIDS and measles. Of the total deaths, over 70 per cent are reported from developing nations. An estimated 14.5 million serious pneumococcal cases are reported globally every year, mostly among children under five years of age, and an estimated 500,000 deaths are from low and middle-income countries.[7] India accounted for a significant portion of these numbers until the advent of the conjugate vaccines.[8]

In addition to *S. pneumoniae*, other bacterial, viral and fungal organisms are also responsible for pneumonia and meningitis in children. Hib is the second most common cause of bacterial pneumonia and meningitis. In addition, *Neisseria meningitidis*, known as the meningococcus, causes significant morbidity and mortality in children and young adults through sporadic meningitis and/or bacteremia.

The pneumococcus alone has over 100 strains, known as serotypes or serogroups, and different serogroups are prevalent in different parts of the world. Both Hib and meningococcus have multiple variants, with their prevalence varying by geographical region. Respiratory syncytial virus (RSV) is the most prevalent viral cause of pneumonia, whereas *Pneumocystis jiroveci*† is a fungus responsible for one-quarter of all pneumonia deaths in infants infected with the human immunodeficiency virus (HIV).

Since the time conjugate vaccines against pneumococcus were first developed in the West in the 1980s, Indian vaccine companies have been making efforts to decode the technology and replicate it in their own ways, especially market leaders like the Serum Institute of India and Biological E.

---

* A serious infection where bacteria get into the bloodstream and can spread throughout the body.

† A type of fungus that can cause a serious lung infection in people with weak immune systems, such as those with HIV.

The Serum Institute collaborated with the US non-profit, Programme for Appropriate Technology in Health (PATH) and launched a vaccine development initiative with a grant from the Bill & Melinda Gates Foundation. This ambitious endeavour was undertaken after many pharmaceutical companies had already failed to develop new pneumococcal vaccines for children. Both the Serum Institute and Biological E. encountered numerous challenges as they aimed to produce this complex vaccine at a lower cost. For instance, they had to decode the patent technologies to come out with a new method to produce the vaccine in India and address the specific serogroups common in Asia, Africa and Latin America.

After conducting research in India and other low- and middle-income nations, PATH and the Serum Institute began to develop a vaccine targeting ten pneumococcal serotypes prevalent in these regions. By the time the indigenous vaccine development took off, the transnational pharma giant Pfizer entered the Indian market with its vaccine CRM197 PnC-7v,* containing polysaccharide antigen against seven Asia-specific serotypes. Intense lobbying enabled the company to offer it to poor countries through the Global Alliance for Vaccine and Immunization (GAVI) at subsidized prices for inclusion in national immunization programmes.[9]

By 2015, clinical trials of the Serum Institute's vaccine started in earnest in the regions where it was desperately needed – Africa, Southeast Asia and India. The Serum Institute led trials in India, while PATH sponsored trials in West Africa, conducted by the Medical Research Council Unit The Gambia at the London School of Hygiene & Tropical Medicine.

The results of the Phase III trials from Gambia found that the vaccine met all necessary standards. With this success, the Serum Institute launched the vaccine under the brand name PNEUMOSIL. The new vaccine obtained WHO's pre-qualification by 2019,

* A specific type of conjugate vaccine made by Pfizer. 'CRM197' is the protein used and 'PnC-7v' refers to it protecting against seven strains of pneumococcus.

indicating its safety and efficacy for use in international programmes administered by UNICEF and GAVI. The Indian government approved the vaccine for nationwide use in December 2020, three years after pneumococcal vaccines were included by India in its Indradhanush immunization programme.

The vaccine was received with open arms and GAVI reported that by 2020, PNEUMOSIL had been used by 185 million children. As demand surpassed supply, the Serum Institute geared up to produce 100 million doses a year, which could further be scaled up to 150 million doses a year in three years. The Serum Institute even offered to supply the vaccine to GAVI at a price of $2 per dose.[10] This undercut GSK and Pfizer as both these transnational giants had been supplying their high-priced vaccines to GAVI through a subsidized programme.

The Bill & Melinda Gates Foundation has called PNEUMOSIL an Indian success story since it was produced in India, by an Indian company, and has been made available globally to low- and middle-income countries at an accessible price. For a three-dose course, the vaccine costs about 30 per cent less than the other vaccines already offered by GAVI.[11]

All this while, Biological E. had been working on a much better vaccine – a pneumococcal polysaccharide conjugate vaccine that could tackle fourteen different strains of the bacteria, a 14-valent vaccine. Developed through its in-house research, the company successfully obtained a US patent by January 2023,[12] a month after it secured approval from DCGI. The vaccine, named PNEUBEVAX14, is comparable to Pfizer's 13-valent Prevenar13 and Merck's 23-valent VAXNEUVANCE.

With a current capacity of 25 million doses a year, Biological E. is scaling up its production to 100 million doses. The project has been generously supported by the Technology Development Board of the Department of Science and Technology, with a ₹1 billion loan. Thus Biological E. too played a significant role in slashing the prices of this crucial vaccine in India as well as in the rest of the world.

It is interesting to note that despite the first pneumococcal conjugate vaccine hitting the market in 2000, it took nine years for a vaccine targeting the strains prevalent in LMICs to be developed.

As India continued its battle against pneumococcal bacteria, the race was closing on the meningococcal vaccine front as well. The gap between Western vaccine giants launching innovative meningococcal vaccines and that of Indian companies developing similar or better versions had greatly reduced.

For instance, within six months of Pfizer announcing that the US FDA had accepted its application for a pentavalent meningococcal vaccine candidate to address serotypes A, B, C, W and Y in December 2022,[13] the Serum Institute's MenFive, addressing serogroups A, C, W, Y and X, was prequalified by WHO.[14] The difference between the two vaccines was that the Serum Institute's vaccine contained polysaccharide antigen against the meningococcal strain X prevalent in Africa, while the Pfizer vaccine provided protection against strain B prevalent in North America.

By the time Pfizer launched the vaccine, after securing the FDA clearance in October 2023 under the brand name PENBRAYA, MenFive was made available across the African continent. MenFive was the result of an arduous thirteen-year journey by the Serum Institute and PATH, with funding from the UK government's Foreign, Commonwealth and Development Office through a partnership forged soon after the Serum Institute's launch of MenAfriVac in 2010.

MenAfriVac was the outcome of the Meningitis Vaccine Project, supported by WHO, to eradicate the meningitis epidemic in sub-Saharan Africa, specifically to target the meningitis A strain prevalent in the African meningitis belt. This project marked the first instance of medical research creating a vaccine specifically for an African disease. The Bill & Melinda Gates Foundation pitched in with a $70 million grant, assisted by PATH.[15]

MenAfriVac offered long-term immunity of ten to fifteen years and was suitable for infants aged one year and above. After successful trials, the vaccine was introduced in Burkina Faso, Mali and Niger in 2010, targeting individuals aged one to twenty-nine in these high-risk countries.[16] The vaccine almost eliminated the A strain of *Neisseria meningitidis* from the African meningitis belt covering twenty-six countries. Before the entry of MenAfriVac, meningitis used to be an annual epidemic in many areas of Africa, claiming tens of thousands of lives every season. Three years after the launch of MenAfriVac, the incidence dropped by 94 per cent in vaccinated areas.[17]

The story of conjugate vaccines does not end there. It also features multinational vaccine companies embezzling charity meant for the poor, and it all started with none other than GAVI, the Vaccine Alliance.

Given that newer vaccines took ages to reach poor countries due to price barriers, GAVI created a special fund. In 2007, the Advance Market Commitment (AMC), a unique funding mechanism to incentivize research, develop and produce vaccines, was launched. Its objective was to expedite the rollout of pneumococcal conjugate vaccines in low-income countries. Six donors came on board – Italy, the UK, Canada, Russia, Norway and the Bill & Melinda Gates Foundation. The donors pledged $1.5 billion to cross-subsidize the vaccine, covering the cost difference between what the poorer countries could pay and the prices set by vaccine makers.

The project was well-intentioned – to ensure the vaccine's early access to poorer countries at affordable prices and thereby save lives. However, vaccine giants took advantage of GAVI's initiative. Greedy for profit, they charged the poorest countries approximately $9 for a full course of vaccine while also receiving an additional $12 per child from the AMC, totalling $21 per full course.

A large number of countries did not qualify as 'low income', and Pfizer and GSK charged them almost $80 per two-dose vaccine supplied through UNICEF. Due to these exorbitant prices, many middle-income countries chose not to include the vaccine in their national immunization programmes.[18]

In effect, by 2019, GAVI paid $1.2 billion to Pfizer and GSK from the AMC fund, leaving just $262 million for all the other vaccine initiatives. These companies enjoyed their duopoly in the GAVI supply and continued to keep the prices high, even as they kept renewing their long-term agreements. For instance, Pfizer signed the first ten-year supply agreement to supply 300 million doses in March 2010 and entered into three more agreements thereafter, extending the commitments up to 2027 for a total of 930 million doses.[19]

Thus, despite clear indications that two major Indian vaccine manufacturers were poised to introduce their vaccines by 2020 at significantly lower price points, GAVI continued signing additional agreements with Western pharmaceutical giants.

The original goal of the AMC was to increase vaccine supply and ensure affordability worldwide. However, this objective was gradually diluted. For the AMC to succeed, it was essential to facilitate the entry of new vaccine manufacturers, particularly from countries capable of producing vaccines at lower costs. Instead, GAVI strayed from its mission, repeatedly renewing agreements with Western pharmaceutical companies at exorbitant prices.

This continued unchecked until Médecins Sans Frontières (MSF) – the global humanitarian NGO – called out the mismanagement in 2019. MSF urged GAVI to stop funnelling subsidies to Pfizer and GSK and reminded the Alliance that it was designed to encourage new producers to enter the market and bring prices down.

In fact, the MSF had been raising concerns for nearly a decade. As early as 2011, it criticized the AMC's allocation of $1.5 billion in pay-outs to towering pharmaceutical companies, arguing that these funds could have been better utilized to accelerate the development of more affordable vaccines. Yet GAVI ignored these warnings, allowing its funds to be drained by vaccine giants for over a decade.[20]

This revealed a troubling paradox: an initiative designed to democratize vaccine access ultimately fortified the dominance of Western pharma giants, sidelining cost-effective alternatives from the Global South. It became a missed opportunity – one that not only siphoned out public funds but delayed access to affordable life-saving vaccines for millions. As the world prepares for future pandemics and emerging health threats, the AMC experience stands as a cautionary tale of how good intentions can be derailed by entrenched interests.

It's a heavy reminder that when global health becomes global business, the poorest pay the highest price.

33

DAUGHTERS OF THE TRIAL

IN 2009, TRAGEDY STRUCK THE TRIBAL HEARTLANDS OF Khammam district in undivided Andhra Pradesh. Five teenage girls, full of promise and barely stepping into adulthood, died under suspicious and harrowing circumstances. Their deaths were hastily labelled as suicides – an easy explanation in a remote and voiceless corner of the country. But their grief-stricken families and relentless civil society groups refused to accept the silence. As they dug deeper, a chilling pattern emerged: all five girls had received a trial vaccine* just days before they died.[1]

What was initially dismissed as a coincidence began to look like a cover-up, raising unsettling questions about medical ethics, consent, and the price paid by the most vulnerable in the name of progress.

While Andhra Pradesh grappled with these tragedies, two similar deaths were reported in the western state of Gujarat, in what initially seemed like an unrelated incident. Most of the affected girls in Andhra Pradesh had been under the care of wardens in special tribal hostels. Due to the remoteness of the region, it took time for news of these deaths to reach mainstream media. When the full picture emerged, it became clear that it was a man-made catastrophe – one involving global pharmaceutical giants conducting vaccine trials on young girls without proper consent or adequate oversight.

---

* A vaccine that is still being tested to check its safety and effectiveness before it is approved for widespread use.

In the preceding months, the US-based non-profit PATH International had convinced the government of Andhra Pradesh that female students from government schools, mostly living in tribal hostels, should participate in a cervical cancer vaccine trial as test subjects. The vaccine, manufactured by Merck & Co. (Merck Sharp & Dohme, MSD), was designed to combat human papillomavirus (HPV), a sexually transmitted infection. It was easy for PATH and MSD to convince the state health department because India's premier medical research agency, ICMR had already endorsed it.

Therefore, on 9 July 2009, the Andhra Pradesh government allowed PATH to begin what was labelled the 'demonstration project to vaccinate women against cervical cancer.' The vaccine was administered to 14,000 girls between the ages of ten to fourteen in three mandals of Khammam – Bhadrachalam, Kothagudem and Thirumalayapalem – in the subsequent months.[2]

On 13 August 2009, the Gujarat government too launched a two-year demonstration project in three blocks of Vadodara District – Dabhoi, Kawant and Shinor. Three doses of the HPV vaccine were administered to approximately 10,000 girls in the age group of 10 to 14 years. The vaccine was called Cervarix, under trial by transnational pharma behemoth GSK.[3]

Everything would have continued as usual if not for the deaths – four in Andhra Pradesh and two in Gujarat – a month later, under suspicious circumstances. All hell broke loose as details of the catastrophe gradually emerged. What unfolded from the trials was alarming for PATH and its vaccine trial partners.

In March 2010, a team of women's groups and health activists who visited Bhadrachalam to assess the situation were shocked to find that the project targeted young girls from economically disadvantaged backgrounds – scheduled tribes, scheduled castes, Muslims and other backward communities. The majority of participants were from tribal boarding schools, which helped the organizers conveniently bypass the need for parental consent. Vaccinations were carried out through camps on school premises, with hostel wardens often granting consent in lieu of parents, raising ethical concerns about the lack of proper consent.

The issue caught the attention of social activists and political parties. Communist Party of India (Marxist) Polit Bureau member Brinda Karat demanded an impartial inquiry and action against those responsible for granting permission to carry out the trials.[4] The trials were soon suspended, and the Ministry of Health and Family Welfare appointed an expert committee to conduct an enquiry. After verifying the facts of the mater, the committee concluded that the deaths were not on account of the use of the vaccine and that there was no violation of any ethical norm in the conduct of the observational study.* This wasn't sufficient to pacify the agitated. Demands for review of the report of the committee followed.

A one-man third-party expert who reviewed the reports for the committee, Y. K. Gupta, head of the Pharmacology Department of AIIMS, did not endorse the report. He looked into the deaths, case by case, and pointed out gaps in the report and autopsy records. He noted that even though it was an observational study, the trials were intended as Phase IV marketing trials,† which were carried out before the vaccine reached the market and generally, the purpose of which was to identify even one adverse event in 10,000 vaccinations.[5]

With pressure mounting among the public and in the Parliament, the Standing Committee on Health and Family Welfare was tasked with examining irregularities, if any, in granting permission to conduct the trials. By April 2010, the Ministry of Health and Family Welfare conceded that the project was a 'post-licensure operational research study',‡ better known as Phase IV post-marketing clinical

* A type of research where investigators observe the effects of a treatment or condition without changing who gets what – they just watch and record data.

† A stage of drug testing that happens after a vaccine or drug is approved. It checks how it performs in the real world over time and looks for rare side effects.

‡ A type of research that studies how well a drug or vaccine works after it has been officially approved for use.

trial. ICMR too admitted that its ethical guidelines had been flouted during the course of the trial.

The Standing Committee, after hearing the officials of ICMR and the Health and Family Welfare, found that consent was obtained from hostel wardens and not from the parents, which was a flagrant violation of norms. In addition, the children or their parents had no idea about the virus, the disease and the vaccine.

What was more shocking was the effort to cover up the victims' deaths.

The Committee found that the deaths were summarily dismissed by the local authorities as unrelated to vaccinations without conducting any in-depth investigations. The causes attributed to the deaths were suicide, accidental drowning, malaria, viral infections, subarachnoid haemorrhage,* etc. In many cases, the reasons for the deaths were pronounced without conducting autopsies. The committee also observed that since some of the deaths were classified as suicides, the potential role of the vaccine causing suicidal thoughts could not be dismissed either.[6]

The Standing Committee Report also pointed out that the trials were initiated independently by PATH, without any go-ahead from the National Technical Advisory Group on Immunization (NTAGI), the agency responsible for granting permissions for vaccinations.[7] The report questioned ICMR's rationale for endorsing the use of the HPV vaccine in an agreement with PATH in 2007, well before the vaccine was approved for use in India in 2008, as well as its decision to include it in the national immunization programme by trespassing into the domain of the NTAGI.[8]

The report identified PATH's actions as clear violations of the human rights of the girls involved, as well as a significant breach of medical ethics. Consequently, the Standing Committee recommended that the National Human Rights Commission (NHRC) and the

---

* A type of bleeding in the brain that can be very serious and cause sudden death. It often needs immediate medical attention.

National Commission for Protection of Child Rights (NCPCR) investigate these human rights and child welfare violations.

Furthermore, the Standing Committee raised serious concerns about DCGI's role in the matter. It criticized the DCGI for failing to intervene despite evident violations of its regulations and pointed out irregularities in the approval processes for clinical trials, marketing and import licenses.[9] Subsequently, responding to a Public Interest Litigation in 2014, the Supreme Court of India summoned the DCGI and ICMR to explain their actions in light of the Parliamentary Standing Committee's report.

Given these findings and the responses of various governmental and judicial bodies, many believe that the CEOs of MSD and GSK, along with PATH, should have been held accountable and prosecuted for the deaths of innocent girls. This would have sent a strong message that India would no longer serve as a testing ground for international pharmaceutical companies.

The poorly designed and inadequately monitored study, using imperfect vaccines, pushed efforts to vaccinate young Indian women against HPV by at least a decade. Vaccinations against cervical cancer by state governments would start only in 2016, with the Punjab and Delhi governments taking the lead. The Government of India would include vaccinations against cervical cancer in the budget provisions in 2024. In fact, by then, almost 25 per cent of global deaths due to cervical cancer were being reported from India, with over 120,000 new cases every year,[10] which analysts suggested as heavily under-reported.

In the middle of this turmoil, efforts to develop an indigenous recombinant vaccine against HPV were going on at the Serum Institute of India. The BIRAC funded the recombinant vaccine project, which was under development almost for a decade, with the Bill & Melinda Gates Foundation joining the project and extending a $62,000 grant in 2016. The Serum Institute had promised the Gates Foundation a vaccine against nine HPV virus types, similar to MSD's Gardasil9, the most advanced vaccine in its category protecting against nine serotypes.[11]

By 2023, the first indigenous vaccine developed by the Serum Institute, covering virus types 6, 11, 16 and 18 received regulatory approval upon completion of safety trials. In comparison to MSD's Gardasil9, given in three doses, the Serum Institute's two-dose vaccine CERVAVAC stood out. Upon its market launch in January 2023, it was priced at ₹2,000 (~$25), much less than its competitors. The company offered it to India's national immunization programme, Mission Indradhanush, at almost one-tenth of the price. The 2024 interim budget made provisions for inclusion of the vaccine in Mission Indradhanush from 2025.

More recombinant vaccines to combat cervical cancer are on the horizon from various Indian companies. Given the size of the market and its gradual inclusion in national immunization programmes, many companies are actively developing newer versions. In fact, nearly 150 countries have included the vaccine in their national programmes, and the demand continues to grow.

The approval and launch of CERVAVAC marked a turning point not just in India's scientific journey but in reclaiming dignity and autonomy in public health policymaking. A decade and half after the Khammam tragedy exposed the darkest corners of global health experimentation, India now stands on the cusp of leading the fight against cervical cancer with its own indigenous solutions. The low-cost, two-dose vaccine developed by the Serum Institute is not only a scientific milestone but also a moral one; proving that ethical research, local innovation and public accountability can work hand in hand to protect lives.

Yet, the scars of the past endure. The loss of young lives in the name of medical progress remains a painful reminder of what happens when profit eclipses ethics, when the most voiceless among us are treated as expendable. As India moves forward, it must carry both the lessons of those failures and the hope of a more just, inclusive healthcare future. From exploitation to innovation, India has rewritten the story of the HPV vaccine, but not without the ghosts of Khammam.

34

PHILANTHROPY, POWER AND THE GLOBAL SOUTH

WHILE THE HPV VACCINE CONTROVERSY IN KHAMMAM exposed troubling gaps in ethical oversight, it was only one chapter in a much larger story of global institutions shaping healthcare trajectories in the Global South. PATH, a global nonprofit working to accelerate health equity through innovation and partnerships, has played a pivotal role in over seventy countries. PATH has been closely monitoring the clinical trial space and actively partnering with companies from developing nations. Its influence has only grown in recent years, despite the 2009 fiasco.

Alongside PATH, the Bill & Melinda Gates Foundation has emerged as one of the most powerful forces in the Global South. Originally founded in 1994 as the William H. Gates Foundation to support healthcare and philanthropic causes, it was renamed in 1999 when Bill and Melinda Gates took the reins and brought epidemiologist William Foege on board as a senior advisor. The foundation opened its India office in New Delhi in 2003, shortly after launching its Washington, D.C. office. It has since expanded its footprint, using its vast financial resources to influence vaccine policies, fund health systems and shape national immunization strategies – particularly across Asia and Africa.[1]

In time, the Gates Foundation has emerged as one of the world's largest philanthropic donors, with its endowment estimated at almost $50 billion and boasting Wall Street investor Warren Buffet among its board members. It is also the largest donor to WHO after the US government. What is more interesting – and worrisome for many – is that the foundation has become one of the largest investors in the growing sectors of biotechnology and biopharmaceuticals.

The foundation began identifying and sponsoring projects in the poorest regions of the world, focusing on healthcare, with vaccines always being a priority. It partnered with PATH and the US VAP on the Rotavirus vaccine project in India, meningococcal projects in Africa, and pneumococcal vaccine projects in Africa and India. Despite its substantial endowment, many countries and societies viewed the Gates Foundation with suspicion, due to Bill Gates' extensive history of operating profit-driven businesses and benefiting at the expense of unsuspecting customers.

Considering its influence on the global healthcare landscape and Gates' ambitious plans for vaccines, the foundation worked out a different strategy as soon as the William Gates Foundation transitioned into the Bill & Melinda Gates Foundation. The first point of the strategy was to ride on established non-profits like PATH, given their deep pockets and their bandwidth to implement projects in poorer countries.

The second strategy was to form global public-private partnerships, in some cases by replacing the existing entities with newer ones, with a seat on the board. This strategy was tested soon after the birth of the foundation, with the formation of a new vaccine alliance to replace the older, purely UN-sponsored agency. Hence emerged the Global Alliance for Vaccines and Immunization, now known as GAVI, the Vaccine Alliance.[2]

Technically, GAVI was born out of the March 1999 Bellagio conference which was convened with the theme of 'Vaccine Development and Delivery: Partnerships for the 21st Century'. The thirty-four participants of the conference – the World Bank, WHO, UNICEF, the Rockefeller Foundation and the Gates Foundation among them – thought a global entity with power to negotiate vaccine prices with manufacturers would help make vaccines affordable for the poor countries.

However, what was not made clear at this stage was that the global vaccine giants were working hand in hand with the Gates Foundation to form such a platform. The full picture came into view after the formation of GAVI in 2000, when vaccine companies were among the board of directors of the new entity. The Gates Foundation bargained for a permanent seat, wielding its financial prowess, with the other permanent members being WHO, the World Bank and UNICEF.[3]

GAVI emerged from the ashes of the Children's Vaccine Initiative (CVI), an alliance formed by UN agencies in 1990 to improve the accessibility of vaccines to the poorest countries. Internal politics and the dogfight between WHO and UNICEF hampered CVI's smooth functioning and led to its untimely death.[4] It is also worth examining the role of the Gates Foundation in the quiet demise of the ten-year-old CVI – and the almost immediate birth of GAVI, where Bill Gates swiftly secured a seat on the board.

Therefore, when the HPV vaccine controversy broke out in India, both the Gates Foundation and GAVI were on the docks. They were accused of pushing the vaccine agenda of pharmaceutical companies because of their direct involvement in the trials. Another allegation was that the Western biotechnology industry was lobbying to bring in more vaccines to India, while the Health Ministry was unable to ensure adequate controls.[5] One such powerful lobby that existed in India for a long time was the Rockefeller Foundation.

The Rockefeller Foundation never had a great reputation in India since its involvement in the rice germplasm controversy in the 1970s.[6] It was seen as exerting significant influence over the 1985 vaccine agenda of WHO and UNICEF, the Expanded Programme on

Immunization (EPI). As a core member of the consultative group – alongside WHO, UNICEF and the CDC – it faced allegations of shaping the EPI vaccination schedule in ways that favored American vaccine manufacturers.

The Organization of Pharmaceutical Producers of India (OPPI), a lobby of transnational pharma giants masquerading as the voice of research-based pharmaceutical companies in India, also came under the radar. With giant vaccine makers such as Pfizer, GSK, Sanofi Pasteur and MSD as patrons, OPPI has been influencing the government and regulators covertly and overtly to benefit US- and Europe-based pharma corporations since the 1960s.

OPPI has been criticized for causing more harm than good to indigenous vaccine technology development and nurturing innovation in the country. Since the days of liberalization in the 1990s, this powerful body has had unfettered access to the corridors of power in New Delhi, often touting the investment potential of its member companies. Three decades since liberalization and despite consistent promises of billions of dollars in investment, none of the global vaccine makers have established a vaccine development or production centre in India, save Sanofi Pasteur, which acquired a locally nurtured vaccine maker, Shantha Biotechnics.

Such lobbies and consultants have been playing their role in pushing the agenda of transnational vaccine makers with the governments and regulatory bodies in India to get access to run clinical trials on Indian subjects – an attractive microcosm of a varied genetic pool,* always in great demand for drug and vaccine testing.[7] Their key role has been to help Western vaccine makers explore the ever-growing Indian market and middle-income groups.

Despite daunting challenges, Indian vaccine companies have emerged resilient, challenging global corporations on their home turf, often without the support of key global healthcare gatekeepers like

---

* The collection of different genes found within a population. A diverse genetic pool helps scientists test how different people might react to a medicine or vaccine.

WHO and UNICEF. WHO plays a crucial role in prequalifying their vaccines for global acceptance, while UNICEF facilitates their inclusion in national immunization programmes, particularly those subsidized by the United Nations.

Facing increasing financial and technological dominance from global vaccine giants, small vaccine makers and public sector companies from developing nations struggled to survive. By the turn of the century, they recognized the need to unite for survival or risk an inevitable extinction. This realization led to a landmark meeting convened by WHO in Geneva on 16–17 March 2000, aimed at defining their role in a rapidly evolving global healthcare landscape.

The discussions culminated in the establishment of a new consortium, comprising vaccine manufacturers from developing nations.[8] Following this, the group again convened formally several months later for its formal inaugural meeting in Bilthoven, Netherlands. At this meeting, the group was officially named the Developing Countries Vaccine Manufacturers Network (DCVMN) International. A steering group, led by representatives from Indonesia, China, Brazil, Egypt, Iran and Cuba, was formed in which Mahima Datla of Biological E. in India, was elected for a three-year term.[9]

The network's primary objective was to supply all EPI vaccines, including HBV and Hib, to GAVI at affordable prices by meeting WHO standards. Member countries of DCVMN committed to scaling up production to ensure consistent supply to UNICEF starting 2005, in addition to meeting their own national demands. The second priority was research and development of new vaccines tailored for developing countries.[10]

This, in fact, was aimed at capturing the market share held by multinational vaccine giants supplying to UNICEF and GAVI. However, DCVMN certainly had an advantage due to the price levels they could offer compared to the vaccine giants. Soon, GAVI began to take notice of the group, and inviting DCVMN as a special invitee to its meetings. These informal collaborations eventually led GAVI to offer a seat on its board to DCVMN. The reason for GAVI's generosity was DCVMN's potential to provide vaccines at affordable prices to poor countries, especially considering that the network was already supplying approximately 60 per cent of the world's vaccine requirements.

Also, because the network's influence was growing among multilateral agencies, funding agencies and vaccine giants from the West. Initially conceived as an organization of public-sector vaccine makers, DCVMN has now evolved into a forum encompassing both public and private vaccine manufacturers from developing countries, with WHO's endorsement, thanks to a set of well-intentioned WHO officials.

Initially led by Indonesian vaccine producer PT Bio Farma, India soon took the lead of DCVMN. An increasing number of Indian companies achieving WHO pre-qualification for global vaccine supply facilitated this transition. By 2005, the organization's headquarters were established in Hyderabad, home to four major Indian vaccine manufacturers – Bharat Biotech, Biological E., Shantha Biotechnics and Indian Immunologicals. By 2024, ten out of forty-six members of the network were Indian companies, with most of them being WHO-prequalified. The DCVMN was emerging as a powerful vaccine coalition, representing the underdogs in a global vaccine landscape dominated by Western players.

Seven years after the founding of GAVI and DCVMN, an initiative was launched at the annual World Economic Forum (WEF) in Davos, stemming from the debate that vaccines kept unused in labs could have prevented the Ebola outbreak in West Africa, which had claimed over 11,000 lives. Therefore, the governments of India and Norway, along with the Bill & Melinda Gates Foundation, the UK-based Wellcome Trust and the WEF joined hands to establish the Coalition for Epidemic Preparedness Innovations (CEPI) as a solution.

Following initial discussions at the 2016 WEF, preparatory meetings were held in London in August and New Delhi the same year. India's Department of Biotechnology, led by Secretary Dr K.

Vijayraghavan, a distinguished biologist, played a key role leading these discussions, leading to the formation of CEPI.

The concept of CEPI originated from Stanley A. Plotkin, renowned for his contributions to the Rubella vaccine development. Plotkin along with British researcher Jeremy Farrar of the Wellcome Trust and Adel Mahmoud, a key scientist behind the HPV and rotavirus vaccines, proposed the establishment of a global vaccine development fund through a 2015 medical journal paper.[11] At the 2017 WEF, CEPI was formally launched with an initial funding commitment of $460 million, with the aim to develop vaccines against six emerging infectious diseases (EID) capable of causing significant epidemics: Middle East Respiratory Syndrome (MERS), Lassa fever, Nipah, Ebola, Marburg fever and Zika.[12]

Since 2019, CEPI has introduced 'vaccine bonds' to strengthen funding, while GAVI has leveraged them to accelerate sovereign pledges. The International Finance Facility for Immunization (IFFIm), in collaboration with CEPI, began financing GAVI's vaccine initiatives.[13] As a natural extension of these developments, India launched the Ind-CEPI Mission in March 2019, allocating approximately $40 million through BIRAC to accelerate vaccine development. Bharat Biotech was the first beneficiary, to advance its Chikungunya vaccine into Phase II/III trials in Costa Rica in partnership with the International Vaccine Institute (IVI) in South Korea.[14]

In the aftermath of the Covid-19 pandemic, CEPI also invested $30 million in the Serum Institute of India to enable rapid vaccine technology transfer during outbreaks for swift global distribution. This investment focused on building infrastructure to facilitate the rapid production and supply of vaccines.[15]

From a bold idea in a journal paper to a global coalition backed by billions, CEPI exemplifies how strategic philanthropy, public-private partnerships and multilateral cooperation can reshape the vaccine development landscape. With India emerging as a key partner through initiatives like Ind-CEPI and the Serum Institute's growing prominence, the country's role in global epidemic preparedness is now firmly established. As the world anticipates the next outbreak, these alliances signal a new era of speed, scale and science-driven solutions. In the race against epidemics, collaboration is the new cure.

35

FROM VIALS TO VOTES

IN THE QUIET VILLAGE OF KONDAMPATTI, NESTLED IN THE rolling plains of Dharmapuri district in Tamil Nadu, life follows the rhythm of the seasons – steady, ritualistic and steeped in tradition. Here, where caste lines ran deep and unspoken rules governed the course of love and marriage, a young couple dared to cross boundaries that had long been forbidden.

She was a spirited daughter of the Vanniyar community, a socially powerful caste group with a long-standing sense of cultural pride and deep agrarian roots. He, gentle and resolute, came from the neighbouring Dalit colony, where generations had endured discrimination but held fast to hope and quiet dignity. Their love blossomed despite the odds, whispered through the rustling paddy fields and evening meetings by temple walls. But love stories like theirs rarely end quietly in places where caste is law and honour is currency.

Ignoring repeated warnings from elders, and defying the weight of history, the couple decided to elope – setting off a chain of events that would shake the village and stain the state's conscience.

When news of their union reached the village elders, simmering tensions erupted. A caste panchayat, convened on 7 November 2012, ruled that the girl must return to her family. When she refused, choosing love over lineage, her father – unable to bear the perceived shame – took his own life.

The consequences were swift and devastating. That evening, a 2,500-strong mob descended on Kondampatti and neighbouring Anna Nagar, torching over 148 Dalit homes, looting property and unleashing terror that would require 300 policemen to contain.

Behind the smoke and ruin stood the shadow of a political machine – Pattali Makkal Katchi (PMK), led by S. Ramadoss, a prominent Vanniyar leader. Although Ramadoss denied accusations that his party had orchestrated violence, the PMK's long-standing opposition to inter-caste marriages and its role in stoking caste tensions placed it squarely under public scrutiny.

Founded in 1989, demanding job reservation for the Vanniyar caste, the PMK had transformed from a fringe movement into a political force. Representing nearly 3 million Vanniyars – about 5 per cent of the state's population – the party's rhetoric often danced on the edge of divisiveness. And in Dharmapuri, that rhetoric had turned to violence.[1]

In the 2004 Parliament elections, PMK secured five Lok Sabha seats, contesting as part of the United Progressive Alliance (UPA). Ramadoss leveraged the victory to negotiate a prominent ministry position in the UPA government, led by Prime Minister Manmohan Singh. Consequently, the Health Ministry was allocated to PMK, and Ramadoss appointed his thirty-five-year-old son, with no prior administrative or political experience, as the cabinet minister for health. Since his son had not contested the 2004 Parliament elections and was not elected to the Lok Sabha, he was swiftly made a Rajya Sabha member with the support of other UPA partners from Tamil Nadu.

Junior Ramadoss, a clinical doctor by training, initially met the high expectations of the healthcare community by implementing strict regulations on tobacco sales and introducing a national alcohol policy. However, he waited for the right moment to strike gold, carefully laying the groundwork for some manoeuvring.

An opportunity arose through the actions of two of his close mates – N. Elangeswaran and P. Sundaraparipooranan, both from Tamil Nadu. Elangeswaran was the serving director of BCG Vaccine Lab, Guindy and Pasteur Institute (PII), Coonoor. He was also a top contender for the coveted post of DCGI. Having risen through the ranks of PMK, Sundaraparipooranan transitioned into an entrepreneur overnight following Ramadoss's appointment as minister.

Elangeswaran, leveraging his role as the head of two PSU vaccine units, manipulated the internal workings of the vaccine industry, while Sundaraparipooranan worked externally to capitalize on it. Shortly after Ramadoss assumed office, Sundaraparipooranan established a company in Chennai called Vatsan Bio Pharma, with himself, his wife, and E. Shanti – the spouse of Elangeswaran – as shareholders. Around the same time, the team also formed Green Signal Bio Pharma, a second company with overlapping interests. By 2006, Green Signal had secured approval from Minister Ramadoss and was positioning itself to enter vaccine production.

In September 2006, a small but telling move was made when vaccine seeds were procured from the BCG Vaccine Lab for a modest sum of ₹105,000. Just a month later, a deal was made to sell its measles vaccine seeds, obtained through questionable means, to PII Coonoor for an astounding ₹32.5 million. This raised eyebrows, especially since PII had no experience nor plans to produce any measles vaccines, and could have obtained the same from the public sector Indian Immunologicals. Both deals were orchestrated and signed off by Elangeswaran, acting in his capacity as the director of the institutes. Further deepening the irregularities, PII agreed to share 70 per cent of the profits from the measles vaccine with Green Signal Bio Pharma.[2] Not long after, PII would send a proposal to the Health Ministry to start measles vaccine production.

Having secured sufficient stock of vaccine seeds, Green Signal began preparing to initiate BCG vaccine production. The company aimed to achieve two objectives: disrupting vaccine production at the BCG Vaccine Lab and establishing its own infrastructure. In July 2007, Elangeswaran, as the director of the BCG Lab, ordered the institute to stop breeding guinea pigs, indirectly halting the vaccine production. Facing a shortage of guinea pigs at the BCG Vaccine Lab, Elangeswaran arranged the transfer of approximately 600 animals from PII. However, the entire consignment went missing mysteriously en route to the BCG Vaccine Lab and, unsurprisingly, was found at 'a private vaccine manufacturer's compound in Mettupalayam'. In a similar turn of events, an entire batch of scientific staff undergoing training at PII abruptly defected to Green Signal Bio Pharma overnight.[3]

In January 2008, the Union Bank of India extended two loans totalling ₹153.6 million to Green Signal Bio Pharma to establish its production facilities. Strangely, it was the BCG Vaccine Lab that stood guarantor to secure the loans. With sufficient vaccine seeds, experimental animals, trained technicians and necessary facilities, Green Signal Bio Pharma was ready to produce its BCG vaccine.

By this time, with the BCG Lab's production halted, the government had to source an alternative supplier for BCG vaccines. The natural choice was Green Signal Bio Pharma. With the Health Minister backing the venture, the decision to redirect BCG vaccine procurement for the Universal Immunization Programme (UIP) seemed inevitable, aligning well with the trio's strategy.

Now came the final nail in the coffin.

Citing a 2007 WHO inspection and its advisory to comply with current GMP, three vaccine production units were abruptly shut down by the Health Ministry in early January 2008. It was unprecedented. Despite the earth-shattering decision, things moved quietly at the ministry. However, even the best efforts of the team could not keep the news under wraps for long.

Perturbed by the unsavoury move, a top government official in the Health Ministry leaked the news to leading business daily *Economic Times* towards the end of January. The news suggested that the Health Ministry had suspended the manufacturing licences of three government-supported vaccine makers – CRI, Kasauli, PII,

Coonoor and the BCG Vaccine Lab. The reason given for the action was 'violating WHO good manufacturing practices'.[4]

The news report also speculated that WHO had recommended suspension of the licenses of these units and was considering dropping India from the list of countries that supplied vaccines to UN agencies like the UNICEF for national vaccination programmes.

When the news broke, the three units were busy producing primary vaccines for India's UIP in addition to supplying to the UNICEF. Each of the three institutes had been leaders in their respective areas of strength. For instance, CRI Kasauli had been producing vaccines against diphtheria, tetanus, pertussis, yellow fever, typhoid and Japanese encephalitis, besides serving as the quality control organization for vaccines and sera produced in the country. PII was the global leader in anti-rabies vaccines and had also been manufacturing the DTP-Hepatitis B (DTP-HB) combo. The BCG Vaccine Lab had been meeting the entire national requirement of tuberculosis vaccine, BCG.

The decision to close down the vaccine production facilities severely disrupted UIP. Many states ran out of vaccine supplies and were not even permitted to retrieve last inventory from the three institutes. The situation was exacerbated by a global shortage of primary vaccines and a lack of realistic governmental plans to address the demand-supply gap.

The government's proposed solutions – a vaccine park* in Chengalpet and mobilizing Hindustan Latex – proved unrealistic and time-consuming.[5] As a result of this mindless overnight decision, the lives of 27 million newborns annually were at grave risk. Reports of infant deaths emerged sporadically from different parts of the country. With government hospitals and primary care centres unable to provide primary vaccines, demand surged in private clinics and hospitals. A vaccine that cost ₹30 under the UIP was sold in private

---

* A specialized area or facility set up to manufacture vaccines at scale using advanced technology and infrastructure.

clinics at ten to hundred times more. Western pharma lobbies began pushing to include expensive imported combo vaccines* in the UIP, even as these vaccines flooded the open market.

The overall result was the worst ever vaccine crisis India had ever faced – a man-made catastrophe driven by profit motives of a few unscrupulous individuals. The UIP faltered in meeting its commitments, forcing desperate parents to turn to private clinics for essential vaccines. Large segments of rural and tribal communities went without vaccinations for an extended period, leading to the deaths of innumerable children.[6] While the fires raged, those in charge looked away – Nero played the flute. No systematic effort was ever made to document the full extent of the tragedy, and the true number of infant deaths caused by the collapse of state vaccination coverage was never officially acknowledged.

Ramadoss, on the other hand, was busy attempting to legitimatize the shutdown. He set up a committee headed by the Director General of Health Services (DGHS) to endorse the decision to close down the units. He asked the committee 'to prepare a road map for smooth transition of the three units from vaccine manufacturing to testing and training centres.' The committee faithfully submitted its report by September 2008, suggesting CRI and PII be deployed to produce yellow fever vaccines and the BCG Lab be used as a facility to certify the quality of BCG vaccines produced by other companies.[7]

Soon after the issue erupted into a controversy, the Parliamentary Standing Committee on Health and Family Welfare launched an investigation. The committee found fault with the suspension decision and recommended that the licenses be reinstated without delay.[8] However, despite repeated appeals, the Ministry failed to act. For over a year, the deadlock continued, and the suspension remained in place until the end of the ministry's term in May 2009.[9]

After the 2009 parliament elections when a new government,

* A single shot that protects against multiple diseases, like the DTP vaccine that protects against diphtheria, tetanus and whooping cough.

excluding the PMK, came to power, the vaccine catastrophe was revisited. A clear picture of this catastrophe emerged only after a new minister assumed charge at the Health Ministry. A committee, led by a former Special Secretary in the Health Ministry, Javed Chowdhury, was formed to investigate the issue. Its report in February 2010 paved the way for the resumption of vaccine production at the three units.[10]

By then, the vaccine shortage had aggravated to unimaginable levels, multiplying unreported, unaccounted infant deaths to unthinkable proportions.

A query raised under the Right to Information Act by an activist showed a shortfall of 170 million doses of diphtheria, measles, tetanus and oral polio vaccines for the year 2009, despite the government procuring some from the private sector and deploying certain quantities of imported vaccines. Rajya Sabha member Brinda Karat pointed out that the crisis had deepened, with the vaccine shortage under the UIP rising to 22 per cent from 15 per cent in 2008.

The Javed Chowdhury committee strongly criticized the government for its long-standing neglect in supporting the three units to upgrade to global quality standards.[11] Despite a growing birth rate and increased demand for vaccines, the Ministry had failed to modernize vaccine production infrastructure, enhance research and development or adapt to technological advancements to boost capacity. A 2007 WHO evaluation did highlight lapses in GMP compliance at some units. Earlier inspections too had identified quality gaps but did not recommend shutting down production. Similarly, later inspections by the DCGI did not call for closure either.

The Parliamentary Committee too had criticized the Ministry of Health for not allocating enough time or budget to address the issues, despite WHO's offer to assist and upgrade technology. Minister Ramadoss defended his actions, citing WHO's criticism of vaccine quality and the need to restructure the DCGI. He tried to explain to a news magazine his rationale for the Ministry's decision: despite warnings since 2004, compliance was not achieved by the units till 2007, leading to WHO asking them to meet standards by December.[12] What he conveniently ignored was the fact that he was the central health minister since 2004, and it was his duty to rectify the deficiencies and gaps.

Despite having all the advantages – political backing, early approvals and strategic positioning – Green Signal Bio Pharma could not exploit the crisis beyond a point. In contrast, established private sector vaccine makers quickly seized the opportunity. They stepped in as the primary vaccine suppliers for the UIP, charging significantly higher prices than the prices offered by public sector units before the suspension.[13]

The interest of the private sector in the unfolding situation was unmistakable, reflected in the remarks of Cyrus Poonawalla of the Serum Institute of India. He told *Down to Earth* that the ministry probably had no choice but to halt operations of the companies because of their mismanagement and substandard production conditions. Nonetheless, he acknowledged that the public sector's inability to modernize its facilities to meet GMP standards was perhaps due to the low vaccine prices offered by the health ministry, which was adversely affecting both public and private players.[14]

Elangeswaran's questionable activities extended well beyond facilitating the establishment of Green Signal Bio Pharma for BCG vaccine production. He engaged with private vaccine manufacturers and offered them vaccine seeds from PII. Polio and DPT seed viruses were distributed free of cost to Bharat Biotech and the Serum Institute of India. As the media began to expose these actions, Elangeswaran deflected blame onto senior Health Ministry officials, accusing them of pressuring him to shut down the two public units under his control to benefit private players. Matters escalated when he publicly named ministry officials during a press interaction in May 2008, crossing a line that prompted the then Health Secretary to recommend disciplinary action. While action appeared imminent, it was quietly stalled – thanks to the tacit backing and behind-the-scenes influence of the minister.[15]

Much later, after the case reached the Supreme Court of India through a public interest litigation, the suspended units were finally revived and modernized to meet WHO's GMP standards. Despite this, the units struggled to restore production to pre-suspension levels, as many experienced staff had left, and the labs and machinery had remained unused for years. More importantly, accountability for the unjust suspension was never established.

The Vaccine Park in Chengalpet, envisioned as an alternative to the three units, received approval from the Cabinet Committee on Economic Affairs (CCEA) a decade and half later in April 2012. With a proposed budget of ₹5.94 billion, the park spans 100 acres near Chennai and was intended to produce 585 million doses of six essential vaccines.[16] The park's management was entrusted to the public sector contraceptive maker HLL Lifecare, which established a wholly owned subsidiary named HLL Biotech (HBL) for the purpose.

However, twelve years and a pandemic later, not a single vial of vaccine has been produced at the park.[17] Designed as a national hub for vaccine research, manufacturing and distribution, the project cost escalated to ₹10 billion over time. Amid the severe vaccine shortage during the Covid-19 pandemic, Tamil Nadu Chief Minister M. K. Stalin requested Prime Minister Narendra Modi to transfer the park's assets to the state government on lease to facilitate Covid-19 vaccine production. The request was never granted.[18]

By then, private sector vaccine manufacturers had secured significant influence – not just in Government procurement but also in national politics. For instance, the Serum Institute donated over ₹500 million to the ruling BJP in 2022 through the Prudent Electoral Trust.[19] Bharat Biotech donated ₹250 million to the main opposition in Andhra Pradesh, Telugu Desam Party, which seized power in the state in 2024.[20] Data from the Election Commission of India for 2023–24 revealed that thirty-seven healthcare companies together purchased electoral bonds worth over ₹9 billion to donate to political parties ahead of the 2024 parliamentary elections.[21]

The vaccine sector had by now morphed into a theatre of political influence, with pharma giants currying favour with their political benefactors through opaque instruments like electoral bonds. Business expediency left many manufacturers with no option but to align with political camps to secure influence, preferential contract and regulatory leeway. Politicians, in turn, found covert partners in some vaccine corporations, leveraging them to build parallel empires of control. The boundaries between the ethics of public office and the ambitions of private profiteering blurred beyond recognition.

What makes this nexus even more sinister was its toll on the public. While power brokers and fixers struck backroom deals, millions of infants were left unprotected – they became victims of manufactured crises. Vaccines were becoming less about public health and more about power, profit and politics.

36

MONKEYS, TICKS AND NEW FRONTIERS

IN JANUARY 1957, A SHADOW OF DREAD FELL OVER THE unassuming Primary Health Centre in Ulavi, at the edge of the dense jungles of Karnataka's Shimoga District. Disturbing reports had begun to surface; of monkeys dying mysteriously, their bodies marked by signs of severe haemorrhage. The alarm deepened when villagers – woodcutters and cattle grazers who had wandered near the sites – succumbed to the same grim fate.

A team of healthcare experts embarked on an urgent investigation. Their pursuit led to a chilling discovery – a deadly virus was on the loose. The serological tests* carried out to identify the virus revealed that the pathogen was unlike anything previously catalogued. As they probed deeper, the team uncovered a haunting backstory. The virus's emergence coincided with deforestation to expand grazing lands for livestock. With their habitat cut down, monkeys were forced to spend more time on the forest floor, bringing them into closer contact with the undergrowth that was teeming with ticks.

The impact on local people was devastating. Infected individuals developed severe haemorrhagic fevers,† with a fatality rate ranging

* Blood tests used to detect the presence of antibodies or viruses, helping to identify infections.

† A group of illnesses that involve fever and bleeding (internal or external), often caused by viruses.

up to 10 per cent.[1] The serene forest had transformed into a silent killer and the once peaceful coexistence between humans, monkeys and their shared environment had been irrevocably shattered by this invisible adversary.

This was around the time the Rockefeller Foundation sought permission from the Indian Government to set up a centre to study viruses spreading mysterious diseases. The centre came up in Pune as the Viral Research Centre (VRC) in 1957 and set off with studying the arthropod-borne viruses, otherwise known as arboviruses, that are transmitted via vectors like mosquitos, ticks and sandflies.

Arboviruses were spreading some of the deadliest diseases without any checks and balances, and it remained a challenge to handle these tough germs. The types of diseases spread by these microbes included yellow fever, dengue, Japanese encephalitis, Zika and West Nile disease. For many of these vector-borne diseases, there wasn't any preventive measure in place till the turn of the century.

So, when this mysterious disease began to spread by April 1957 in the jungles of Kyasanur, the VRC was alerted. The VRC team found that people living in villages adjacent to the forest were experiencing alarming symptoms, many leading to death. The team observed that those who had ventured into the forest and encountered dead monkeys were the ones falling ill.[2] Therefore, it was concluded that the disease was yellow fever, which was the sole known disease prevalent in the woods, capable of affecting both monkeys and humans.

The VRC team breathed a sigh of relief as there had been a vaccine available for yellow fever since the 1930s. It was developed by the Rockefeller Foundation and its scientist Max Theiler, the only Nobel Prize for developing a viral vaccine to date. The 17D virus vaccine, introduced in Brazil in 1938, marked a turning point in the fight against yellow fever, a disease that has been prevalent in thirty-four African countries and thirteen countries in Central and South America, killing approximately 30,000 to 60,000 people a year.

The Theiler vaccine had been in use for over eight decades as a safe and effective preventive measure. WHO's guidelines regarding the vaccine have remained unchanged because of the continuity and severity of the disease. More significantly, the vaccine is still produced using the original methods – by passing through embryonated chicken eggs and stored as a frozen homogenate.[3]

A VRC team began gathering mosquitoes from different elevations within the forest since yellow fever is spread by mosquitoes. The team struggled to find many mosquitoes that fed on humans during the daytime. In the meantime, the results of the blood samples that had been sent to its centre in Pune were out. The outcome: the germs found in the blood samples were from the same group of viruses that cause yellow fever, but not exactly the yellow fever virus.[4] Moreover, the mosquito samples did not show the presence of any viral material.

When the month-long investigation hit a roadblock, someone observed the monkey carcasses on the jungle slopes. Noticing a lot of ticks feeding on their decaying flesh, the team decided to take a chance and collect some tick samples. This decision proved consequential. Confirming their worst fears, a couple of staff members who had collected the ticks fell ill on the third day.

That was the turning point. The investigation concluded with identifying the virus in the tick samples collected from the monkey carcasses and establishing the mode of transmission.

There started the real hunt for a preventive measure, a vaccine for the disease that came to be known as the Kyasanur Forest Disease (KFD). The VRC took it upon itself to develop a vaccine and after nearly a decade of work, a team led by C. N. Dandavate declared success. By this time, the VRC was taken over by ICMR, and the Rockefeller Foundation had wrapped up its work in India. The vaccine was developed using a virus strain isolated from the infected and after conducting field trials in Shimoga district, it was ready for deployment by 1969. After successful trials, vulnerable populations were vaccinated annually thereafter.[5] In the absence of any effective treatment available, vaccination remained the only public health intervention.

For over four decades, the vaccines worked reasonably well. The intramuscular administration of the formalin-inactivated* KFD vaccine was found to reduce the rate of incidence. Since the vaccine-induced immunity is short-lived, a booster dose is given some six months later and thereafter annually for five years.

Despite having strong preventive measures in place, the disease became a major public health concern not just in Karnataka, but also in neighbouring states of Tamil Nadu, Maharashtra, Kerala and Goa, covering the entire southern stretch of the Western Ghats region. The spread was slow and gradual, akin to the pace of a moving tick, in contrast to the swift flight of vectors like mosquitoes.

However, strong data emerged showing the recurrence of the disease among vaccinated people, indicating a decline in the efficacy of the current vaccine. The virus strain used in the current vaccine – strain P9605, originally isolated in 1965 – had undergone several passages in mice as part of laboratory trials. Therefore, the formalin inactivated vaccine seems to be ineffective against current strains of the virus in circulation.[6] Studies have shown 2.24 per cent diversity† in the currently circulating strains of KFD virus in contrast to strain P9605.[7]

In 2022, ICMR put out an open tender calling parties to develop a new vaccine with higher efficacy and safety, based on a new strain of virus isolated from the recent outbreaks.[8] Not many contenders came forward at the first instance and a second expression of interest was floated a while later. The muted response from the private sector was likely due to the limited commercial potential of a vaccine targeted at a geographically confined disease affecting remote tribal populations. Eventually, the Hyderabad-based public-sector vaccine company Indian Immunologicals was given the job, and the development work is currently underway.

KFD is not the only villain from the arbovirus group that was

---

* A vaccine made from a virus that has been 'killed' using the chemical formalin so it can no longer cause disease but can still trigger immunity.

† Genetic variations among virus strains, which can affect how well vaccines work against them.

creating havoc in the country. Many more were detected in subsequent decades, dengue being the worst public health problem. Dengue, caused by four different virus types, DEN-1, DEN-2, DEN-3 and DEN-4, is structurally similar to other arboviruses. It consists of a single-stranded RNA enclosed in a nucleocapsid,* all within a lipid envelope† derived from the host cell membrane. It has three different proteins, a core protein, a membrane-associated protein and an envelope protein, the latter being responsible for key functions like virus neutralization‡ and interaction with receptors.[9]

Globally, over 2.5 billion people are at risk of contracting dengue, and about 50–100 million are infected annually with its life-threatening complications, dengue haemorrhagic fever and dengue shock syndrome. The first dengue epidemic was reported in India in the early 1960s in the eastern region and it became a notifiable disease in 1996.[10]

Sanofi Pasteur was the first to come up with a vaccine in 2015: a live attenuated yellow fever/dengue tetravalent vaccine, marketed under the name Dengvaxia. Dengvaxia was invented in 1997 by researchers from Saint Louis University, Missouri. A biopharmaceutical company, which later became Acambis Inc., obtained rights to the vaccines developed at SLU, along with that of Japanese encephalitis and the West Nile virus. Acambis and Sanofi Pasteur teamed up to conduct human trials in Asia, Africa and Latin America. When Acambis was acquired by Sanofi in 2008, the rights of Dengvaxia were secured by Sanofi.

However, it has not been licensed in India due to a lack of sufficient data. What prevents this vaccine from entering the Indian market is the 1964 Declaration of Helsinki, which necessitated conducting clinical trials in or near the communities where interventions will be

* The combination of the virus's genetic material (RNA or DNA) and the protein shell that protects it.

† A fatty outer layer some viruses steal from the host cell, which helps them infect new cells.

‡ When antibodies or vaccines stop a virus from infecting cells.

used – especially in LMICs – to ensure relevance, respect for local context and equitable benefit.[11]

Soon after Dengvaxia, the US National Institutes of Health (NIH) too developed a vaccine, TetraVax-DV, while the Japanese pharma major Takeda developed its tetravalent dengue vaccine, DenVax. Both are currently in the last phases of efficacy trials and regulatory approvals.

Considering the enormous size of the dengue market, a number of players entered the vaccine development scene in India – some backed by global support while others were purely indigenous efforts.

The NIH's live-attenuated dengue vaccine, TetraVax-DV has been licensed to Panacea Biotec, the Serum Institute of India, Biological E. and Indian Immunologicals, granting them non-exclusive rights for clinical development and marketing.[12] Using the NIH virus seeds, Panacea developed a process to produce the vaccine viral substance, and quickly moved to clinical trials, with financial support from the Technology Development Board of the Ministry of Science and Technology.[13]

By the time Covid-19 virus struck the world, the Serum Institute had completed phase I clinical trials, establishing the safety and immunogenicity of its tetravalent live attenuated vaccine in adults. The study carried out in Australia showed 80 per cent efficacy against the Den-1 serotype and 100 per cent efficacy against Den-2 serotype. On the other hand, Biological E. never explored the rights procured from the NIH. Instead, it entered into a pact with Takeda to produce its tetravalent live attenuated vaccine QDENGA, at a rate of 50 million doses a year.[14] The fourth effort was made by the Indian Immunologicals which has been developing the live attenuated tetravalent dengue vaccine candidate using the licensed seeds from NIH. The vaccine is being supported for clinical trials by the National Biopharma Mission.

In the meantime, a completely indigenous effort was made by a team of scientists from the International Centre for Genetic Engineering and Biotechnology (ICGEB), New Delhi, who developed the DSV-

4 dengue vaccine. In 2016, Mumbai-based Sun Pharma entered into an agreement to acquire the technology of the DSV-4 vaccine from ICGEB. DSV-4 is a recombinant virus-like particle (VLP)-based vaccine and not a live attenuated one. It was developed using *Pichia pastoris*, an approach similar to the one used in the development of hepatitis-B vaccines.[15] With the support of the National Biopharma Mission, the candidate is undergoing Phase I clinical trials.[16]

Another major threat among arboviruses is chikungunya, a debilitating disease that has rapidly spread in recent history. Though the chikungunya virus has been present in India for decades, the first recorded outbreak occurred in Calcutta in 1963. Since then, the country has experienced several outbreaks of varying severity.

One of the most significant outbreaks of chikungunya was in 2006. Starting in the southern state of Kerala, it soon spread across the country, affecting millions of people across various states, leading to widespread suffering.

In the national capital, the outbreak reached alarming proportions, overwhelming hospitals and healthcare facilities. Patients flooded emergency rooms, seeking relief from the intense joint pain and other debilitating symptoms caused by the virus. Hospitals were ill-equipped to handle the surge in cases, leading to long waiting times, shortages of medical supplies and overcrowded wards.

Since then, India has experienced several chikungunya outbreaks, in 2010, 2016 and in 2019. These outbreaks also served as an opportunity for the Indian healthcare system to test its preparedness and resilience in managing large-scale public health emergencies, which would soon prove valuable when responding to Covid-19.

Chikungunya transmits through *Aedes aegypti* and *Aedes albopictus* mosquitoes. While the illness is usually not fatal, it can cause severe joint pain, fever, rash and other debilitating symptoms. The worst aspect of chikungunya is its ability to cause prolonged and intense joint pain, which can last for weeks to months and in some cases, even become chronic. This pain can severely limit mobility and quality of life, making simple tasks like walking or holding objects extremely difficult. Perhaps the most tragic aspect of chikungunya is its ability to affect vulnerable populations, including the elderly, young children and individuals with underlying health conditions. For these groups, the complications of chikungunya can be particularly severe and may result in long-term disability or even death.

Researchers have been exploring various vaccine platforms, including live-attenuated vaccines, inactivated vaccines and VLP vaccines. Several chikungunya vaccine candidates have shown promising results in preclinical trials and early-stage clinical studies.

Bharat Biotech has been developing an inactivated vaccine, Chikavax in collaboration with the ICMR which is currently undergoing Phase II/III clinical trials with support from the Coalition for CEPI. The DBT has been funding the Bharat Biotech project under the Ind-CEPI Mission for the Global Chikungunya Vaccine Clinical Development Programme (GCCDP). The target is an affordable chikungunya vaccine that meets WHO pre-qualification standards to distribute to LMICs.

A live-attenuated vaccine, Chikavax has shown promising safety and immunogenicity in preclinical testing and Phase I clinical trials in India. Thereafter, Bharat Biotech teamed up with Seoul-based International Vaccine Institute (IVI) for Phase II/III randomized, controlled trials across nine locations in five countries – Costa Rica, Panama, Colombia, Thailand and Guatemala.[17]

Amongst other vaccine candidates in the pipeline, the live attenuated CHIKV vaccine, developed by Austrian biotech firm Valneva with CEPI's support, has completed Phase III studies and is close to getting regulatory approvals in the US and EU. Independent of CEPI, the VLP vaccine project of the US Emergent Biosciences is in Phase III trials and received a US Department of Defense grant for a post-licensure trial in the endemic region of Thailand.[18]

After years of efforts to develop a vaccine, Merck abandoned its plans in 2023, following its acquisition of Themis, a company with a promising chikungunya vaccine candidate under trial – V184 – in a $366 million deal in 2020. Themis had been developing this measles-vectored vaccine for many years with the support of CEPI. While the candidate had completed Phase II trials, Merck suspended further trials after an internal assessment of its pipeline prioritization.[19]

There are many other infectious diseases for which vaccines are urgently needed and are feasible to develop. Unfortunately, many of these illnesses are ignored by pharma giants due to prioritization based on market viability, high development cost, time overruns and lack of incentives from national governments or international agencies.

For several diseases categorised as 'travel vaccines' – Zika, Marburg and West Nile – there have been concerted efforts to develop effective solutions. While some vaccines are already available, others are expected to enter the market soon. National governments increasingly require their citizens to be vaccinated against these endemic threats before traveling to high-risk destinations, as part of strengthened border health protocols.

Efforts are underway to find travel vaccine solutions for Middle East respiratory syndrome coronavirus (MERS-Cove), severe acute respiratory syndrome (SARS) virus, Cytomegalovirus (CMV) and Respiratory syncytial virus (RSV). Interestingly, it is not the major transnational vaccine giants but smaller, agile biotech firms that are leading these efforts.

For instance, among the nine vaccine candidates currently in development for the deadly Zika, none are being spearheaded by the 'big four' vaccine makers – Merck (MSD), GSK, Sanofi and Pfizer. Instead Valneva, Moderna, Themis, GeneOne and Inovio are driving such innovations. The complete absence of large players reflects their focus on markets that promise a 'reasonable return' on investment, often leaving neglected diseases and low-income geographies to smaller, mission-driven developers.

The cost of developing a new vaccine can range anywhere from $500 million to $1 billion, depending on the complexity of the vaccine candidate and the target microbe.[20] Even after investing substantial capital, there is no guarantee that a vaccine developer will achieve a good return on its investment. The reality is only about 7 per cent of projects progress to the pre-clinical stages and eventually obtain a license.[21]

Regardless of who initiates vaccine development, the most critical factor today is the ability to produce vaccines at scale, rapidly and at affordable prices. Gradually, it has become clear which players are best positioned to meet these demands – a fact reflected in the evolving global vaccine production landscape.

Most part of the last century, UNICEF sourced nearly all its vaccines from developed countries. By 2000, that share had dropped to 53 per cent. In 1992, developed nations accounted for 25 per cent of polio vaccines, 90 per cent of measles vaccines, 85 per cent of yellow fever vaccines and 79 per cent of hepatitis B vaccines procured globally.[22] By 2020, the tide had turned significantly: small and medium vaccine manufacturers from developing countries were involved in 181 non-Covid-19 vaccine projects, ranging from novel candidates for dengue, chikungunya and Zika to more complex vaccines like HPV and pneumococcal conjugates.[23]

The rise of India as a low-cost vaccine manufacturing powerhouse has been the game-changer. By offering affordable pricing and fulfilling large national immunization contracts, Indian vaccine firms have disrupted the traditional business model of large Western pharmaceutical companies, which relied heavily on 'reasonable return on investment' calculations. As a result, many of these legacy players have scaled back or exited the vaccine space altogether.

Data from ClinicalTrials.gov, a US-based platform that tracks clinical trials, reveals that vaccine R&D among major Western firms has declined compared to the surge seen in the 1980s and 1990s. Fewer vaccine trials targeting new infectious diseases are now being sponsored by big vaccine companies, and this number has not been rising.[24] While this retreat may seem concerning, it has paved the way for a promising shift.

A new generation of vaccine manufacturers from the Global South are steadily filling the void, not just as suppliers but as innovators. In parallel, emerging biotech firms from the West – once considered tier-2 and tier-3 players – are also stepping up. Together, they are redefining the future of vaccine development: one that is decentralized, more equitable and driven not solely by profit, but by purpose and public health priorities.

The next era of vaccines may no longer be led by the traditional giants – and that may be precisely what the world needs.

37

EBOLA, ANTHRAX AND BIOTERRORISM

DECEMBER 2013. IN A RAINFOREST VILLAGE OF MELIANDOU IN southern Guinea, Emile Ouamouno, a two-year-old toddler who loved playing in muddy fields among chickens and goats, returned home sick after a typical day of playing with his friends.

That night, he developed a high fever and chills, and his mother observed that he was vomiting constantly and passing black stool.* Days later, on 6 December, Emile died. His mother, who had been caring for him, suffered from severe bleeding, both orally and rectally, and passed away by 13 December. A fortnight later, Emile's three-year-old sister also died after experiencing high fever, vomiting and black diarrhoea. Their grandmother, who had nursed them, passed away on New Year's Day. By then, many villagers who had visited the sick began exhibiting the same symptoms. The mystery illness quickly spread to neighbouring villages as friends and relatives from other areas attended the grandmother's funeral.

A midwife from Meliandou unknowingly transmitted the disease to her relatives in a nearby village and then to a healthcare worker treating her. The infected healthcare worker was taken to a hospital in Macenta, eighty kilometres away. There, a doctor who cared for him contracted the disease and unknowingly infected his brothers in Kissidougou, 133 kilometres away. The chain of transmission from

* Very dark-colored feces, often a sign of internal bleeding in the stomach or intestines.

healthcare workers spread like wildfire, fuelling an outbreak that would soon spiral out of control,[1] not just in Africa, but around the world. The death toll soon crossed 5,000 worldwide, including a few in the United States.

Once the disease spread to developed nations like the US, alarm bells began to ring. The disease was identified as Ebola, also known as Ebola virus disease (EVD) and Ebola haemorrhagic fever (EHF). It was the deadliest of all recorded viral diseases, considering its virulence, mortality, transmission, lack of treatment and outbreak dynamics.

Ebola was first reported in 1976 in South Sudan and Congo. A viral haemorrhagic fever infecting humans and other primates, it was caused by deadly viruses of at least five different types known by their place of origin – Zaire, Sudan, Reston, Bundibugyo and Taï Forest. The most dangerous among these were the Zaire ebolavirus and the Sudan ebolavirus.[2]

Warnings such as 'Do not touch the dead', 'If somebody is sick, leave them to death', and 'Dare touch a patient, get infected and killed' – issued by overwhelmed healthcare workers – did little to help contain the disease. Instead, they fuelled a climate of fear and panic.

By August 2014, WHO declared the outbreak a public health emergency of international concern.[3] A month later, WHO called the Western African epidemic 'the largest, most severe, most complex public health emergency seen in modern times.'[4] However, the global community did not rise to the occasion in response. Both WHO and the UN were criticized for their sluggish, inadequate response, while Western nations were faulted for failing to support a war-torn region in the midst of a crisis with global implications.[5] Many Western governments, preoccupied with domestic priorities and skeptical of the epidemic's potential to cross borders, underestimated the urgency and scale of international intervention required.

Amid this grim chapter, a rare glimmer of hope emerged. As the outbreak finally began to retreat after claiming thousands of lives, results from a two-year trial of a recombinant Ebola vaccine –

developed in real time during the crisis – offered promising efficacy against the strain driving the epidemic.

The initiative had come from an unexpected quarter – Canada. The Public Health Agency of Canada (PHAC) had been working on the vaccine since the last decade of the twentieth century. By 2003, PHAC's National Microbiological Laboratory in Winnipeg succeeded in developing a workable candidate and applied for a patent, before starting the trials. Three back-to-back animal trials funded by the Canadian and the US governments followed. These trials concluded that a single intramuscular injection of the vaccine induced completely protective immune responses in non-human primates, such as crab-eating macaques against Ebola and Marburg viruses.[6,7]

As more studies were conducted, in 2010, PHAC quietly licensed the rights of the vaccine to a company linked to the US Defense Threat Reduction Agency (DTRA) for a paltry sum of $205,000 and minimal royalties.

The company, Bioprotection Systems, a subsidiary of Newlink Genetics connected to the US Department of Defense, turned out to be wheeler-dealer. When the next outbreak occurred in Guinea, the largest Ebola outbreak ever, Newlink had no vaccine in production and no human trials underway. With WHO committed to offering vaccines to key resources dealing with the disease, the Canadian government ended up donating 1,000 doses from its stockpile of 1,500.[8] In fact, four valuable years were lost due to the rights being handed over to an unsuitable entity, one that lack the capacity to run trials or to produce vaccines at scale. Calls to hand over the rights to a company that could produce and test the vaccine grew louder and more urgent. It was then that the American pharma giant Merck & Co. acquired the rights from Newlink for $50 million.[9]

The Phase II clinical trial started in March 2015 in Guinea, focusing on frontline health workers, while the Phase III trial was carried out as a 'ring vaccination'* in which people who had contracted Ebola virus were vaccinated. When the results were out in December 2016, the vaccine was found to be almost 100 per cent effective.[10] The US FDA and European Medicines Agency (EMA) approved the Merck vaccine named ERVEBO in 2019 after another large-scale ring vaccination study in Congo during an outbreak. The results showed 97.5 per cent success in stopping the transmission.[11] Subsequently, it was deployed for commercial use.

In 2020, Janssen Pharmaceutical, a Johnson & Johnson company, too came out with a version of the vaccine. China and Russia came out with their versions quickly, given the potential of misusing the virus as a bioterrorism weapon. India had an altogether different play. India's leading vaccine maker, the Serum Institute of India had been partnering with the Oxford Vaccine Group of the University of Oxford for different vaccines for a while. One such partnership was for an Ebola vaccine, funded by the UK Department of Health and Social Care (DHSC).

As the Oxford team, led by Professor Teressa Lambe, prepared for the clinical trials of the vaccine candidate in Oxford and Tanzania, the Serum Institute was brought on board with a plan to quickly manufacture the vaccine in the event of new outbreaks. The Serum Institute was supported by Professor Sandy Douglas of the Jenner Institute for scaling up manufacturing. So, when the 2022 Uganda outbreak happened, the Serum Institute's manufacturing facility was pressed into service. It produced 40,000 doses in less than sixty days and shipped them to Kampala.[12]

Long before this achievement by the Serum Institute, the Ella Foundation, founded by the promoters of Bharat Biotech, had claimed a breakthrough in developing a vaccine using the adenovirus, which causes mild flu. The team engineered a human adenovirus to contain an optimized synthetic gene† based on the virus from the 2013–16 Ebola outbreak.

---

* A strategy where people who have been in contact with an infected person and their contacts are vaccinated to stop the disease from spreading.

† A lab-made version of a gene that is adjusted for better performance, often to trigger a stronger immune response in the body.

The Ebola virus, with a ribbon-like structure, sports a coat dotted with spike-like proteins called glycoprotein. The development of immune responses against this protein holds the key in offering protection, and the Ella vaccine works on using controlled production of the glycoprotein.[13] Merck's vaccine, on the contrary, contained a gene for the surface protein of the Sudan ebolavirus stitched into vesicular stomatitis virus (VSV), a livestock pathogen that rarely causes harm in humans.[*14]

The Ella Foundation left it to the Government of India to take over the work; to advance or sponsor it to run trials and establish it as a commercial vaccine. Because the virus has been contained in the Western African region and considering the poor purchasing power of the people there, pharmaceutical companies have shown little interest beyond supporting the national efforts. National governments showed limited interest, primarily due to potential use of the virus as a weapon of bioterrorism.

The fact that the US, Russia and China were involved in developing and stockpiling the vaccine was to safeguard national security concerns. With the Serum Institute demonstrating its ability to manufacture large volumes rapidly, the Indian government appeared less inclined to support a second vaccine. However, interest of the Indian defence establishment in acquiring the Ella Foundation vaccine cannot be ruled out.

No evidence has yet emerged in the public domain about the Gwalior-based Deference Research and Development Establishment (DRDE) acquiring the vaccine from the Ella Foundation. The DRDE, a specialized agency of the DRDO, has been involved in preparing countermeasures for many of the deadly bacteria and viral agents. In fact, India has long established a dedicated biological cell at the armed forces headquarters, along with directories of nuclear, biological and chemical (NBC) warfare. A Biosafety Level 2 (BSL-

* Since it rarely causes illness in humans, scientists use VSV as a harmless carrier to deliver parts of dangerous viruses like Ebola in vaccines.

2) laboratory was also established at the Institute of Preventive Medicine, Hyderabad to strengthen the country's capacity to respond to potential bio-terror attacks.[15]

The urgency of such preparedness became starkly clear in 2001 when the world was confronted with the real possibility of biological warfare. Soon after the 9/11 attacks, letters laced with anthrax germs began appearing in the US post, sending shockwaves across global security and public health systems. Five Americans were killed and seventeen were infected with the gram-negative bacteria in what became the worst biological attacks in US history.[16]

In no time, a similar threat reached India. On 30 October 2001, an envelope containing some powdery substance, later suspected to be anthrax, was received at Rashtrapati Bhawan, the official residence of the President of India in New Delhi. This followed similar letters reaching the then Home Minister L. K. Advani, the Ministry of Health, the Law Ministry and other government departments. By then, the National Institute of Communicable Diseases, the nodal agency, had been flooded with close to 100 such letters from different parts of the country for examination.[17] Eventually, none of these letters were found to contain anthrax spores* of any kind.

Anthrax is a rare but serious illness caused by *Bacillus anthracis*, mainly affecting livestock and wild game. Humans can get infected through contact with sick animals, contaminated meat or by inhaling spores, but it is not transmitted from person to person. Symptoms vary but primarily include skin sores, vomiting and shock. Prompt antibiotic treatment can cure most infections, though inhaled anthrax is harder to treat and can be fatal. While rare in the developed world, anthrax remains a concern due to its use in bioterrorism.

The attack in the US and Indian mail scares brought home a serious concern – the lack of countermeasures in case of a real attack. India did not have a stockpile of anthrax vaccine or an indigenously

* Tiny, tough versions of the anthrax bacteria that can survive harsh conditions and can be inhaled, making them dangerous as biological weapons.

developed vaccine against the bacillus. It took another eight years for an anthrax vaccine to be made available in the country. Since 2009, Emergent BioSolutions – the developer of BioThrax, the only US FDA-approved anthrax vaccine – has been offering the vaccine in the country after receiving market authorization from the DCGI. Biological E. has since been distributing this vaccine in India.[18]

The market authorization for BioThrax vaccine was followed by the 2008 National Disaster Management Guidelines from the Indian National Disaster Management Authority (NDMA). The agency specified the management of biological disasters and recommended certain measures, such as having a ready supply of anthrax vaccines for deployment in the event of an outbreak.

BioThrax, originally known as Anthrax Vaccine Adsorbed, was developed in the 1950s by the United States Public Health Service and was first licensed for human use in 1970. The US Department of Defense and Department of Health and Human Services were the main buyers with almost 10 million courses (60 million doses) consistently produced in the US Strategic National Stockpile for mass vaccinations in case of any bio-terrorist attack using anthrax spores.

Originally produced by the Michigan Department of Public Health, the ownership of vaccine production changed hands after the State of Michigan converted the unit into a private enterprise known as the Michigan Biologic Products Institute (MBPI) in 1990. By 1998, MBPI was acquired by BioPort Corporation of Lansing, Michigan for approximately $24 million. BioPort changed its name to Emergent BioSolutions in 2004.

The US stockpile was an answer to Russia's stockpile of biological weapons, including anthrax and Ebola microbes. Since 1979, the Soviet Union had preferred anthrax spores as a bioweapon and had also developed an effective vaccine by 1960. The Soviet STI-anthrax vaccine was the first vaccine created in a biological warfare facility and the country had been using this biowarfare technology for the benefit of public health.

After the collapse of the Soviet Union, the anthrax spore stockpiles were not completely destroyed, but kept by the Russian agency for biological weapons, Biopreparat, which has been operating with relative autonomy and had the Ministry of Defence as its sole customer. By 1998 February, reports that the Russians had developed a new anthrax strain by genetic engineering sent shockwaves around the world. The US was naturally worried about the effectiveness of its vaccine against this new strain, and there was no way to assess its efficacy without obtaining a sample of the new strain.

Therefore, when the anthrax letter bomb incidents in the US and the hoaxes in India occurred, many Indian groups swung into action – private firms, government institutes, defence labs and academic institutes. The group that eventually succeeded was a team of researchers from the School of Biotechnology at the Jawaharlal Nehru University (JNU), New Delhi.

The team combined a protective antigen protein and a protein present in the outer layer of the anthrax spore.[19] The Department of Biotechnology supported the project and funded JNU to set up a Biosafety Level-3 laboratory at the School of Biotechnology. In fact, a few weeks after the letter bomb scare in the capital, the minister in charge of Science and Technology, Murali Manohar Joshi, made an announcement that the JNU team had been working on a recombinant anthrax vaccine since 1995, which would be produced by Panacea soon.[20]

However, it took another two decades of conducting animal and human trials and receiving regulatory approvals for the vaccine to be ready for a market launch. It was only in 2009 that a peer-reviewed primate study was published by the JNU team.[21] It is common knowledge that vaccine development is a long cycle, either by the government or by private entities. The International Federation of Pharmaceutical Manufacturers & Associations projects the cycle for the development of a novel vaccine to be ten to fifteen years.[22] For academic institutions like JNU, such cycles can be longer given the constraints of funding.

Panacea participated in a global competitive bidding by the US Department of Health and Human Services (HHS) for supplying 25 million doses of recombinant anthrax vaccine even as the development and clinical trials were on, but it was summarily rejected.[23] Ever since, Panacea has faced a lot of troubles in the Western market, given its possession of a technology that can be associated with biological weapons. It has been on the radar of US agencies including the Biomedical Advanced Research and Development Authority, the Department of Defense's Biological Threat Reduction Programme and so on.

The US Centres for Disease Control (CDC) considers germs responsible for anthrax, botulism, plague, smallpox, tularemia and viral haemorrhagic fevers such as Ebola, Marburg, Lassa and Machupo as agents that can be used as biological weapons for mass destruction.[24] The Office of Chemical and Biological Weapons Affairs (CBW) monitors all firms and entities in possession of any agents with potential as a bioweapon.

Aside from Panacea, several Indian vaccine manufacturers too have faced significant hurdles – including restrictions on cross-border movement of goods and personnel, as well as delays in obtaining clearance for procuring advanced machinery and equipment from the West. These challenges stem primarily from concerns that their technology could, in theory, be weaponized.

The US strictly enforces the Biological Weapons Convention (BWC), which prohibits the development, stockpiling, acquisition, retention or production of biological agents and toxins for non-peaceful purposes. As a result, Indian vaccine companies have often found themselves caught in the crosshairs, with executives and consignments facing rigorous screening and monitoring by US border control agencies. According to US authorities, such scrutiny is necessary to enforce its ban on the transfer or acquisition of biological agents, toxins, weapons and delivery systems. However, once a company falls under the scrutiny of these agencies, it remains indefinitely in the spotlight.

The threats posed by viruses like Ebola and bacteria like anthrax are not just public health emergencies; they are tests of global solidarity, scientific readiness and political will. If the Ebola epidemic revealed the consequences of delayed action and neglected R&D, the anthrax scares highlighted the importance of anticipating the unthinkable.

As the world continues to battle unpredictable outbreaks and silent biological threats, it must ask itself whether it is prepared – not just to respond, but to anticipate, innovate and act decisively.

PART V

GLOBAL LEADERSHIP
(2011–2025)

38

THE QUEST FOR CANCER VACCINES

IN MARCH 2024, *NATURE* CARRIED A STRIKING HEADLINE: 'Cutting-edge CAR-T cancer therapy is now made in India – at one-tenth the cost'.

Just a month later, the President of India Droupadi Murmu formally launched the therapy, hailing it as the country's first homegrown gene therapy for cancer. Developed by a team of Indian scientists and cleared by regulators in late 2023, the therapy marked a watershed moment in Indian biomedical innovation.

At the centre of this revolution was an unassuming but determined thirty-five-year-old scientist: Alka Dwivedi.

Dwivedi and her team had achieved what many thought impossible – they had indigenously redesigned the most cutting-edge, patented cancer therapy of the West, capable of curing advanced blood and lymph cancers, and slashed its price by nearly 90 per cent without compromising on efficacy or safety.

It was the kind of medical breakthrough that might have made Dwivedi a household name anywhere else. But lost among the 1.4 billion people of India, she was barely recognized outside her circles, save some mentions in the *Hindu* and *India Today*. The Indian media was busy covering political turmoil and parliamentary elections when the news broke, while social media was captivated by the Ambani wedding, celebrity airport looks and influencer feuds. Dwivedi's achievement – one that could save countless lives around the world for decades, if not centuries – was drowned out by clickbait content and election drama.

Dwivedi's journey to this milestone was as remarkable as this cancer vaccine itself. Raised in the narrow lines of dusty Mirzapur in rural Uttar Pradesh, she completed her schooling and early university in Mirzapur. She then pursed biotechnology for her master's at a little-known university in Nagpur. A brief internship at IISc, Bangalore during her master's opened her eyes to the world of serious scientific research.

She gained some industrial exposure at Japanese life sciences firm Daiichi Sankyo in Gurgaon, followed by a year-long stint at the Indian Agricultural Research Institute (IARI), New Delhi. There, she worked on plant-nematode interactions using RNA interference – her first real brush with genetic engineering. After a year at IARI's iconic Pusa campus, she joined IIT Bombay's Biosciences and Bioengineering Department.

That's where she met Dr Rahul Purwar, an immunologist trained at Harvard Medical School and Hannover Medical School. Together, they set their sights on cancer immunotherapy – often referred to as 'cancer vaccine' because it helps the body to generate own immunity against cancer cells. Their objective: bring the Western designed CAR-T cell therapy to India and make it accessible to Indian patients. They got medical support from Dr Gaurav Narula and Dr Hasmukh Jain, two expert oncologists at the nearby Tata Memorial cancer hospital.

CAR-T cell therapy, hailed as a breakthrough in oncology, involves extracting a patient's T-cells, genetically engineering them with synthetic receptors (CARs) and reinfusing them into the body to hunt and destroy cancer cells. This 'living drug' has achieved astonishing success in treating blood cancers like leukemia and lymphoma since its advent, especially in children.[1] But the cost was prohibitive – up to ₹30–40 million (roughly $500,000) per patient even as cancer has been emerging as one of the worst killers in the modern world.[2]

Over the past decades, the incidence of cancer has been steadily rising across the globe. In 2022, the most commonly diagnosed cancers were lung cancer (2.5 million cases), breast cancer in women (2.3 million) and colorectal cancer (1.9 million). Lung cancer was the leading cause of cancer-related deaths, claiming approximately 1.8 million lives in a single year, followed by colorectal (900,000 deaths) and liver cancers (760,000 deaths).[3] In 2020, there were an estimated 19.3 million new cancer cases and 10 million deaths due to cancer worldwide.[4] By 2022, the number of new cases increased to an estimated 20 million. According to WHO, one in five people develop cancer during their lifetime – about one in nine men and one in twelve women dying from the disease.[5]

According to the National Cancer Registry Programme, the official source for India's cancer data, approximately 1.46 million new cancer cases are diagnosed each year in the country.[6] The WHO India data for 2022 reported 192,000 new breast cancer cases, 82,000 new lung cancer cases, 127,000 new cervical cancer cases, 70,000 new colorectal cancer cases and 213,000 new cases of head and neck cancers. In India, nearly 917,000 people die from cancer every year, with 75,000 deaths attributed to lung cancer, 98,000 to breast cancer, 80,000 to cervical cancer, 80,000 to oral cancer and 58,000 to stomach cancer.[7] Besides this alarming data, a large number of cases go unreported beyond the coverage of cancer hospitals and in rural areas.

The incidence of cancer has been on the rise due to growing environmental pollution, over-use of plastics and chemicals and increasing dependence on processed and packaged food. The affected patients have been desperately seeking a cure. One of the reliable solutions that emerged in the West in the new millennium was CAR-T.

The concept of CAR-T originated in Israel in the late 1980s and was brought to clinical fruition by renowned oncologist Carl June's team in the US, with the launch of the first human trial in 2011. CAR-T cell therapy took immunotherapy to a highly personalized level – a patient's own T-cells are extracted and genetically altered to recognize cancer. When infused back into the patient, these tailored cells seek out and destroy malignant cells with heightened precision.

In 2017, US FDA approved two CAR-T therapies – Kymriah (Novartis) and Yescarta (Gilead) – that made headlines for their remarkable success in treating certain leukemias and lymphomas, especially in children. The therapy marked a new era of 'living drugs'* that are custom-made to each patient's cancer. Despite its promise, high costs and complex logistics made CAR-T therapy inaccessible for most of the world.

When Dwivedi arrived at IIT Bombay in 2015, CAR-T trials in the US were gaining momentum. But in India – where nearly 1.5 million new cancer cases were being reported annually – the therapy was out of reach for most. When she witnessed cancer patients lining up daily at the nearby Tata Memorial Hospital, the mission became a personal one for Dwivedi, setting her on track to develop a safe, effective and affordable version of CAR-T therapy in India, by India, for India.

Dwivedi led the technical process – designing the CAR and producing the viral vector that delivers cancer-fighting genes into a patient's T-cells. But resources were scarce. A better equipped bioengineering lab was still under construction at IIT Bombay, and a variety of equipment had to be imported. Every step was a struggle. More significantly, researchers with know-how and hands-on experience were hard to come by.[8] The silver lining was that the project had received key support from Tata Trust in the beginning with ₹1.76 million and later from National Biopharma Mission through BIRAC, which sanctioned ₹191.5 million to fund the Phase I/II clinical trials.[9]

A breakthrough came in 2017 after Dwivedi spent time at the US National Cancer Institute, where she picked up critical know-how in CAR-T cell manufacturing and viral vector development.

* A nickname for treatments like CAR-T, where a patient's own cells are modified and used as medicine.

Returning to Mumbai, she cracked key challenges in CAR and vector production and began generating CAR T-cells in the lab. Animal trials showed promising remission rates. The project soon received a regulatory green light for clinical trials on cancer patients.[10]

By 2021, the team had built a GMP-grade facility at IIT Bombay – one that met WHO standards for sterility and safety. Clinical trials began shortly after, enrolling informed patients from Tata Memorial battling advanced leukemia and lymphoma.[11]

4 June 2021 marked a historic milestone in India's cancer care journey. At the Bone Marrow Transplant unit of Tata Memorial Centre (TMC) in Mumbai, the country's first CAR-T cell therapy was successfully administered to patients by Narula and team. The results were stunning. Nearly three of four patients responded to the therapy, and almost half of them went into complete remission. Even more encouraging was the reduced toxicity. By tweaking the therapy design, the team managed to minimize dangerous side effects, making treatment safer and more tolerable.[12]

Just as important was how they did it. Every component – from viral vectors to cell-processing systems – was made in India. No costly imports. No reliance on foreign patents. The result: a world-class CAR-T therapy at one-tenth the cost of its Western counterparts. In October 2023, the therapy – branded NexCAR19 – received approval from India's Central Drugs Standard Control Organization, becoming the country's first sanctioned CAR T-cell product.

By mid-2024, more than 150 patients had received NexCAR19. The team expects that number to cross 500 by 2025. Construction is underway on a larger manufacturing facility on the outskirts of Mumbai, with the goal of producing 1,200 treatments annually.[13] The new site will house high-efficiency labs for vector and CAR T-cell production, along with expanded quality control units to accelerate turnaround time. The team dreams of bringing down the cost of the therapy to as little as ₹10,000 one day.[14]

But their ambition doesn't stop there – nor at India's borders. The team's startup ImmunoACT, after enlisting as many as eighteen hospitals across twenty-eight cities in India, has signed up with the Government of Mexico and is exploring partnerships in other low- and middle-income countries, where access to cutting-edge cancer care remains elusive.

From a modest lab at IIT Bombay to global recognition, the journey of Alka Dwivedi and her colleagues has redefined what is possible in Indian science. In 2024, the *Bulletin of the World Health Organization* published a rare feature-length interview with her. The same year, *TIME* featured her, along with nineteen other emerging healthcare personalities from around the globe, on its TIME100 Health list – a fitting tribute to a mission driven by science, equity and unrelenting hope.

CAR-T-cell therapy came at a time when there wasn't any cure for blood and lymph cancers. In fact, the concept of a 'cure' for cancer often depends on the type of cancer, its stage at diagnosis and individual patient factors. One cannot develop a preventive vaccine for most forms of cancer – except for virus-induced ones – because vaccines are meant to prevent diseases caused by identifiable external agents, and cancer is typically not caused by such agents.

Two vaccines are in use in the category of preventive cancer vaccines – able to stop cancer before it begins, by training the immune system to recognize and eliminate viruses that are known to trigger cancer development. These vaccines are not trained to target cancer cells, but rather the pathogens causing viral infections that can eventually lead to it. By preventing such infections, the vaccines significantly reduce the risk of associated cancers.

The most prominent example is the HPV vaccine, which protects against high-risk strains like HPV-16 and HPV-18 that are responsible for majority of cervical cancer cases. Distributed by the Serum Institute as Cervavac, Merck as Gardasil and GlaxoSmithKline as Cervarix, these vaccines also guard against other HPV-induced cancers of the anus, throat, penis, vulva and vagina. Indian regulators approved Cervarix for cancers of the cervix, vulva, vagina and anus in women and for anal cancer and genital warts in men.[15] It also helps prevent pre-cancerous changes in these areas, which can lead to cancer if left untreated. With strong efficacy in preventing both cancer and precancerous lesions,* of late the HPV vaccine has been integrated into many national immunization programmes globally.

Another vital example is the hepatitis B vaccine (HBV), which prevents infection from the hepatitis B virus – a key cause of liver cancer (hepatocellular carcinoma). Like the HPV vaccine, HBV doesn't target cancer itself but cuts off its root cause by preventing chronic viral infection. Its widespread use has led to a sharp decline in liver cancer rates, particularly in high-prevalence regions such as India. Endorsed by WHO, HBV plays a central role in global liver cancer prevention efforts.

In such conventional vaccines against bacterial and viral infections, non-infected people are exposed to a weakened or an inactivated form of the threat which allows the immune system to recognize the specific markers, or 'antigens,' of the pathogen and mount a defensive response in advance. Unlike bacteria and viruses, which are easily recognized as foreign by the body's immune system, cancer cells closely resemble normal, healthy cells. Additionally, each person's tumour is unique and has its own set of specific antigens. For these reasons preventive vaccines, which are effective only against infectious diseases, are not feasible against most cancers. Researchers realized long ago that more advanced methods were needed to fight cancer. That led to the development of targeted cancer vaccines and cancer immunotherapies.

Targeted vaccines are designed to stimulate the immune system to attack cancer cells that express specific tumour-associated antigens,† aiming to destroy malignant cells while sparing normal ones. On the other hand, cancer immunotherapies, also sometimes referred to as 'cancer vaccines', are therapies that boost or direct the immune system to recognize and fight cancer. Often called 'immunotherapeutic

---

* Abnormal tissue changes that aren't cancer yet but can become cancer if not treated.

† Markers found on cancer cells that help the immune system recognize and attack them.

vaccines', they trigger an immune response specifically against cancer cells, offering promising avenues for treatment, not prevention.

There are several types of immunotherapy: some use lab-made antibodies to block cancer's defense mechanisms (like checkpoint inhibitors*), while others involve boosting immune cells taken from the patient by modifying them in a lab and putting them back in the body to fight cancer (like CAR-T cell therapy). Certain therapies use proteins or genetic material (like DNA or mRNA†) to teach the body to recognize cancer, much like a vaccine. Others use harmless viruses to deliver cancer-fighting instructions or even directly kill cancer cells.

To deliver cancer-fighting instructions into the body, researchers have developed various methods, including using modified viruses to carry antigens directly to tumour sites and trigger an immune response. The immune system responds when an altered virus, or viral vector, is introduced into the body. Another approach involves using the whole cancer cell, rather than a specific cell antigen, to make the vaccine. These cancer cells are modified in the laboratory to make them more recognizable to the immune system, prompting an immune response. This method uses cancer cells from the patient or a donor, or grown in the laboratory.

A notable example of this method is PROVENGE, a sipuleucel-T vaccine developed by the US-based cellular therapy firm Dendreon, designed to treat advanced prostate cancer. In this treatment, specific immune cells called antigen-presenting cells (APCs)‡ are collected from the patient's blood. These cells are then exposed in the lab to a protein found on prostate cancer cells,

---

* Drugs that remove the 'brakes' from the immune system, helping it fight cancer more effectively.

† Messenger RNA (abbreviated mRNA) is a type of single-stranded RNA involved in protein synthesis. mRNA is made from a DNA template during the process of transcription.

‡ Immune cells that show other immune cells what to attack, sort of like showing a 'wanted poster' of the invader.

which trains them to recognize and remember this protein. Once reintroduced into the patient's body, these activated cells work with the immune system, especially white blood cells called T cells and B cells, to destroy the malignant cells.

The third approach involves developing vaccines using special proteins or small protein pieces like peptides found in cancer cells. The genetic codes of these cancer cell proteins are copied in the labs and replicated in large quantities. These are then used to train the immune system to recognize and respond to cancer cells.

The fourth approach uses fragments of genetic material DNA or RNA found in cancer cells to make vaccines. Once injected into the body, these fragments instruct body cells to make proteins that trigger an immune response against the cancer.

In the early 1990s, Japanese immunologist Tasuku Honjo made a discovery that first set the course for the future of cancer treatment. He identified a protein called PD-1, a kind of molecular 'brake' that prevents the immune system from attacking the body's own tissues. Around the same time, American scientist James P. Allison was exploring another immune checkpoint called CTLA-4.* Both researchers realized that cancer cells were exploiting these brakes to hide from immune attack. Their work led to the development of immune checkpoint inhibitors – drugs that release these brakes and allow T-cells to fight cancer. This groundbreaking approach became the foundation for therapies like Keytruda from Merck & Co. and Opdivo from Bristol-Myers Squib,† now being used to treat cancers such as melanoma, lung and bladder cancer. For this pioneering work, Allison and Honjo were awarded the 2018 Nobel Prize in Physiology or Medicine.[16]

Another frontier in targeted cancer vaccines is personalized neoantigen vaccines. These vaccines are created by sequencing an

---

* CTLA-4 and PD-1are both proteins that act like brakes in the immune system. Cancer can use them to hide from being attacked.

† Keytruda and Opdivo are brand names of checkpoint inhibitor drugs that help the immune system attack cancer.

individual's tumour to identify unique genetic mutations – called neoantigens – present only in the cancer cells. This vaccine trains the immune system to recognize and attack cells with these neoantigens. One of the most promising trials in this space has been by Moderna and Merck. They combined Moderna's personalized mRNA-based neoantigen vaccine (mRNA-4157/V940) with Merck's checkpoint inhibitor – monoclonal antibody pembrolizumab branded as Keytruda.[17] This combination showed encouraging results in reducing recurrence in end-stage melanoma patients, sparking widespread excitement about the potential of tailored cancer vaccines.

Yet another major advance was Tumour-Infiltrating Lymphocyte (TIL)* therapy, which harnesses the immune system's natural response to cancer. In this method, T-cells that have already migrated into a tumour are harvested, multiplied in large numbers in the lab, and then reinfused into the patient. These 'ready-to-fight' immune cells have shown promising results in patients with melanoma, and clinical trials are underway for other cancers of cervix and lung. Unlike CAR-T therapy, which requires genetic engineering, TIL therapy uses the body's own anti-tumour response, amplified and redirected for therapeutic effect. In March 2024, the first TIL therapy – for advanced melanoma – secured the FDA approval.[18]

As researchers refine these techniques, TIL therapy continues to offer hope as a potent weapon in the growing arsenal of cancer immunotherapies.

Another innovation in cancer immunotherapy involves dendritic cell-based vaccines. Dendritic cells, a type of immune cells, help the immune system recognize and attack abnormal cells. The dendritic cell vaccines stimulate the immune system to attack the cancer cells. Two dozen vaccines, based on dendritic cells against breast cancer, are currently under various stages of development in different labs.[19] Even though dendritic cells-based vaccines were

* TILs are immune cells that have already entered a tumour to try and fight it. They are collected, multiplied in the lab, and put back in the body to boost the fight against cancer.

first attempted twenty years ago, clinical trials are progressing at a slow pace. These trials focus on various types of cancers, including carcinoma (epithelial cells covering organs and tissues), melanoma (skin cancer arising from melanocytes), glioma (cancer of the brain or spine originating from cells supporting nerve cells), sarcoma (cancer of connective tissues like bone, muscle, cartilage, fat or blood vessels) and lymphoma (cancer of the lymphatic system).[20]

One notable example of such vaccine, or more accurately an immunotherapy, that recently entered the final stages of clinical trials was based on a work initiated by Chandrima Shaha and her colleague Anil Suri at the NII, New Delhi way back in 1988.[21] It took three decades for Suri and his collaborator T Rajkumar from the Cancer Institute, Adyar, Chennai to develop this work into a meaningful outcome – a dendritic cell (DC)-based vaccine/immunotherapy targeting cervical, ovarian and breast cancers. It is named ASPAGNII.[22]

The story of ASPAGNII began unexpectedly, in the realm of reproductive biology. When Shaha began her research on antisperm antibodies* at the newly established NII in the 1980s, under the guidance of renowned immunologist T. P. Talwar, she was investigating the immunological roots of infertility. Drawing on her prior work with the Population Council in New York, Shaha focused on isolating sperm antigens† that could potentially be used in anti-fertility vaccines.

Her methodical experiments involved collecting fresh human semen samples, purifying the sperm and immunizing rabbits to generate antibodies. These antibodies were then extracted, refined and analyzed using techniques such as gel electrophoresis‡ and

---

* These are immune system proteins that mistakenly attack a person's own sperm, potentially leading to infertility.

† Tiny molecules on the surface of sperm that the immune system can recognize. Scientists study them to create fertility or cancer vaccines.

‡ A lab technique used to separate proteins or DNA based on their size using an electric field.

Western blotting.* Her goal was to identify specific antigenic proteins involved in fertility, a mission that demanded immense patience and precision.

Nearly a decade later, her colleague Suri carried this research forward and reported the discovery of a protein called SPAG9 (Sperm-Associated Antigen 9). The SPAG9 gene – located on chromosome 17q21.33† in humans and chromosome 11 in mice – was initially thought to be active only in testicular tissue, where it played a role in sperm development.[23] However, Suri's work revealed a surprising twist: SPAG9 was also expressed in several cancerous tissues, especially epithelial ovarian cancer.‡[24] This opened up a new avenue – repurposing what was once a fertility antigen into a novel target for cancer vaccines.

In time, SPAG9 became the core of ASPAGNII, the immunotherapy that carried forward decades of Indian research into a real-world application. From infertility studies to oncology, the story of SPAG9 exemplifies how fundamental research in one field can serendipitously pave the way for breakthroughs in another.

During this long testing period, the duo conducted clinical trials at the Cancer Institute, Adyar on a large number of cervical cancer patients. In the process, Suri set up the Centre for Cancer Immunotherapy at NII to undertake clinical trials funded by the Department of Science and Technology. ICMR joined the team, offering support to conduct clinical trials among Stage IV§ ovarian cancer patients. With backing from the Department of Biotechnology, the team had also been conducting a Phase II randomized controlled

---

* A lab test used to detect specific proteins in a sample, often after gel electrophoresis.

† A specific location on the long arm (q) of chromosome 17 in the human genome, specifically within the 21.33 band. Chromosomes are like instruction books in each cell, and this refers to a certain 'page and line' in the book.

‡ A common type of ovarian cancer that begins in the outer layer (epithelium) of the ovary.

§ The most advanced form of cancer, where it has spread to other parts of the body.

clinical trial* to evaluate the effectiveness of ASPAGNII among certain types of recurrent breast cancer.[25]

SPAG9 was licensed to Syngene International, a subsidiary of Bangalore-based Biocon Limited, promoted by entrepreneur Kiran Mazumdar-Shaw, way back in 2017.[26] Touted as a promising breakthrough in India's cancer vaccine research, SPAG9 held promise to treat multiple tumour types. However, little has been heard from Syngene regarding its clinical progress or market readiness, suggesting either scientific hurdles, regulatory delays or limited commercial prioritization.

Meanwhile, a different therapy approach has gained traction – repurposing established vaccines. BCG vaccine, which provides protection against tuberculosis, has been found to be effective in treating early-stage bladder cancer. It has been widely used since 1990, when the US FDA approved it for high-risk non-muscle invasive bladder cancer. Similarly, the MMR vaccine has shown potential in treating certain cancers, with studies indicating that vaccine-derived viruses can activate the tumour immune microenvironment,† leading to a multifaceted antitumour immune response.[27]

In addition to repurposing licensed vaccines, researchers have explored the use of live virus strains being used in vaccines or their genetically modified derivatives as cancer immunotherapy agents. For instance, the polio virus strain used in oral and inactivated polio vaccines (OPV/IPV) has been adapted into a modified virus known as PVSRIPO, which is being tested in clinical trials for glioblastoma, fast-growing brain cancer originating from glial cell. While this builds on a known vaccine strain, it functions more as a vector than a repurposed vaccine.

Similarly, the YF17D strain of the yellow fever vaccine – renowned for its robust immune-stimulating properties – is being evaluated in

---

* A carefully designed medical study where participants are randomly assigned to receive either the new treatment or a standard one, to compare which works better.

† The mix of cells, signals and conditions around a tumour that can either help or block the immune system's attack on the cancer.

preclinical models as a potential cancer immunotherapy platform, though it has not yet reached clinical deployment. Other notable examples include Talimogene laherparepvec (T-VEC), a genetically modified herpes simplex virus approved for treating advanced melanoma, and Pexa-Vec, based on a modified vaccinia virus – both designed to selectively infect and kill cancer cells while stimulating systemic anti-tumour immunity. These approaches represent a growing class of virus-based immunotherapies.

What had long confounded researchers and oncologists was the realization that a one-size-fits-all approach to cancer prevention was implausible, due to the diverse origins of malignancy in cancer cells. While some cancers are induced by viral infections, most arise from genetic predispositions or environmental interference on the body's physiology. By the last decade of the last millennium, the hope for a universal cancer vaccine had largely diminished.

Then, in 2000, breaking news from Duke University in the US reignited the hope that the development of a universal cancer vaccine might be within reach. As reported in *Nature Medicine*, preliminary laboratory studies offered the first functional evidence that developing a 'universal' cancer vaccine was scientifically viable. Indian-origin researcher Smita Kesavan Nair identified a polypeptide component called telomerase (TERT) which she called 'an attractive candidate' for the purpose. She explained that TERT is found to be a broadly expressed tumour rejection antigen and is silent in normal tissues but found to be reactivated in more than 85 per cent of cancers.[28]

In healthy cells, the telomerase complex found in ribonucleoprotein shows minimal activity, whereas it is highly active in over 85 per cent of tumours. Therefore, a promising approach for a universal cancer vaccine involved stimulating the immune system to target and destroy tumour cells by focusing on this polypeptide component.

Way back in 1995, Nair also pioneered the use of mRNA (messenger RNA) as a therapeutic tool for cancer vaccines. Her research team was also the first to develop a cancer vaccine by extracting dendritic cells with mRNA from the patient's tumour and then reintroducing the modified cells back into the patient. Nair's team demonstrated the feasibility of using dendritic cells as an effective platform for delivering RNA to cancer patients in 1996,[29] and the technology was licensed to a cancer therapy firm in North Carolina, Argos Therapeutics Inc. This study was the first to prove that RNA could be utilized as a vaccine and scaled up for mass production in clinical applications.[30]

On the Indian landscape, two key projects are currently underway at IISc. At the Organic Chemistry Department, young scholar Keerthana Thekke Veettil's six-year-long research under N Jayaraman focuses on a new method of synthetically made Tn Glycolipid hitchhiking a ride in the bloodstream. In her approach a synthetic Tn glycolipid – mimicking a cancer-specific marker – is chemically tagged to bind albumin in the bloodstream, which naturally carries it to lymph nodes where it activates immune cells to recognize and remember the Tn antigen. This primes the body to mount a targeted immune attack if actual tumour cells bearing the antigen are encountered later. This approach makes it a promising method for cancer vaccines. The study, gaining attention from cancer innovators worldwide, is expected to utilize albumin-mediated delivery for various cancers and immunotherapies.[31]

The second project is being led by Purusharth I. Rajyaguru from the Biochemistry Department. His work on sodium azide-induced translation repression and RNA granule assembly could lead to innovations in cancer vaccines and immunotherapies. By studying how RGG-motif proteins regulate mRNA dynamics and stress responses, his research provides insights into the molecular mechanisms cancer cells exploit for survival. These processes could help develop novel cancer vaccines that enhance antigen presentation and immune recognition of tumour cells. Beyond cancer, these insights into RNA regulation and stress responses can drive advancements in mRNA-based solutions for other diseases as well, expanding the potential of mRNA technology in biomedical applications.[32]

These groundbreaking studies, both in India and globally, highlight the remarkable strides being made in the field of cancer vaccines. As the world moves toward personalized medicine, mRNA-based cancer vaccines represent a transformative shift in how we understand and treat cancer. The ability to tailor vaccines to the unique genetic profile of a patient's tumour offers the promise of a more effective, less invasive treatment strategy. With each milestone, from the pioneering efforts of Indian-origin Nair's team to the cutting-edge research at institutions like IISc, the foundation is being laid for a future where cancer can be fought not with broad-spectrum therapies, but with individualized vaccines that empower the immune system to target and eliminate cancer cells more precisely.

However, while the potential of these innovations is immense, the road ahead remains complex. As promising as personalized cancer vaccines are, challenges persist in scaling these therapies for widespread clinical use. The integration of new delivery methods, the refinement of RNA technologies and the need for extensive clinical trials to ensure efficacy and safety will require both scientific rigour and global collaboration. But the persistence of researchers around the world, from India to the United States, signals that we are closer than ever to a breakthrough that could redefine cancer prevention.

What once seemed like an insurmountable challenge is now within reach, and the next decade could very well witness the rise of cancer vaccines that bring us closer to the ultimate goal: real and effective prevention.

39

AIDS VACCINES

IN 1985, A THIRTY-TWO-YEAR-OLD MICROBIOLOGY RESEARCHER at Madras Medical College was searching for a thesis topic when her professor, Suniti Solomon, suggested an unusual idea – to screen people in the city for Human Immunodeficiency Virus (HIV).

It had been four years since the US CDC first reported clinical evidence of what would later be known as acquired immunodeficiency syndrome (AIDS). The CDC report marked the beginning of a global epidemic that, over the next two decades, would spread across the world, triggering panic among vulnerable groups, especially sex workers. Soon, researchers across the globe began identifying the virus in their respective geographies.

At the time, Hollywood star Rock Hudson had just announced that he was suffering from AIDS, shaking the Western world into a harsh new reality – promiscuous behaviour could prove lethal. India, too, had launched its own hunt for the virus. Hundreds of blood samples from Bombay's red-light districts were tested at the National Institute of Virology (NIV), Pune – all returned negative.

Compared to Bombay, Madras was viewed as more conservative, making the likelihood of finding a positive case seem highly improbable. Some news magazines even joked that by the time the virus reached Madras, Americans would already have found a cure.

So when Solomon suggested the topic, her student Sellappan Nirmala was sceptical. After much persuasion, however, she decided to give it a shot. With no established red-light areas in the city, Nirmala tracked down unseen sex workers by scouring the streets and a government shelter home. The blood samples she finally collected were sent to Christian Medical College (CMC), Vellore, for ELISA testing.*[1]

Heading the virology department at the CMC, Jacob John took care of the sample tests. Out of the 300 odd samples, six tested positive – all collected from the shelter home. The findings raised alarm, prompting the immediate involvement of ICMR.

Since its identification, AIDS had become one of the most dreaded diseases in India. The HIV virus attacks the immune system, progressively weakening the body's ability to fight off infections and diseases. As the disease progresses, individuals may experience a range of debilitating symptoms, including opportunistic infections,† cancers and neurological disorders. Witnessing the deterioration of a loved one's health, leading to their eventual death, was devastating for those left behind.

For Solomon and Nirmala, their worst fear had come true – the virus had finally arrived on the Indian shores. Struggling to accept the results, the team decided to collect one more set of samples from the six individuals who had tested positive and sent them to the US CDC for confirmation using Western blot tests. When the results came, all six were confirmed to be positive.

ICMR confidentially shared the grim news with Prime Minister Rajiv Gandhi and Tamil Nadu Chief Minister M. G. Ramachandran. A few days later, M.G.R.'s health minister H. V. Hande announced the findings in the state assembly, making headlines across major newspapers the following day. The initial reaction from the public was one of disbelief, with many questioning the accuracy of the tests while others doubted whether the virus was truly AIDS.

---

* A laboratory test that detects antibodies in blood. It's commonly used to screen for viruses like HIV.

† Infections that occur more often or are more severe in people with weakened immune systems, like those with HIV/AIDS.

Notwithstanding the initial knee-jerk reaction, HIV/AIDS soon escalated into a full-blown epidemic in India, spreading rapidly and penetrating every corner of the country. The speed and scale of transmissions were staggering. By the early 2000s, AIDS had turned into a devastating global pandemic, infecting over 63 million people worldwide, with over 38 million living with HIV at any given time. Around 1.7 million new infections were reported in 2019. India emerged as the AIDS capital of the world by reporting the highest number of HIV infections, with around 5.2 million cases. This continued until 2006 when revised estimates nearly halved that figure. Nevertheless, over 2 million people in India still live with HIV and the disease – which is treatable but remains incurable – continues to claim a large number of lives in India.

Discrimination and social exclusion have made HIV/AIDS one of the most feared and stigmatized diseases. Misconceptions about the disease, its modes of transmission and the populations most affected by it have fuelled fear, prejudice and the marginalization of those living with the virus. It has also discouraged potential patients from seeking testing, treatment and support, exacerbating the spread of the disease and hindering efforts to address it effectively.

To prevent large-scale devastation, extensive screening and prevention programmes were initiated in Tamil Nadu very early on. When cases were reported from other regions, these programmes were extended to other parts of the country as well. Despite facing discrimination initially, Solomon rose to be a beacon of hope in India's fight against the virus, setting up programmes and institutes to counter the deadly virus. When this author met her at her office cum residence in 1994 to prepare a report for the Press Trust of India, she expressed hope that a vaccine would soon be developed.

Since the early days of the AIDS epidemic in the 1980s, there was optimism that a vaccine would soon be developed. Researchers around the world explored all possible avenues. After traditional vaccine approaches such as whole killed, live attenuated, subunit, peptide-based* and recombinant vaccines failed to yield any results, novel approaches like pseudovirions and virus-like particles – which resemble HIV but can't replicate or cause infection – were also explored. Scientists even pursued 'combined vaccines', which use a mix of different vaccine types within a single immunization schedule. Yet another option was to use Heat Shock Protein (HSP) for vaccination – proteins produced by cells in response to extreme stress like heat shocks to help stimulate the immune system. Among these approaches, DNA vaccines† and vaccines with DNA constructs emerged as front-runners till the advent of mRNA technology.[2]

Studies in primates showed that peptide-based vaccines might not effectively create broad protection against HIV. Using recombinant technology, researchers developed second-generation vaccine candidates, such as recombinant canarypox virus vectors.‡ Studies in mice and primates found that DNA vaccines can trigger immune responses against HIV-1. One promising approach was a DNA vaccine cassette§ that expresses multiple HIV genes, which has been shown to generate broad immune responses to different HIV strains,¶ a key requirement for a successful HIV vaccine.

However, this hope was soon tempered by numerous setbacks. Obstacles included HIV's vast genetic variability due to the lack of a proofreading mechanism** in reverse transcriptase,†† which allowed for rapid mutations during replication. Additionally, the absence of a

---

* Use short chains of amino acids (parts of proteins) from the virus.

† A vaccine made from small, lab-created pieces of DNA that tell the body to make parts of the virus, so the immune system learns to fight it.

‡ A vaccine method using a harmless bird virus (canarypox) altered to carry HIV genes to trigger immune response.

§ A specially designed piece of DNA carrying multiple viral genes for use in vaccines.

¶ Different genetic versions of HIV. Subtype B is common in Western countries; subtype C is common in India and Africa.

** A feature in most normal cell processes that checks for and fixes errors during DNA copying. HIV lacks this, leading to high mutation rates.

†† An enzyme used by HIV to copy its genetic material inside human cells. It's error-prone, which causes mutations.

suitable animal model, with chimpanzees proving inadequate, further hindered progress.

When the Indo-US Vaccine Programme, designed to develop vaccines against various infectious diseases, was extended for five more years in 1986, AIDS was added to the list of diseases for which vaccines would have to be developed collaboratively. Joining the effort were the Department of Biotechnology (DBT); the All India Institute of Medical Sciences (AIIMS); the National Institute of Communicable Diseases (NICD); CMC; and the National AIDS Research Institute (NARI).

The push for an indigenous HIV vaccine in India stemmed from concerns that vaccines developed in the West might not be effective against the different HIV subtypes prevalent in India. While subtype B was common in Western countries, subtype C was the dominant one in India. Therefore, Indian researchers aimed to develop a vaccine that could address local HIV-1 and HIV-2 strains and their diverse subtypes. Believing that a DNA vaccine cocktail containing gene sequences from prevalent subtypes would be the most cost-effective and straightforward approach, Indian scientists dabbled in that strategy for a while.

In 1999, the Indian government launched an ambitious project under the DBT to develop and manufacture 'home-grown' vaccines against several communicable diseases, including AIDS, with a funding of $4 million over a period of three years.[3] Research at AIIMS, New Delhi was focused on a modified pox virus construct expressing genes of the HIV-1 subtype-C and was expected to be ready for animal trials within twelve months, with clinical trials expected to begin within four years. On a visit to New Delhi, Jean-Louis Excler, senior director of International AIDS Vaccine Initiative (IAVI), responsible for several vaccine candidates in India, the US, Europe and Africa, expressed his concern that while DNA vaccines showed promise in animals, there was no proof that they would be effective in humans. Excler suggested that India could save on development costs by testing the canary pox virus-based HIV vaccine, already developed by Sanofi Pasteur in collaboration with the US Military HIV Research Programme (MHRP) and VaxGen.

By the late 1990s, Indian scientists were exploring various vaccine strategies, including DNA vaccines and recombinant viral vectors, to create a vaccine that could target the diverse subtypes of HIV present in India. Most of the projects received support from organizations like the NIH and UNAIDS. To work with international partners, ICMR set up a dedicated agency, the NARI, which is currently known as the National Institute of Translational Virology and AIDS Research (NITVAR).

By the turn of the millennium, intensified efforts in India's quest to develop an HIV vaccine began. In 2003, India conducted its first Phase I clinical trial of an HIV vaccine candidate. The vaccine, developed by IAVI in collaboration with NARI, was a recombinant modified vaccinia Ankara (MVA)* virus expressing HIV-1 genes. The trial was to assess the safety and immunogenicity of the vaccine candidate in Indian volunteers.[4]

Around the same time, Phase I trials for another significant DNA vaccine candidate, ADVAX, developed by IAVI and the Aaron Diamond AIDS Research Centre (ADARC), were underway. The trial was conducted at the Tuberculosis Research Centre in Chennai to evaluate the safety of the DNA vaccine in healthy volunteers. In 2006, the TBC-M4 vaccine developed by Therion Biologics Corporation in collaboration with IAVI and NARI, entered Phase I trials in Pune.[5] This candidate used a recombinant modified *vaccinia Ankara* vector to deliver HIV-1 subtype C genes. Despite showing a promising safety level, it disappointed the researchers in immunogenicity, leading them to reassess its potential.[6,7]

In parallel, a recombinant Adeno Associated Virus (rAAV) vector† vaccine developed by the US-based company Targeted Genetics using genes from the South African HIV strain was cleared

---

* A weakened version of the smallpox virus used as a vaccine base to deliver HIV genes.

† A harmless virus modified to deliver HIV genes as part of a vaccine. It doesn't cause illness but helps train the immune system.

for trials in India. Approved by Indian regulatory authorities, Phase I trials were planned at NARI in Pune as part of a multinational study. Despite concerns about the genetic difference between HIV strains, researchers noted over 90 per cent similarity in key regions, making it a viable candidate for India. The rAAV vaccine showed robust immune responses in animal models, but like many HIV vaccine candidates of that era, it did not progress significantly beyond early-phase trials.[8]

Yet another Indian effort came from Pradeep Seth's team at the AIIMS, New Delhi. This candidate used a DNA-based approach, with a prime-boost model involving a DNA vaccine followed by the MVA vector as a booster.[9] It was a fully indigenous effort aiming for safety and cost-effectiveness. Although it was ready for human trials around the same time as the MVA and rAAV candidates, it too struggled to gain regulatory clearance and sufficient momentum. Seth also stirred controversy when he tested the vaccine that had not yet received regulatory approval for human testing on himself, perhaps inspired by the legends of Louis Pasteur and other vaccine stalwarts. While Dr Seth defended the act as scientifically motivated, Samiran Nundy, editor of the *Indian Journal of Medical Ethics*, described it as reckless and driven by emotion rather than protocol.[10]

Then came the now infamous 'STEP Study' by Merck in 2009.[11] Although the study was primarily conducted in the United States, it included sites in India as well. The trial was called off when interim analyses showed that the vaccine did not prevent HIV infection nor did it reduce the viral load among infected individuals. Instead, it made the vaccinated people more susceptible to be infected with the virus.[12]

By 2012, Indian researchers shifted focus towards mosaic vaccines, which are designed to provide broader protection against diverse HIV strains. NARI and the Transnational Health Science and Technology Institute (THSTI) collaborated with international bodies like IAVI to explore these innovative vaccine designs.

From 2013 onwards, Indian researchers became involved in

global trials such as HVTN 100 and HVTN 702, which tested modified versions of the RV144 vaccine regimen. Although these trials were primarily conducted in South Africa, Indian scientists closely monitored the results for potential applicability in India.

The RV144 trial conducted jointly by the US military and the Thai Ministry of Public Health, though controversial, marked a significant milestone as the first and only HIV vaccine to provide protection, albeit at a modest 31.2 per cent. Notably, during the initial six months following peak response, the vaccine demonstrated a higher rate of protection at 60.5 per cent. However, its efficacy diminished due to the rapid decline of a weak antibody response. Further analysis indicated that the CD4+ T cells stimulated by the RV144 vaccine displayed reduced susceptibility to HIV infection, likely contributing to its protective efficacy.[13]

Later, India joined the trial of the Tat Oyi vaccine, developed by Biosantech, a French biotech company. This therapeutic vaccine, targeting the Tat protein of HIV, was tested for its ability to reduce the viral load in already infected individuals. The trials conducted in India were part of a broader international effort to assess the vaccine's therapeutic potential.[14]

Yet another important study was done at IISc on macaques, which showed that early immunization with broadly neutralizing antibodies (bNAb) significantly reduced the probability of HIV infection. Researchers from IISc's Chemical Engineering department designed a bNAb model that can trigger a long-lasting reduction in the viral load.[15] It also predicted that early bNAb therapy enhances the stimulation of the host's immune cells, providing a stronger defence compared to Antiretroviral Therapy (ART), which is the standard treatment for HIV.[16] The model was the first quantitative description of HIV dynamics under bNAb therapy and elucidated the mechanisms observed in the macaque study, supporting the potential of bNAb as a promising alternative to ART.

The 2020s have been marked by a significant leap in HIV vaccine research, fueled by breakthroughs in mRNA technology following the global success of Covid-19 vaccines. Pharmaceutical giant Moderna, in collaboration with IAVI, initiated clinical trials in 2022 for mRNA-based HIV vaccines aimed at inducing broadly neutralizing antibodies (bNAb). Central to this new wave was the concept of germline targeting, which involves priming the immune system through a carefully sequenced series of immunogens to eventually produce bNAb. Early-stage trials like IAVI G001 (2021) have shown promise by successfully triggering the desired B-cell precursors in humans.[17]

However, the journey remains challenging. For instance, the Imbokodo trial, which tested a different approach (Ad26 vector + gp140 protein), was discontinued in 2021 after failing to demonstrate efficacy.[18] Nonetheless, these efforts have significantly advanced the scientific tools and knowledge base – ranging from AI-assisted vaccine design and structural biology to rapid prototyping – laying the groundwork for potentially transformative breakthroughs in the years ahead.

Indian institutions like NARI, THSTI and IISc have consistently remained at the forefront of the global quest to develop a vaccine capable of eliciting strong cellular immunity, a crucial factor in controlling HIV infection. Their work increasingly draws from advanced technologies such as mRNA and viral vectors, reflecting the cutting-edge nature of ongoing research. In collaboration with IAVI, THSTI established the HIV Vaccine Translational Research (HVTR) Laboratory in Faridabad near New Delhi in 2012. This lab focuses on developing bnAbs against HIV-1 subtype C, prevalent in India. Despite its efforts to design preventive vaccines capable of eliciting immune responses against diverse HIV strains, none have progressed to trials. In 2019, THSTI was awarded a grant by the University of Oslo and IAVI from the Research Council of Norway for accelerating bnAbs research.

India's journey in HIV vaccine development has been marked by persistent efforts, scientific rigour, significant collaborations and notable trials. From early trials of indigenous DNA and MVA-based candidates to recent explorations in bNAb and mRNA strategies, Indian researchers have made considerable progress even in the face of immense challenges – ranging from the virus's staggering genetic diversity to the absence of optimal animal models.

Globally, the effort to develop an HIV vaccine remains one of the most ambitious undertakings in modern science. The 2023 failure of Janssen's Mosaico trial – the eighth major candidate to falter in advanced clinical stages – was a sobering reminder of the virus' complexity and adaptability. Despite the enormous investments of time, intellect and funding over four decades, a licensed HIV-1 vaccine continues to elude us.

Yet, the pursuit endures. With each setback, science grows sharper; with each trial, knowledge deepens. India's contributions – both independent and collaborative – will be instrumental in shaping the next chapter of this journey. As research turns increasingly toward personalized immunology and precision vaccine design, the dream of a safe and effective HIV vaccine remains within reach. Four decades, eight failed trials, countless breakthroughs – a vaccine remains elusive but the science, like hope, never stops evolving.

40

THE LONG ROAD TO MALARIA VACCINES

ON THE NIGHT OF 25 MARCH 1971, THE STREETS OF DHAKA, the capital of erstwhile East Pakistan, wore an eerie silence. Most people had abandoned the streets early and taken shelter in their homes, anticipating trouble. The uneasy calm was soon broken by the ominous creaking of tanks as heavily armed Pakistani soldiers rolled out of Dhaka Cantonment by midnight, attacking anyone in their path. This brutal crackdown, ordered by Pakistan's President Yahya Khan, continued for several days.

Operation Searchlight was a brutal campaign targeting the Bengali self-determination movement, which sought independence from West Pakistan. Tanks and armoured vehicles rumbled through the city, and gunfire echoed as soldiers attacked students, intellectuals and anyone suspected of supporting the burgeoning movement. Amidst the chaos and bloodshed, a sense of defiance began to grow. Unwilling to submit to tyranny, a guerrilla movement – Mukti Bahini – emerged, composing of military personnel, paramilitary forces and civilians from East Pakistan. With tacit support from India, these brave men and women took to the forests and villages, launching hit-and-run attacks on the moving Pakistani military convoys. With steely resolve, they fought for their dream of an independent Bengali-speaking state.

Supporting the creation of an independent Bangladesh came at a heavy price for India. By sending men and machines, India had diverted resources meant for health and education of its citizens. Many internal priorities suffered, and ongoing projects went dry. One such casualty was the two-decade-old project of Malaria control.

Around the same time, the Arab–Israeli Yom Kippur War of October 1973 had triggered an oil embargo by the Organization of Arab Petroleum Exporting Countries (OAPEC), leading to quadrupling of oil prices and significant economic disruptions globally. With the oil prices shooting up, the cost of DDT and other insecticides too shot up, forcing the Indian government to cut down the spending on mosquito control programmes.

Adding to these woes, malaria-causing mosquitos began to develop resistance to DDT and similar chemicals. By the middle of 1972, India was once again gripped by the deadly scourge that had killed people in droves two decades ago – malaria. The number of cases almost doubled from 1.3 million in 1972 to 2.5 million by 1975.[1]

Malaria had plagued India for centuries, and efforts to combat it had been just as long-standing. Indian scriptures from the Vedic period dating back to 800 BC describe malaria as the 'king of diseases'.[2] Indian-born British researcher Ronald Ross emerged as a malaria warrior in the modern era when he identified the mosquitoes carrying the causative agent while working in Hyderabad under the British Indian Medical Service in 1897.[3] Many efforts followed to combat the disease, mostly by controlling the parasite carrier, *Anopheles* mosquitos.

In recent decades, Indian scientists turned their focus to understanding the parasite itself. A major breakthrough came from the laboratory of Prof. G. Padmanaban at IISc, Bengaluru. His research revealed that *Plasmodium falciparum* synthesizes its own heme – even though it lives inside human red blood cells, which are already rich in heme. Padmanaban's team showed that the parasite imports functional enzymes from the host cell to complete its heme biosynthesis. This discovery offered critical insight into parasite biology and positioned the heme synthesis pathway as a promising target for new antimalarial drugs. His research also showed that combining curcumin – an active component of turmeric – with artemisinin, an antimalarial drug derived from sweet wormwood prevented malaria relapse and neurological symptoms in mice, and can be used to achieve complete cures as shown in laboratory studies.

When the 1972 crisis hit India, the country was still recovering from the massive malaria outbreak of the 1950s. Systematic control measures had brought some relief, but the emergence of a new endemic in different parts of the country raised fresh alarms. Fortunately, fatalities between 1972 and 1975 were far fewer compared to the estimated 800,000 deaths in 1952.

Malarial parasite had long evaded the clutches of advanced science and its powerful tool, the vaccine. The primary challenge in tackling malaria with a conventional vaccine lies in the fact that it is not caused by a bacteria or virus, but by a single-celled protozoan parasite.* The organism belongs to the *Plasmodium* species and requires multiple hosts to complete its life cycle, humans being one of them. The various species of malaria-causing parasites that infect humans include *P. falciparum, Plasmodium vivax, Plasmodium ovale, Plasmodium malariae, and Plasmodium knowlesi,* with *P. falciparum* being the most common and dangerous.

It became increasingly challenging to confront the beast with the emergence of drug-resistant strains of the parasite, making it evident to the healthcare community that a vaccine would be the only sustainable solution. Unlike most other disease-causing agents, the malarial parasite undergoes multiple life stages – first in human liver, then in blood, and finally within the mosquito where it reproduces. This complex life cycle posed a significant challenge, leaving researchers uncertain about which stage to target or whether a multi-stage approach would be more effective.

* A tiny, single-celled organism that lives in other organisms and causes disease. In malaria, this is the Plasmodium parasite.

Adding to this complexity is the fact that a prior malaria infection does not provide sterile immunity, meaning it fails to offer complete protection against future infections. In malaria-endemic regions, most reinfected individuals experienced only mild symptoms due to partial immunity developed from previous infections. This became the starting point for advanced vaccine research. It gained momentum with a breakthrough in the new millennium on the sequencing of the *Plasmodium* genome, which significantly aided efforts to confront the organism through a vaccine.[4]

The earliest efforts towards vaccine development were based on the concept of immunizing with live attenuated sporozoites* – using weakened parasites to trigger an immune response without causing illness. A pivotal study in 1967 demonstrated that mice, immunized with radiation-attenuated† *Plasmodium berghei* sporozoites, were protected against further infection.[5] However, it took thirty-five years for this research to advance to the next stage, with scientists adapting the method for humans through gamma radiation of sporozoites.

Human subjects exposed to bites from these mosquitoes received sporozoites which, upon reaching the liver cells, couldn't mature. This triggered an immune response without causing the disease.[6] Although this approach proved impractical and costly for large-scale use, it validated the concept and encouraged further research. Scientists built upon the insights from this 2002 study and progressed to numerous potential malaria vaccines. Instead of pursuing a live attenuated vaccine, new approaches focused on isolating specific antigens and delivering them using advanced technologies.

Given the parasite's life cycle, researchers explored three distinct vaccine strategies: pre-blood stage, blood stage and transmission blocking. The pre-erythrocytic (pre-blood stage)‡ vaccine targeted

---

* The early, infectious form of the malaria parasite that is injected into humans by a mosquito bite.

† Weakened using radiation so the parasite can't cause disease but can still stimulate the body's immune system to respond.

‡ A stage in the malaria parasite's life before it reaches the blood. This includes its early

the infectious phase to block sporozoites from entering liver cells or eliminating infected liver cells. The challenge here was the narrow window of an hour, within which sporozoites reached the liver after a mosquito bite. While most pre-erythrocytic vaccines are in early trials, two vaccines have reached the market after successful field trials. The first one has been under development since 1987 and was tested in endemic countries starting in 2019.

The vaccine is developed on the core mechanism that CSP protein (from the sporozoite stage) when fused to HBsAg enhances its immunogenicity. When an adjuvant is added it further boosts the immune response. This approach helps the immune system recognize and mount a defence against the malaria parasite before it can infect liver cells.[7]

The Phase III trials of this vaccine across eleven African countries showed 56 per cent efficacy against clinical malaria and 47 per cent against severe malaria in children aged five to seventeen months. The vaccine was less effective in infants aged six to twelve weeks, reducing episodes by one-third.[8] It is being deployed as a crucial public health tool, particularly benefiting children in high-transmission regions where mortality rates are significant.[9] In less than a year of WHO authorization, it was rolled out in Ghana, Kenya and Malawi under the brand name Mosquirix, and crossed a million vaccinations by April 2022.[10]

The second pre-erythrocytic vaccine, R21/Matrix-M, was developed through a collaboration of the Jenner Institute at Oxford University, the Serum Institute of India and the US-based company Novovax. This vaccine, which uses Novavax's saponin-based adjuvant technology, received support from the European and Developing Countries Clinical Trials Partnership (EDCTP), the Wellcome Trust and the European Investment Bank (EIB).

The R21/Matrix-M vaccine has shown higher efficacy and safety in Phase II trials, particularly among children who have received a

development in the liver.

booster dose a year after an initial three-dose regimen. Initially aimed at generating strong T-cell responses* against liver-stage malaria antigens, the vaccine now also targets high-level antibodies against the sporozoite stage.[11] It provided up to 77 per cent protection in phase III trials, significantly higher than RTS,S vaccines, making it a better candidate for malaria prevention.[12]

The efficacy of the R21/Matrix-M vaccine is notably higher among younger children, though it declines slightly in older children. Further studies are being carried out to understand the age-related difference. Despite its high efficacy, there are concerns about the vaccine's variable effectiveness in seasonal versus standard malaria transmission sites. Phase III trials showed a trend of higher efficacy in seasonal sites, and a booster dose helped maintain efficacy.

The Serum Institute began producing it soon after the Covid-19 crisis, stockpiled 25 million doses and created a capacity to produce 100 million doses a year. In May 2024, the Serum Institute shipped its first batch of 43,200 doses to the Central African Republic.[13] The R21/Matrix-M vaccine has been claimed by its developers as a significant advancement in malaria control, with the potential to reduce malaria-related mortality and morbidity and contribute to global malaria eradication efforts.

The second type of vaccines, erythrocytic vaccines or blood-stage vaccines, aim to prevent the rapid invasion by the parasite and its asexual reproduction in the red blood cells. Once the invasion starts in the blood stage, symptoms begin to appear and lead to the bursting of red blood cells, causing severe damage to the body. At this stage, a large number of parasites, merozoites,† are released in the liver – almost 40,000 per infected liver cell – which then move into the blood stream and multiply further. Erythrocytic vaccines containing proteins from the surface of the merozoite would help develop

* The activation of T lymphocytes, a type of white blood cell, in response to antigen, and their subsequent proliferation and differentiation.

† A stage of the malaria parasite that is released from the liver into the blood, where it multiplies and causes illness.

immunity and attempt to reduce the multiplication of merozoites. No blood-stage vaccine has reached the deployment stage, though many are undergoing Phase I and II trials.

The third type of vaccines, known as a transmission blocking vaccine (TBV), targets sexual reproduction of the parasite in the gut of the mosquito. Unlike the conventional vaccines, in this indirect approach the vaccine kills the vector carrying the parasite, the *Anopheles* mosquito. This vaccine does not protect the individual from the parasite itself but it stops the spread of the parasite.

One TBV vaccine candidate, Pfs25-EPA, is under development through a collaboration between the Laboratory of Malaria Immunology and Vaccinology of the US National Institute of Allergy and Infectious Diseases and the Centre for Vaccine Research of Johns Hopkins University. It works on the concept that if the body can develop antibodies against the Pfs25 antigen,* a mosquito taking a blood meal will ingest some of these antibodies, eventually killing the parasite.

With sufficient progress on all three fronts, the next logical step in malaria vaccine research was to combine vaccines of all three types and create a powerful tool. PATH's Malaria Vaccine Initiative (MVI), which works with industry, governmental and academic stakeholders, has been developing on one such combination vaccine targeting multiple lifecycle stages.

Given the widespread presence of *P. falciparum*, most vaccine initiatives have been focusing on this parasite. However, India faced a peculiar challenge as every second malarial infection in the country was caused by *P. vivax*. This highlighted the need for a vaccine targeting this species to control malaria *in toto* in India.

Known to attack the youngest red blood cells, known as reticulocytes, *P. vivax* presented yet another challenge in developing a reliable long-term culture system to facilitate research. After its genome was decoded and published in the new millennium, *P. vivax*

* A specific part of the malaria parasite that helps it reproduce inside the mosquito.

vaccine research gained momentum.[14] Researchers at the International Centre for Genetic Engineering and Biotechnology (ICGEB), New Delhi, in collaboration with Department of Biotechnology and the MVI of PATH, have been leading the effort. Together, they formed an entity by the name of Multi Vaccines Development Programme* for developing four different types of malarial vaccines, with three targeting *P. falciparum* and one targeting *P. vivax*.

For the *P. vivax* blood stage vaccine, Syngene, a subsidiary of Biocon, produced the vaccine candidate (PvDBPII)† and carried out the first phase clinical testing, while the adjuvant used in this vaccine was provided by the Infectious Disease Research Institute (IDRI), US. The work took off to a great start with funding for toxicology studies and Phase I clinical trial from the Biotechnology Industry Research Assistance Council (BIRAC) of DBT. The momentum slowed down during the Covid pandemic, but it regained pace thereafter.

By 2023, researchers found that the antibody responses from the vaccinated individuals in trials were linked to reduction in parasite multiplication. These findings suggested that the immune response generated by the PvDBPII vaccine could protect against malaria. Additionally, the antibodies were effective against multiple variants of the parasite, indicating broad protection.[15]

Despite these strides in the development of malaria vaccines, research is still at a crucial phase with several promising clinical trials still ongoing or at the point of completion. Therefore, the daunting task remains at hand – deploying a safe and reliable vaccine with high efficacy within the current decade.

The biggest challenge in vaccine development for malaria has been achieving sustained protective efficacy, given that antibody and cellular responses are often found to diminish within a year. Experts

---

* A project led by Indian and international groups to develop several malaria vaccines at once, targeting different parasite species and stages.

† A vaccine candidate targeting a part of the *P. vivax* parasite that helps it invade human cells. The name stands for *P. vivax* Duffy Binding Protein II.

agree that crunching timelines or compressing vaccine development into a few months is not a viable approach for malaria. The parasite's complex lifecycle, its ability to evade the immune system and centuries of scientific struggle make malaria a far tougher opponent, notwithstanding recent rapid vaccine development successes like the H1N1.

In 2009, pharmaceutical companies and government organizations quickly developed a vaccine in response to the 2009 H1N1 (swine flu) pandemic. By April of the same year, the US CDC initiated the development of candidate vaccines and created a comprehensive rollout plan. The first vaccine doses were administered by August and within a few months, over 127 million doses distributed. Several H1N1 vaccine types were developed, including live attenuated, inactivated unadjuvanted and inactivated adjuvanted vaccines. Indian companies too developed several vaccines. Notable among them were NasoVac, a nasal spray developed by the Serum Institute and HNVAC, an inactivated, cell culture-derived one from Bharat Biotech.

The malaria vaccine journey is a race against time, suffering and death. Malaria, once etched into ancient scriptures as the 'king of diseases', continues to haunt the poorest and most vulnerable across the globe. Every scientific breakthrough inches us closer, but the battle is far from over. The world awaits a vaccine that not only works but endures. And for that, the science establishment must be relentless, its commitment unwavering, and the global resolve stronger than ever. In the meantime, malaria continues to remind us that science, no matter how fast it runs, must sometimes walk patiently through complexity.

41

mRNA: A CENTURY OF CHALLENGES

THE FLUORESCENT LIGHTS BUZZED OVERHEAD, CASTING A sterile glow over the photocopy room near a busy lab at the University of Pennsylvania (UPenn). Katalin Karikó stood waiting, frustration creasing her brow. The photocopier, normally a reliable workhorse, sputtered and jammed, refusing to cooperate. Papers spilled from the tray, printed with her research on an unusual topic – mRNA. Just as Karikó was about to give up, a shadow fell across the scattered papers. Glancing up, she saw Drew Weissman, another researcher holding a similarly haphazard stack of papers.

Katalin Karikó's journey to mRNA research began in a Hungarian town, far from the halls of elite science. The daughter of a butcher, she dreamt of becoming a scientist – an aspiration shaped by a world where such figures were unfamiliar to her. Arriving in the United States in her twenties, she embarked on a long and unconventional path. For decades, she navigated the fringes of academia at UPenn, shifting from job to job and being at the mercy of seniors to grant her projects to work on and make a living.

She was consumed by her work on messenger RNA (mRNA), confident that mRNA could be deployed to instruct cells to make their own remedies to fight infections. Her husband Bela Francia, however, wasn't convinced about her work. 'You are not going to work, you are going to have fun,' Francia, the manager of an apartment complex, would tell her when she went to university. Looking at the time she spent in the lab and her earnings, he calculated that she was earning about a dollar an hour.[1]

As Karikó and Weissman collected their papers, a sense of camaraderie hung in the air. 'Fascinating work you have there,' Weissman said, glancing at Karikó's research notes on the tray. Intrigued by the unfamiliar topic of mRNA, he started asking questions to which Karikó, usually reserved about her research, found herself responding with an unexpected passion.[2] Weissman asked if it was possible to develop a vaccine against HIV using mRNA. Karikó responded to the challenge with a firm, 'I can do it.'

What began as a casual conversation quickly turned to their research work.[3] Karikó spoke passionately about using mRNA to instruct cells to fight diseases. Weissman shared his work on vaccines. It soon became clear – their goals were not just compatible, but complementary. Karikó's expertise in mRNA could potentially solve the challenges Weissman had been facing in vaccine development.[4] The encounter unwittingly set the stage for a collaboration that would change the course of their careers and ultimately, the future of medicine.[5]

However, her mRNA path hit a roadblock when they began collaborating. Though mRNA was successful in instructing cells in the lab to make proteins, it did not work as such inside living beings. Karikó and Weissman realized that it was because mRNA caused an immune overreaction,* whereas another form of RNA in the human body called transfer RNA (tRNA) did not. They found a molecule called pseudouridine in tRNA that enabled it to evade the immune response. This molecule is also naturally present in human mRNA. When pseudouridine was added to mRNA, they found it not only protected the mRNA from the immune system but also significantly increased its efficiency,† directing the synthesis of ten

* When the body's defense system responds too strongly to something it thinks is harmful.

† Efficiency is about maximizing the benefits of an intervention like vaccine while minimizing cost, time etc. It's about doing things right in the most economical way.

times more protein in each cell.[6,7] This breakthrough demonstrated that modifying mRNA with pseudouridine allowed it to alter cell functions without triggering an immune response, opening up numerous potential applications.

Despite these promising findings, grant reviewers dismissed their mRNA project submissions and advised them against pursuing it further. Their work struggled to find acceptance, repeatedly rejected by leading scientific journals until finally, a modest journal *Immunity* published it in 2005, barely stirring the waters of the scientific community.[8]

Undeterred, the duo pressed on, soon achieving a breakthrough when they successfully induced a monkey to produce a specific protein by injecting it with mRNA for erythropoietin,* a crucial factor in red blood cell production. The results were astounding – the monkey's red blood cell counts soared. This triumph hinted at vast possibilities: using mRNA to produce any protein drug, from insulin to innovative diabetes treatments, and to transform the way vaccines worked till then.

From Louis Pasteur's time, vaccines have been designed in two fundamental ways – by using live attenuated microbes or by using killed microbes. In the first method, a live microbe is weakened and then injected into the human body to generate antibodies to fight against the pathogen, whereas in the second method, inactivated bacteria or virus is inserted into the body to create body immunity to fight the disease-causing organism.

Then came toxoid vaccines, which use inactivated toxins from the pathogen to target the toxic activity created by the organism. Here, pathogens are not targeted; instead, their toxic activity is targeted. Toxoid vaccines are widely used against tetanus, diphtheria and pertussis. This followed the advent of subunit vaccines, marking a shift in vaccine development. Unlike earlier vaccines, subunit vaccines used only a fragment of the cell to fight the pathogen. The evolution

---

* A natural protein made by the kidneys that tells the body to make more red blood cells.

of subunit vaccines was a revolution in vaccine making – made from a piece of the pathogen, not from the whole organism.

Soon came polysaccharide vaccines, conjugate vaccines and protein-based vaccines. Polysaccharide vaccines are made from long chains of sugar molecules (polysaccharides) that make up the surface capsule of certain bacteria, whereas conjugate vaccines link or 'conjugate' the polysaccharide to a protein carrier. For instance, Haemophilus influenzae type B (Hib) vaccine is a conjugate vaccine, pneumococcal vaccine is of polysaccharide or conjugate types and hepatitis B vaccine is a recombinant protein one.

Then the concept of DNA vaccine emerged during the 1990s, with the first successful demonstration of such vaccines in animals in 1993, when plasmid DNA produced an immune response in mice. Throughout the decade, several DNA vaccines for humans entered early-stage clinical trials, including against HIV, cancer and various infectious diseases. Later, DNA vaccines for veterinary use, such as those against West Nile virus in horses, received approval.

Next was the development of viral vector vaccines. These vaccines use a harmless virus to carry and deliver the genetic information of the antigen to host cells, enabling the immune system to produce a response. They act as delivery systems carrying genetic information so that the immune system can fight the pathogen. The best example of viral vector vaccine is the Ebola vaccine.

Ebola, in fact, has served as a test case for most emerging vaccine techniques, including virus-like particle-based vaccines, DNA-based vaccines, whole virus recombinant vaccines, incompetent replication originated vaccines and competent replication vaccines.*[9] Researchers, therefore, used mRNA technology to develop vaccines against some of the most difficult challenges like Ebola and Zika towards the end of the 2010s.

Therefore, when Karikó and Weissman proposed injecting mRNA

* Incompetent means the virus used in the vaccine can't make copies of itself in the body. Competent means it can, though in a controlled way.

to instruct human cells to produce viral components rather than relying on the traditional method of injecting a piece of a pathogen itself, it marked the beginning of a new era in vaccine development – one that was swifter and more adaptable. However, the duo could not have imagined that a global pandemic was looming – and that a historic vaccine would be developed using their technology, earning them the Nobel Prize in Physiology/Medicine in 2023.

When the time arrived to transition their work from the lab to the industry, pharmaceutical companies and venture capitalists remained unimpressed, dismissing the duo's proposals for funding. Dejected but determined, they formed a company, RNARx within the framework of the University to develop their concept further. They secured a small business grant of $100,000 from the US government to conduct animal trials.

By the end of 2009, when some parties began to show interest in the technology, UPenn began negotiating a licensing agreement with RNARx. Unable to close the agreement, UPenn opted for a swift payout instead. In February 2010, exclusive patent rights were granted to a small lab-reagent supplier in Madison, now known as Cellscript, for as little as $300,000. This nondescript company would go on to reap hundreds of millions of dollars in sub-licensing fees from Moderna and BioNTech – benefactors of the duo's findings and the first ones to develop mRNA vaccines* for Covid-19 in subsequent years.[10]

BioNTech was formed in 2008 by researcher couple Ugur Sahin and Özlem Türeci, who met during their early medical careers in Germany. They were both deeply interested in cancer research and immunotherapy, which brought them together professionally and personally. BioNTech received a seed investment of €150 million from two venture capitals – MIG Capital and AT Impf – but it wasn't until 2009, with the acquisition of two small firms

* A modern vaccine made using a tiny instruction manual (mRNA) that teaches the body to make a protein found on a virus or cancer cell, triggering an immune response.

with proprietary technologies, that the company began gaining momentum.

Around the same time, seeing the potential of mRNA technology, an assistant professor at Harvard Medical School, Derrick Rossi, started following the work of Karikó and tried to simulate the technology in his lab. One fine day in 2010, Rossi shared his findings on mRNA with his colleague, Timothy Springer. A biotech entrepreneur himself, Springer quickly recognized its commercial potential and brought it to the attention of Robert Langer, a biomedical engineering professor at MIT and a serial inventor with 1,400 patents. This led to several meetings and the formation of a new biotech firm to explore the possibilities of mRNA technology. It was named Moderna, a portmanteau of words 'modified' and 'mRNA'. By 2017, the company raised a capital of $2 billion, only to focus on mRNA vaccine research.[11]

BioNTech has been closely observing the formation of Moderna, recognizing the emergence of a viable competitor in the mRNA space – a technology they had been developing, though it had struggled to mature. Without wasting much time, BioNTech made the next big move – poaching the mother of mRNA technology Karikó from UPenn, who joined BioNTech as a senior vice president in 2013.

Karikó joining the team enthused the company and boosted the researchers' morale. For the next five years, BioNTech carried out extensive research on mRNA, initiating collaborations and commercialization on multiple fronts. In addition to filing several patents, they also formed a collaboration with French vaccine company Sanofi Pasteur in 2015. Pfizer was also keeping a close watch on these developments and reached out to BioNTech to explore a multi-year collaboration to develop an mRNA-based vaccine for influenza.

By 2019, Sanofi expanded its collaboration to deploy mRNA technology in cancer therapies by investing €80 million. Since then, there has been no looking back for BioNTech. A few months later, Fidelity Management & Research led an investment round for the company generating $325 million funds and by September, the

Bill & Melinda Gates Foundation pitched in with $55 million to work on HIV and tuberculosis vaccines.[12]

The very next month, the company shifted its headquarters from Mainz in Germany to Cambridge, Massachusetts and raised another $150 million by listing its shares at the NASDAQ as American Depository Shares.[13] With its coffers overflowing, the company recruited key personnel and geared up its manufacturing lines. By end of 2019, BioNTech was all set to embark on what would become the world's fastest vaccine development programme during one of the worst pandemics that would hit the world.

Coincidently, it had been exactly thirty-two years since Robert Malone, a graduate student at the Salk Institute for Biological Studies in La Jolla, California, had combined strands of mRNA with fat droplets, creating a molecular mixture, and reported that when human cells were exposed to this genetic blend, they absorb the mRNA and produce proteins.[14] It is also worth noting that mRNA was discovered in the 1960s and the technology of sending mRNA to cells was established in the 1970s, yet it took a global pandemic and 7 million deaths for the first mRNA vaccine to be developed and taken to the market.

There were many hurdles in this long but strenuous path – the journey from mRNA technology to a deployable mRNA vaccine.

The primary hurdle was the rapid degradation of mRNA inside the body before it could effectively deliver the message to initiate protein production in cells. This was overcome through advancements in nanotechnology, particularly the creation of lipid nanoparticles.* These nanoparticles enveloped the mRNA, acting as protective bubbles, facilitating their entry into cells without degradation. Once inside, the mRNA could ensure the production of certain proteins. In the case of SARS-CoV-2, it was a spike protein.† The subsequent

* Tiny fat bubbles used to protect and carry mRNA into cells. They act like padded envelopes for fragile genetic instructions.

† A spiky structure on the coronavirus surface that it uses to enter human cells. Vaccines target this so the body can block the virus before it enters cells.

processes alert the body's immune system to the presence of a 'foreign molecule' which is nothing but the newly produced protein, triggering the immune system to respond.

Just before the arrival of SARS-CoV-2, mRNA vaccines with lipid envelopes were deployed against the Ebola virus. mRNA vaccines have also demonstrated immunity against influenza, Zika and rabies when deployed as lipid-encapsulated or as non-encapsulated optimized mRNA. Weissman had published a work titled 'mRNA Vaccines – A New Era in Vaccinology' in 2018 in the *Nature Reviews Drug Discovery* journal.[15]

Despite these strides in mRNA research, India was yet to adopt this frontier technology at its research institutes or universities. In fact, Indian scientists didn't pay great attention to it until mRNA emerged as a saviour at the peak of the Covid-19 pandemic. When the rebirth of the saviour vaccine technology was happening in the West in the aftermath of the pandemic with great fanfare, India was working on vaccines using inactivated virus, combined with a strong adjuvant to generate immunity. These Indian efforts, led by ICMR and the National Institute of Virology (NIV), were based on the traditional killed virus method. By using a whole-virion inactivated vero cell-derived platform,* a killed version of the SARS-CoV-2 virus was employed – one that cannot replicate but can only elicit an immune response. Bharat Biotech was selected as an industry partner in May 2020 after the virus was isolated by NIV. The result was COVAXIN.[16]

However, the first vaccine that was made available to Indians was from the Serum Institute, using viral vector technology. Named 'COVISHIELD' by its developer, the Oxford-AstraZeneca team, the vaccine used the modified version of a chimpanzee adenovirus (ChAdOx1) as a vector to deliver the genetic material into human cells. The genetic material carried by the adenovirus vector encoded

---

* A vaccine method using the whole virus that's been killed and grown in lab cells (vero cells). It can't cause disease but still teaches the body to fight it.

the spike protein of the SARS-CoV-2 virus. Once inside the cells, the genetic material produced the spike protein of the virus. The presence of spike protein triggered the body's immune system to recognize it as 'foreign', prompting an immune response, including the production of antibodies and the activation of T-cells. As a result, when a vaccinated person later encountered the actual SARS-CoV-2 virus, their immune system was primed to recognize and fight the virus more effectively, thereby providing protection against Covid-19.[17]

The Russian Sputnik V vaccine, manufactured by Dr Reddy's Laboratories in collaboration with the Gamaleya Research Institute, utilized the non-replicating viral vector technology using a human adenovirus vector (rAd26 and rAd5).[18] Much later in the game, Biological E. arrived at the scene with a vaccine based on the recombinant protein subunit platform developed by Texas Children's Hospital Centre for Vaccine Development and Baylor College of Medicine in Houston, Texas, along with Dynavax technologies based in Emeryville, California. The vaccine was named Corbevax and its development was led by Peter Hotez.[19,20]

By then, the Serum Institute of India had launched its second vaccine named Covovax under license from the US firm Novavax which used a protein subunit technology.[21] The last in the series was ZyCoV-D vaccine developed by Zydus Cadila. It was a DNA vaccine that used a genetically engineered plasmid containing the DNA sequence encoding the spike protein of SARS-CoV-2. It was touted as the first successful DNA vaccine for humans.[22]

Notwithstanding all these development efforts, there weren't any mRNA vaccine in India's bouquet of offerings till 2024, as India had not been making any significant strides in mRNA technology. The exception was some work at the IISc, Bangalore, where Associate Professor Purusharth Rajyaguru's team focused on a yeast protein to break down RNA granules, which decides the course of action of mRNA. This research with implications in neurodegenerative diseases like Amyotrophic Lateral Sclerosis (ALS) and Frontotemporal

Dementia (FTD) has been progressing for a while.[23] However, in the wake of the Covid-19 pandemic and soon after the global attention on mRNA, following quick offerings from BioNTech and Moderna, several Indian companies and research institutions jumped into the mRNA fray.

In May 2022, CCMB, Hyderabad announced the development of mRNA vaccine technology and emphasized that the institute has been developing a potential mRNA vaccine candidate for SARS-CoV-2 completely indigenously.[24] The idea for an indigenous mRNA vaccine took shape at the Atal Incubation Centre of CCMB soon after mRNA vaccine gained significance early in the Covid-19 pandemic. Engaged initially with RT-PCR testing and viral genome sequencing,* CCMB expanded its efforts to include virus neutralization technologies. Once it was clear that mRNA vaccines have been successful globally, the team moved to re-engineer† Moderna's Covid-19 vaccine since a lot of its information was publicly available.

The CSIR supported the initiative, leading to a collaborative project involving half a dozen Indian institutions such as Institute of Genomics and Integrative Biology (IGIB) in New Delhi, Indian Institute of Chemical Biology (IICB) in Kolkata, Indian Institute of Chemical Technology (IICT) in Hyderabad, Institute of Microbial Technology (IMTECH) in Chandigarh, National Institute for Interdisciplinary Science and Technology (NIIST) in Thiruvananthapuram and Institute of Himalayan Bioresource Technology in Palampur.[25]

After streamlining the formulation process, the vaccine was tested for antibody generation through standard experiments and quantified neutralizing antibody titers. Utilizing CCMB's facility with live SARS-COV-2, it was successfully proven that the vaccine-generated antibodies had the ability to neutralize the live virus. Animal testing

---

* A scientific method used to read and understand the complete genetic instructions (DNA) of an organism.

† In biotech, to modify or recreate a product, often using scientific or technological know-how.

at the IISc, Bangalore validated that vaccinated animals were protected from the coronavirus infection. Since early 2023, CCMB has been engaging private firms to transfer the technology to carry out human trials.[26]

Around the same time, in a parallel but less visible effort, a little-known Indian grant-making organization, Ignite Life Science Foundation, awarded an undisclosed grant to a collaborative team of scientists from IISc's Department of Bioengineering and THSTI, Faridabad to build an indigenous mRNA vaccine platform. Though the grant was announced with a focus on developing thermostable mRNA vaccines suitable for tropical, low-resource settings, nothing was heard from the team afterwards.[27] THSTI has been working on RNA modifications to improve vaccine stability and reactogenicity to reduce unintended immune responses.

Among the drug companies, Gennova Biopharmaceuticals, a subsidiary of Emcure Pharmaceuticals, emerged as a leader in mRNA technology in India. Its mRNA Covid-19 vaccine, GEMCOVAC-19, has undergone preclinical and early clinical trials with promising outcomes. Gennova has forged partnerships with international collaborators in leveraging innovative lipid nanoparticle (LNP) technology to enhance the delivery of mRNA, a crucial component for mRNA delivery.

A significant innovation is its freeze-drying technology, which allows the vaccine to be stored at 2 to 8 degrees Celsius. This is in contrast to other mRNA vaccines that require storage at sub-zero temperatures, making GEMCOVAC-19 suitable for tropical countries like India. This storage stability facilitates broader and more practical distribution, aligning with efforts to democratize mRNA vaccines globally. The initiative garnered support from the Department of Biotechnology and received clearance from the Drugs Controller General of India (DCGI) to run Phase II/III trial as early August 2021.[28] Gennova's early commitment to mRNA technology positioned it at the forefront of mRNA vaccine innovation in this part of the world.

Biological E. obtained the mRNA technology through a partnership with Providence Therapeutics, a Canadian biotechnology company. In August 2021, Biological E. had signed a deal with Providence to license its mRNA vaccine technology, allowing it to use Providence's mRNA platform to develop and manufacture mRNA vaccines, including a Covid-19 vaccine.[29] Almost a year later, the company was selected to receive mRNA technology from the technology transfer hub of WHO's Product Development for Vaccines Advisory Committee (PDVAC).[30]

The Serum Institute of India too forged a partnership with a Belgian company, Univercells in January 2024 to develop cancer therapies using mRNA, in combination with its recombinant BCG vaccine. Other companies aiming to develop mRNA technology for vaccine and therapies include Bharat Biotech, Reliance Life Sciences, Dr Reddy's Laboratories, Zydus LifeSciences and Biocon.

While mRNA vaccines have opened new frontiers in immunization, research around the world is rapidly advancing toward next-generation technologies that promise to overcome the limitations of current platforms. Scientists are now exploring self-amplifying RNA (saRNA) vaccines, which require significantly lower doses, and circular RNA (circRNA) constructs that offer greater stability and longer-lasting protein expression. These innovations could improve efficacy, cost, and access – especially in resource-constrained settings.

Other promising areas include microneedle patch vaccines for painless, heat-stable delivery; AI-designed antigens for broader protection against rapidly mutating viruses; and lipid-polymer hybrid nanoparticles for more precise immune targeting. Meanwhile, intranasal* and oral mRNA vaccines are under development to stimulate mucosal immunity, a critical line of defense for respiratory infections. As the field evolves, India must stay at the forefront not

---

* A vaccine given through the nose instead of an injection, often as a spray, aiming to trigger an immune response in the respiratory tract.

only by replicating what has worked globally, but by investing in these frontier innovations and adapting them to local needs.

The road ahead to establish a safe and reliable mRNA technology and other emerging vaccine technologies in India is much more challenging than simply re-engineering the process. It needs resources, patience and determination – qualities that Karikó demonstrated throughout her life journey.

To ensure that India does not remain dependent on global suppliers for cutting-edge vaccines and therapies, the development of indigenous mRNA platforms and emerging platforms is both a strategic and scientific imperative. The groundwork laid by early public-private efforts – from CCMB's academic rigour to Gennova's translational expertise – has opened up the possibility for India to emerge as a credible global hub for vaccine technology innovation. But scaling from lab-scale breakthroughs to commercial success requires deep investments in infrastructure, talent pipelines and regulatory preparedness.

Beyond infectious diseases, the promise of mRNA and new vaccine technologies extends to cancer immunotherapy, rare diseases and even personalized treatments. India's ecosystem is only beginning to tap into this vast potential. The convergence of synthetic biology, delivery science and genomics presents an unprecedented opportunity. With the right mix of public support and private risk-taking, India could help shape the next era of global vaccinology.

India's emerging vaccine technology journey has just begun – not only to vaccinate, but to innovate too.

42

FROM MONKEYS TO MAITRI

AT THE PEAK OF THE FIRST COVID-19 LOCKDOWN IN MAY 2020, scientists from ICMR embarked on an unusual mission – a wild monkey chase. To be precise, they were chasing Rhesus macaques.* This was despite the country having at least 500,000 Rhesus macaques in the wild, some of which strayed into human settlements, leading to man-monkey conflicts.

Researchers from the National Institute of Virology (NIV), Pune reached out to multiple zoos and organizations breeding Rhesus monkeys for animal experiments, hoping to source at least twenty Rhesus macaques that could potentially aid in the fight against Covid-19. But their efforts yielded no success.

India, like the rest of the world, began its vaccine chase as soon as it became evident that the pandemic was here to stay and the only way out was through the development of a vaccine. Unfortunately, India did not have access to frontier technologies like mRNA and therefore decided to take the traditional approach – designing a vaccine using killed viruses.

Serious discussions within ICMR commenced in all earnestness in the early days of April, a week or two after the announcement of the first lockdown on 24 March 2020. A few key calculations

* A type of monkey commonly used in medical research because their biology is similar to humans in many ways.

influenced India's decision to develop its own Covid-19 vaccine. First, Western nations leading early vaccine development would not be able to meet global demand, as every country would be rushing to secure enough doses for their population or even double that number. Second, given India's tropical climatic conditions, no vaccine that required cold chain storage and transportation would be a fitting solution for the country. Third, having an indigenous option would reduce the dependence on foreign exchange and foreign suppliers at such a crucial time.[1]

Pride also played a significant role. At a time when the government was promoting India as the 'pharmacy of the world' – with the country developing, re-engineering and mass-producing drugs and vaccines of all kinds while meeting nearly 50 per cent of the global vaccine demand – failing to develop a Covid-19 vaccine would have raised questions about India's standing in the biopharma sector. In other words, developing a home-grown vaccine at the quickest pace would demonstrate India's prowess in the sector.

With pressure mounting from the Government, ICMR decided to bite the bullet. But the challenge was figuring out how. Looking for collaborators for a joint development, ICMR could think of three to four vaccine makers with large capacity and ability to scale to up production in a short period.

Top of the list was the Serum Institute, but it had already announced plans for a live attenuated vaccine with Codagenix, an American biotech company, as early as February, while the virus was spreading in Europe.[2] As the world crossed 3 million infections and 200,000 deaths by the end of April, half a dozen Indian companies were working on vaccine development, mostly with international partners. By then, the Serum Institute had joined the Oxford collaboration, which included Jenner Institute at the University of Oxford, Oxford University Hospitals NHS Foundation Trust, Public Health England (PHE) and the UK Vaccines Taskforce.

It was quite possible that as the stakes grew higher, British–Swedish pharma company AstraZeneca may have feigned its inability to scale up production. Thereby, a volume player like the Serum Institute was brought on board. The Oxford-AstraZeneca vaccine, known technically as ChAdOx1 nCoV-19, was based on a replication-deficient simian adenovirus vector* that contained the genetic material of the SARS-CoV-2 spike protein. This technology was chosen for its ability to elicit a strong immune response without the virus replicating in the human body.

Another player Bharat Biotech had started working with the University of Wisconsin-Madison and US-based firm FluGen, and even talked about producing 300 million doses of vaccine in a while. On 2 April, the partnership announced that it would develop an intranasal vaccine named CoroFlu by inserting SARS-CoV-2 gene sequences into FluGen's flu vaccine candidate M2SR, a self-limiting version of the influenza virus,† to induce immune response against Covid-19.[3]

Despite this development, Bharat Biotech was seen as the best bet by the ICMR for its plan, considering that it had completed a large facility for polio vaccine production and a BSL-3 laboratory just a few months ago which could be re-purposed for Covid-19 vaccine production to meet the volume requirements. In addition, it was manufacturing sixteen different vaccines and had collaborated with ICMR on developing a Japanese encephalitis vaccine and a rotavirus vaccine.

The ICMR institution NIV, Pune had moved to in vitro studies as soon as the virus strain was identified and isolated. By the time controlled laboratory studies and mice experiments were completed, with large primate studies were set to begin, a total lockdown was declared. That's when the monkey chase began.

With the lockdown in place, troops of monkeys that usually

* A harmless virus from monkeys that's modified so it can't reproduce. It carries genetic material from another virus (like Covid-19) to help the body build immunity.

† A genetically modified flu virus used as a base in experimental vaccines. It doesn't spread in the body and is designed to safely stimulate immunity.

descended on villages bordering forests vanished into the jungles. As people stayed indoors, food waste and fruit scraps disappeared from the streets, leaving the primates with little reason to venture out. Monkey trappers in the villages struggled to locate the troops, making it nearly impossible to capture any for research.

The NIV scientists turned to nearby zoos in search of alternatives. Across the world, animals were dying in zoos and experimental breeding centres due to food shortages and the inability of curators to attend to them during the lockdown.[4] In Indian zoos too, only old or malnourished macaques remained. For its primate studies, the NIV team needed young, healthy baboons with strong immune responses – a search that was proving increasingly difficult.

Eventually, help came from the Maharashtra Forest Department. A specialized team was deployed for the search, venturing deep into the jungles and scanning large swaths of forest. They managed to trap the required number of Rhesus macaques from somewhere near Nagpur, ending the long chase. The team of officials and local trappers spent twenty days in the forest to catch twenty monkeys, averaging one monkey a day![5]

By early May, ICMR signed the partnership with Bharat Biotech and announced their plan to develop a vaccine under the name COVAXIN. ICMR was to isolate the SARS-CoV-2 virus from a large number of samples and carry out virus passage testing and confirmation, electron microscopy studies and the next generation virus sequencing.* Bharat Biotech agreed to fund the candidate vaccine development at ICMR, oversee Phase I and II clinical trials, recruit a clinical research organization for trial monitoring and conduct pre-clinical safety and toxicity studies in small animals.

Perhaps remembering the raw treatment meted out to the IISc team during hepatitis B vaccine development in 1998, the ICMR team put it on paper that Bharat Biotech would recognize the

* A modern method of reading the complete genetic code of a virus quickly and accurately to understand how it behaves or mutates.

contribution of the government partner by printing the name of ICMR-NIV on the vaccine boxes when they went to market. ICMR Director-General Balram Bhargava divulged to *The Hindu* that the Memorandum of Understanding (MoU) also stipulated that Bharat Biotech would pay 5 per cent of the net sales as royalty to the ICMR, in addition to prioritizing in-country supplies.[6]

Thus kicked off an unusual partnership, perhaps the quickest one forged between a private entity and a government organization in India in recent times. Continuing the work already started by NIV team and other ICMR teams, the joint Bharat Biotech-ICMR team developed three inactivated vaccine candidates named BBV152A, BBV152B and BBV152C. The first two had the same adjuvant, a substance that is added to the vaccine to enhance the immune response, while the third one had a different adjuvant. The last two candidates had six micrograms each of inactivated SARS-CoV-2 mix, and the first one only had three micrograms of the virus mix.

Once it was tested on mice and rabbits and found to be effective in generating high levels of neutralizing antibodies,* it was then tested on simian hamsters.† The candidates were found to be offering adequate protection to these animals too by clearing the virus load from the lower respiratory tract and reducing the virus load in the upper tract. Of the three, the first one with three micrograms inactivated virus strain was found to be the most effective.[7]

After the hamsters, it was the turn of Rhesus macaques. Monkeys were grouped in sets of five to run the vaccine experiment. While one group was given a placebo, the other three groups were given vaccine candidates deep into their lungs by direct injections. When they were exposed to the virus, the vaccinated ones cleared the virus from their lungs and nasal passages within seven days of infection. Unlike

* Special proteins made by the immune system that block viruses from infecting cells.

† Likely refers to laboratory hamsters used as test animals for research. 'Simian' may be a mistaken label here as hamsters are not primates.

the placebo group,* the vaccinated ones did not develop pneumonia, thereby confirming the findings.[8]

Relying on these findings, by the end of June 2020, Bharat Biotech secured approval from the DCGI to conduct Phase I and II clinical trials, crucial phases of vaccine development.[9] Phase I trials primarily focused on evaluating safety, tolerability and initial immune response in a small group of healthy volunteers. Phase II trials expanded the study to a larger group to further assess safety, determine the optimal dose and gather preliminary data on the vaccine's efficacy.

The approval and rollout of COVAXIN sparked significant debate due to several contentious issues. One of the primary concerns was the vaccine's approval without the completion of Phase 3 efficacy trials. Gagandeep Kang, a prominent virologist, expressed her apprehensions openly, stating, 'I would not take the vaccine without efficacy data.' She emphasized the importance of transparency and the potential risks of undermining public trust in vaccines.[10] The term 'clinical trial mode' used during the vaccine's approval added to the confusion. Kang noted that she had 'never seen anything like this before', highlighting the ambiguity and lack of clarity in the regulatory process.[11]

Furthermore, the absence of publicly available efficacy data at the time of approval led to divisions within the scientific community. A group of scientists issued a statement urging for the release of Phase 3 trial data before mass administration, emphasizing the need for transparency to maintain public confidence.

The government's decision to approve COVAXIN was perceived by some as being influenced by political considerations, aiming to promote self-reliance at the cost of science. However, the Union Health Ministry refuted these claims, asserting that the approval process adhered to scientific norms. These controversies also underscored the challenges faced during the pandemic in balancing

---

* A group in a clinical trial that receives a harmless, inactive substance instead of the real vaccine, used to compare effects and measure true efficacy.

rapid vaccine deployment with rigorous scientific evaluation, and the importance of maintaining public trust through transparency and adherence to established protocols.

By the time vaccine development progress updates from Moderna, Pfizer-BioNTech and AstraZeneca-Oxford were trickling in, other vaccines from Janssen in the US, Sputnik in Russia and Sinopharm and Sinovac in China were entering human trial phases. To keep pace with the global vaccine trials, the ICMR and Bharat Biotech recruited twelve sites across the country to conduct randomized, double-blinded, placebo-controlled trials.*

Even as the Phase I trial were set to start, Bhargava wrote to the dozen institutes participating in the trials on 2 July that 'it was envisaged to launch the vaccine for public use latest by August 15, 2020.'[12] As the letter leaked to the media, criticism mounted.[13] None other than the Indian Academy of Sciences, India's foremost science body, issued a statement. It read, 'any hasty solution that may compromise rigorous scientific processes and standards will likely have long-term adverse impacts of unforeseen magnitude on citizens of India.'[14]

ICMR's move to launch the vaccine by 15 August was considered more of a political move than one guided by science, and rumours were rife that it was intended to pave the way for the Prime Minister to announce the vaccine launch in his upcoming independence day speech. With criticism mounting, ICMR issued a clarification that Bhargava's letter was meant to cut unnecessary red tape without bypassing any necessary process and speed up the impending trials.[15] The statement laid the controversy to rest to some extent.

As many as 755 individuals participated in the Phase I trials that started in July and the Phase II trials which began shortly after. Both phases concluded with remarkable results, with the vaccine demonstrating safety and a strong immune response. To lend

* A rigorous method for testing vaccines where participants are randomly assigned to groups, neither they nor the researchers know who got the real vaccine or placebo, to eliminate bias and ensure reliable results.

credibility to the studies, the results were published in peer reviewed international journals by early 2021.[16] This was followed by the results of Phase II trials and the three follow up studies.[17]

The efforts to prove the three 'E's of vaccine trials – Efficacy, Effectiveness and Efficiency – were nearing completion. In a vaccine/drug trial, 'efficacy' results show the vaccine's performance under ideal conditions, while 'effectiveness' demonstrates its working in a real setting. Efficiency, on the other hand, is about its cost versus its benefits. BBV152 succeeded on all fronts with flying colours.

Contrary to the raised speculations, nothing related to the Covid-19 vaccine happened by 15 August – no announcement, no declaration.

In fact, by the time the Phase I and II trials were over and results were analyzed, it was almost Diwali. The complete lockdown was long over, and the country was going through the 'unlock' phases. The nation was gradually returning to normalcy with the number of cases and casualties decreasing. Around the world, the UK was preparing to grant Emergency User Authorization (EUA)* to the mRNA vaccine of Pfizer-BioNTech. The US FDA was considering mRNA vaccines of Pfizer-BioNTech and Moderna for EUA. Russia had already begun administering Sputnik vaccine without waiting for the Phase III trials to be over.

India too was reviewing its regulatory pathways to respond swiftly. Since 2019, India had a provision allowing the deployment of drugs and vaccines for emergency use without waiting for the completion of the Phase III trials. Provisions in the New Drugs and Clinical Trials Rules, 2019 could be interpreted to grant such approvals for public use in case of emergencies. Therefore, by invoking such a provision, the government began considering deploying the vaccine for public use. Accordingly, Bharat Biotech approached the DCGI for emergency use authorization by the end of December.

* A fast-track approval that allows the use of unapproved medical products during emergencies (like pandemics) when there are no adequate, approved alternatives.

The Subject Expert Committee (SEC)* of CDSCO met on 1 and 2 January 2021 and made recommendations to the DCGI on Bharat Biotech's accelerated approval request. Accordingly, the DCGI cleared the case on 3 January.[18] In the same meeting, DCGI also cleared the application of the Serum Institute for its COVISHIELD vaccine.

COVISHIELD had undergone rigorous clinical trials, starting with early-phase trials in the UK, followed by Phase III trials in multiple countries, including the UK, Brazil and South Africa. These trials demonstrated the vaccine's efficacy and safety, leading to emergency use authorizations (EUA) in several countries, including the UK. ICMR co-funded the Indian clinical trials of COVISHIELD in partnership with the Serum Institute. Phase II and III clinical trials were conducted at fifteen locations across India on 1,600 participants who had enrolled by 31 October 2020.

Seeing the approvals for COVAXIN and COVISHIELD, Pfizer wasted no time in approaching the DCGI, seeking emergency authorization for its BNT162b2 mRNA vaccine. The SEC met in the early days of February and rejected its application to recommend for approval. The committee noted reports of palsy, anaphylaxis† and other severe adverse events coming from some countries upon administering the BNT162b2 vaccine. Since it wasn't clear whether these adverse events were connected to the vaccine or not – and the documents submitted by Pfizer did not spell out how the vaccine would generate safety and immunogenicity in the Indian population – the committee did not recommend its application for DCGI approval.[19]

This effectively closed the door to global vaccine players, reserving the Indian Covid-19 vaccine market exclusively for domestically developed or manufactured vaccines like COVAXIN and COVISHIELD. Later however, during the peak of the second

* A group of scientists and medical experts in India who evaluate clinical trial data and make recommendations about drug or vaccine approvals.

† A severe, potentially life-threatening allergic reaction that can occur quickly after exposure to something (like a vaccine or drug).

wave in May–June 2021, when the country faced a severe vaccine shortage, the Indian government would approach Pfizer and Johnson & Johnson seeking their vaccines. This decision also placed immense pressure on the two leading domestic manufacturers to scale up swiftly and meet national demand.

Both Bharat Biotech and the Serum Institute were alerted to prepare for the launch soon after Independence Day. By November 2020, the Serum Institute had manufactured 40 million doses under a manufacturing and stockpiling license from the DCGI.[20] Bharat Biotech too produced a few million doses and kept a stockpile. With two vaccines and sufficient cold storage facilities, the Indian government announced a nation-wide launch of its vaccination campaign from 16 January, immediately after the harvest new year. The plan was to start with 30 million healthcare workers and frontline warriors. This would be followed by vaccinating all people above the age of fifty and those with co-morbidities* under fifty, which meant another 270 million.[21] The Serum Institute and Bharat Biotech were ordered to make available a stock of 300 million vials in the coming months.

Parallel to the rollout of the vaccines, the Ministry of Health and Family Welfare also launched a digital vaccination management system named Co-WIN. It was meant to assist the programme managers on vaccine session allocations, verification of beneficiaries and generate digital certificates for the vaccinated. Despite initial hitches, Co-WIN also took off across the country.

Almost a month before India's launch, the US and Canada had launched the Pfizer-BioNTech vaccine, a week after its launch in the UK. France, Germany and Italy had launched it on 27 December 2020. China launched its own vaccine in the middle of January. In effect, India was almost a month behind most of the G7 countries, and China and Russia, in introducing a vaccine. People were getting impatient with the delay.

---

* The presence of additional diseases or medical conditions in a person – like diabetes or heart disease – which may worsen the risk of complications from Covid-19.

In addition, when the announcement of the pan-India introduction of COVAXIN was made, it raised concerns about granting emergency approval for an under-trial vaccine. Many questioned its legitimacy and the need to rush it when another vaccine was already available. The All India Drug Action Network, a healthcare watchdog, expressed concern due to the absence of efficacy data and a perceived lack of transparency. It even suggested that the move might undermine confidence in India's scientific decision-making process.[22] The DCGI, V. G. Somani, defended the decision by declaring the vaccine was safe, and that only typical side effects like mild fever, pain and allergies were expected.[23]

By this time, Covid-19 had escalated to unprecedented levels, emerging as a catastrophe of unknown magnitude. The country crossed 10 million infections and 150,000 deaths. India stood just behind the US in terms of the number of daily new cases.

In the meantime, the Phase III trials to test COVAXIN's effectiveness and safety in a large, diverse population commenced across twenty-one test sites in November – on 26,000 individuals between twelve and ninety-eight years of age. Touted to be the largest of such trials ever conducted for a vaccine in India, it included almost 2,500 people aged above sixty years and 4,500 people with co-morbidities.

The results of the Phase III trials were also promising, demonstrating an efficacy of 100 per cent to prevent severe Covid-19 infections and 78 per cent to prevent asymptomatic disease.[24] However, the global scientific community wasn't convinced. A report in *Science* analyzing these published studies expressed concern about the potential of an inactivated whole virus vaccine to prevent SARS-CoV-2 infection.[25]

Despite these reservations, support came from the West. Two professors from Emory University's School of Medicine in Atlanta called the study a significant advancement in the Covid-19 vaccine landscape in the *Lancet Infectious Diseases* journal. It also hoped that Bharat Biotech's extensive experience in producing and distributing vaccines to LMICs would help address global vaccine disparities.[26] It was clearly indicating COVAXIN as a solution to the looming vaccine equity challenge.

By July, Bharat Biotech concluded Phase III trials with its final analysis of efficacy-related data. The final tally showed 77.8 per cent effectiveness against symptomatic Covid-19, with twenty-four confirmed cases in the vaccinated group versus 106 in the placebo group. It also proved to be 93.4 per cent effective against severe symptomatic Covid-19. Safety analysis showed only 12 per cent of the vaccinated experiencing commonly known side effects and less than 0.5 per cent reporting serious adverse events.

The Phase III data also demonstrated 63.6 per cent protection from asymptomatic Covid-19 and 65.2 per cent protection against the B.1.617.2 Delta variant which was getting reported in the second wave.[27] Though the Delta variant was first identified in India in late 2020, it would be declared as a variant of concern by WHO by May 2021 after observing its high transmissibility and potential for increased severity of illness.

The Chinese vaccines – CoronaVac developed by Sinovac and BBIBP-CorV from Sinipharam – also employed the same approach of ICMR-Bharat Biotech vaccine – using an inactivated virus. But COVAXIN showed better results. The key to this success was one crucial factor – the adjuvant used in the vaccine preparation. Instead of the commonly used adjuvant of aluminium hydroxide or alum, a new adjuvant namely Algel-IMDG* was used in COVAXIN. Though the original intention was to avoid the undesirable inflammatory response of aluminium hydroxide, the replacement offered an unexpected outcome – enhanced vaccine efficacy. In the long run, it helped build the reputation of COVAXIN.

The WHO granted Emergency Use Listing (EUL) to COVAXIN on 3 November 2021, nearly seven months after the company

---

* A novel adjuvant used in COVAXIN instead of traditional aluminium-based ones. It enhanced vaccine effectiveness while reducing inflammation-related side effects.

submitted its Expression of Interest. This delay, longer than that experienced by other vaccines, raised concerns and speculations. Several factors contributed to the prolonged approval process. WHO's Technical Advisory Group requested additional clarifications from Bharat Biotech to conduct a final risk-benefit assessment. Experts pointed out that Covaxin's phase 3 trial data had not been published in a peer-reviewed journal at the time, and there were concerns about the wide confidence intervals in efficacy estimates, especially among older adults.

Additionally, WHO conducted a post-EUL inspection of Bharat Biotech's manufacturing facilities between 14 and 22 March 2022, identifying deficiencies in GMP. As a result, WHO suspended the supply of COVAXIN through UN agencies and asked Bharat Biotech to address these gaps.

While some speculated that lobbying by transnational pharmaceutical companies might have influenced the EUL delay and suspension, there is no concrete evidence to support such claims. WHO officials emphasized that the timeline for EUL depends largely on the completeness and quality of data submitted by the manufacturer.

It was a mammoth task for the government to vaccinate 1.4 billion people in the shortest possible time, making it one of the largest such exercises anywhere in the world. In addition to the Task Force led by the Principal Scientific Adviser K. Vijayraghavan to accelerate R&D for Covid-19 drugs, diagnostics and vaccines, a National Expert Group on Vaccine Administration for Covid-19 (NEGVAC) was formed to devise a comprehensive vaccine administration plan. It was co-chaired by V. K. Paul, Member (Healthcare) in NITI Aayog, the government's primary public policy think tank, and the Health Secretary. Committees, task forces and control rooms were structured under NEGVAC at state, district and block levels. Additionally, the central government created an empowered group on Covid-19 vaccine administration to ensure the efficient use of technology and an inclusive, transparent and scalable vaccination process.

An existing digital network called the electronic Vaccine Intelligence Network (eVIN)* played a crucial role in identifying beneficiaries and establishing a vaccine distribution network across the country. Developed indigenously, eVIN had digitized vaccine inventories and had been monitoring the cold chain temperature via an app set up on smartphones. Originally launched in 2015, this technology provided a stable and readymade platform for the Covid-19 vaccination campaign. Alongside, the Co-WIN app helped schedule vaccine appointments, coordinate administration of the vaccine and generate vaccination certificates.

While both COVISHIELD and COVAXIN were pivotal to India's vaccination strategy, COVISHIELD's rollout was swifter and more extensive initially. The fact that COVISHIELD was developed in collaboration with AstraZeneca and the University of Oxford, with clinical data from multiple countries, helped build trust in its efficacy and safety from early days. The Serum Institute's vast manufacturing capabilities allowed for the rapid production and distribution of COVISHIELD, ensuring wide availability across the country, in addition to offering consignments for Government of India's Vaccine Maitri programme.† COVISHIELD, due to its initial head start, became the dominant vaccine in the early phases. COVAXIN's acceptance was slow to come, only picking up in the later stages of vaccination.

The vaccination drive that began in January 2021 faced numerous difficulties in its early days, including vaccine hesitancy, logistical hurdles and supply chain issues. Despite the challenges, the drive ramped up significantly with the creation of mass vaccination centres and mobile units. Co-WIN too played a crucial role. The drive gained momentum by involving both the public and private sectors and launching awareness campaigns. In about ten months of its vaccination drive, India crossed the 1 billion vaccine dose milestone

* A digital system used to manage vaccine stocks and monitor storage temperatures to ensure vaccines remain effective.

† India's humanitarian initiative to supply Covid-19 vaccines to other countries in need.

and within one year, 70 per cent of the adult population had been fully vaccinated, with 93 per cent receiving at least the first dose.[28]

While India was accelerating its vaccination programme with increasing confidence, the picture elsewhere in the world was more uneven. Vaccine equity was emerging as a concern globally as the rich countries with plenty of resources were placing orders for vials several times the size of their population, whereas the developing nations were struggling to find resources and channels to source vaccines even as thousands were dying of the disease.

Tedros Adhanom Ghebreyesus, WHO Director-General, minced no words when he stated that the world was on the brink of a catastrophic moral failure. By January 2021, while 40 million vaccine doses had been administered across forty-nine high-income countries, a low-income country had received just twenty-five doses. 'Not 25 million; not 25 thousand; just 25,' remarked Ghebreyesus, highlighting the stark inequity in vaccine access.[29]

This was despite WHO forming a global initiative named COVAX as part of the ACT (Access to Covid-19 Tools) Accelerator to ensure equitable access to Covid-19 vaccines, in collaboration with GAVI, CEPI and UNICEF in April 2020. The poor delivery to poor countries was in spite of rich countries committing ample supply to COVAX. This was when Ghebreyesus stated that the price of this catastrophic moral failure would be the lives and livelihoods of people in the world's poorest countries.

For months, the ACT Accelerator and COVAX worked hard to ensure equitable vaccine distribution, overcoming numerous barriers. They secured 2 billion doses from five producers by September 2020, with more options, and aimed to start deliveries from February 2021.

However, concerns had arisen about COVAX's vaccine acquisition and whether high-income countries would honour their commitments. As vaccines began to be deployed, rich countries placed orders to Pfizer and Moderna for huge quantities with advance payments. In July 2020, the US entered into a $1.95 billion agreement with Pfizer for 100 million doses and later secured an additional 100 million doses from Moderna. The EU made huge advance purchases, including 300 million doses from Pfizer and 160 million from Moderna. Other rich countries such as Canada (56 million), Japan (120 million), the UK (40 million) and Israel entered into advance purchase agreements with these vaccine manufacturers.

For quite a while, it was reminiscent of a chaotic fish market where vaccine companies were accepting orders from anyone who could pay higher amounts. Clearly, equitable vaccine access was at risk. Alarmed by this trend, Ghebreyesus raised his voice at the 148th meeting of the WHO executive board to point out that some countries and companies were undermining COVAX by prioritizing bilateral deals, increasing prices and delaying WHO approvals. This, he said, was to create vaccine hoarding, market chaos and prolonged pandemic impacts.[30] WHO sent a strong message that vaccine equity was crucial not only morally but also strategically and economically for the world.

Amid this growing imbalance, India seized the moment to assert its vaccine leadership and reaffirm its longstanding commitment to the Global South. With two domestically produced vaccines in its kitty, India launched the Vaccine Maitri (Friendship) initiative – just a week after starting its national vaccination drive. Beyond humanitarian aid, the move was a bold statement of its emergence as a responsible global public health leader, seeking to build solidarity with LMICs across Asia, Africa and Latin America.

While the initiative served a strategic purpose in enhancing India's diplomatic ties with recipient countries, it led to a huge vaccine crisis within the country. It also raised questions about prioritizing exports over domestic needs, especially when India's own Covid-19 cases had been surging since April 2021.

Eventually, when the second wave of Covid-19 peaked in India in May, the government had to pause the Vaccine Maitri initiative to focus on addressing the domestic vaccine requirement. This affected the supply to other countries and dented India's image, albeit briefly. The supplies resumed later as the situation improved. By the time

Covid-19 cases began to drop in June 2023, India had distributed 300 million doses to ninety-four countries, of which at least 234 million doses were against payments. Only 52 million doses were routed through COVAX for LMICs and 15 million doses as grants sent to neighbouring countries.[31]

India's arch-rival, China did not miss the opportunity either. Leveraging its geopolitical clout, China sought to assert its dominance in the field despite being a non-player in the global vaccine industry. Early on, China distributed more vaccine doses than India, providing crucial support to several countries and bolstering its international image as a reliable partner. However, as concerns grew over the efficacy of Chinese vaccines against newer variants, countries like Indonesia, Thailand and the Philippines began switching to alternatives. This shift cast a shadow over China's vaccine diplomacy, painting it in a poor light. While China's vaccine diplomacy faced growing skepticism, the broader global response revealed that vaccines had become more than just tools of public health – they were instruments of soft power, strategic influence and ethical test cases in a divided world.

The global vaccine story was never just about health – it is a complex interplay of diplomacy, competition and moral reckoning. The Covid-19 crisis exposed the best and worst of global cooperation. On one hand, scientific breakthroughs and collaborative platforms like COVAX demonstrated humanity's capacity to unite under pressure. On the other, vaccine nationalism, supply hoarding and broken promises revealed deep fractures in global solidarity. The moral urgency voiced by WHO had to compete with realpolitik, commercial interests and national pressures.

India's dual role – as both a recipient and supplier of vaccines – offered a unique vantage point. The Vaccine Maitri initiative showcased a commendable effort to bridge equity gaps, though not without cost. The temporary suspension during the second wave illustrated the fine balance between national imperatives and global responsibility. Yet, India's eventual comeback, delivering vaccines to nearly 100 countries, solidified its emerging role as a leader in global health.

The race for vaccine diplomacy may not have had a clear winner, but it raised an important question for the future: Will the world build a more equitable system for global health security? Or will we return to business as usual, forgetting the crisis and the lessons learnt? The Covid-19 vaccine story leaves behind more than data – it leaves a legacy, a warning and a blueprint for what must change.

43

PATENTS, POWER AND A DIVIDED WORLD

AS THE THREAT OF COVID-19 WANED, ON 20 JUNE 2022, the Central Bureau of Investigation (CBI), India's premier anti-corruption enforcement agency, set a trap for the Joint DCGI, S. Eswara Reddy in New Delhi.

Reddy had served as DCGI from February 2018 to August 2019, when he was replaced by his colleague V. G. Somani after a tough fight for the top slot. Reddy thereafter continued as the joint DCGI. As the second-highest officer in the DCGI, Reddy was responsible for overseeing the approvals of drugs and vaccines trials. Acting on a tip-off from a senior official within the DCGI, the CBI placed Reddy's residence under surveillance in June, suspecting that certain influential individuals were planning to deliver a 'reward' for recommending a Phase III trial application during a recent SEC meeting. Disguised in plain clothes, the officers waited outside Reddy's residence in central New Delhi.

After a long wait, a sedan pulled up and two sharply dressed men entered the house. The CBI officers emerged from their parked vehicles and discreetly trailed them. When a transaction unfolded inside Reddy's drawing room, the agents swiftly intervened, seizing ₹400,000 in cash that Dinesh Dua, director of Synergy Network India Private Limited, was said to have sent for Reddy.

Reddy, Dua and one Guljit Sethi, Director of Delhi-based Bioinnovat Research Services, were arrested. Subsequent searches of their residences, and that of L. Praveen Kumar's, Associate VP of Biocon Biologics Limited, Bangalore, resulted in the seizure of apparently incriminating documents and items.[1]

According to court filings, Reddy had allegedly agreed to expedite the approval process for Biocon's Phase III trial waiver* for its insulin aspart injection† in exchange for a 'reward' of ₹900,000.[2]

The charge against Reddy was that after assuring Dua on 15 June of a favourable outcome at the SEC meeting, he altered the meeting minutes of 18 May 2022. Specifically, he changed the term 'data' to 'protocol', purportedly to secure a Phase III trial waiver for Biocon's insulin aspart candidate.[3] Despite his reinstatement, six months later, the government granted the CBI sanction to prosecute Reddy.

It comes as little surprise that Biocon officials chose a shortcut, likely after exhausting righteous avenues to resolve their pending file. Under the provisions of the Similar Biologics Guidelines, 2016,‡ and the New Drugs and Clinical Trials Rules (NDCT), 2019,§ the company was entitled to a waiver since the required trials had already been conducted elsewhere. Those familiar with this regulatory body attest that expediting processes through unofficial channels has long been the norm, even when applicants were fully compliant.

It's widely known that large corporations and their representatives receive preferential treatment and privileged access to senior officials at the FDA Bhawan on Kotla Road, New Delhi. Relationships between consultants, agents and officers are deeply entrenched. Despite the anti-corruption clean-ups by the BJP government since

---

* An exemption from conducting certain clinical trials, usually allowed if similar data from other countries is already available.

† Insulin aspart is primarily used to manage type 1 diabetes, a condition where the body fails to produce insulin, and it is used occasionally for type 2 diabetes.

‡ Rules for approving 'biosimilar' drugs – cheaper versions of biologic medicines that are proven to be highly similar to already approved ones.

§ The legal framework that guides how new drugs and clinical trials are regulated in India.

2014, little has changed in key offices like that of CDSCO, the parent body of the DCGI. Notably, small and medium enterprises have made progress in drug and vaccine innovation in spite of, rather than because of, a regulatory system plagued by red-tape and maintained by officials who purportedly facilitate illegal gains and foster a culture of opacity.[4]

During the Covid-19 pandemic, however, directives were issued to the DCGI to prioritize clearance of all files related to Covid-19 drugs and vaccines, bypassing bureaucratic delays. This sense of urgency led Pfizer, in December 2020, to believe it could also secure Emergency Use Authorization for its mRNA vaccine along with COVAXIN and COVISHIELD. Pfizer's confidence also hinged on provisions outlined in the NDCT Rules, which allowed waivers for Phase III trials if such trials had already been conducted elsewhere, replacing the previous requirement for a 'bridge trial'.* But there was a catch: As per Rule 101 of the NDCT Rules, the DCGI was to notify the countries where such clinical trials could be conducted.[5]

Pfizer's strategy was clear: securing emergency authorization from the Indian regulator would potentially help validate its vaccine for acceptance in most countries, including recognition by bodies like WHO and UNICEF. Although the BNT162b2 vaccine had been available in the US market since December 2020, it had not yet received approval from the FDA. By the end of 2020, the UK and Bahrain were the only countries to have granted emergency approval for the Pfizer-BioNTech vaccine. The FDA would only approve it in August 2021.[6]

When Pfizer's case was presented before the DCGI, approval for the vaccine was withheld. The application was kept pending by seeking additional details about the vaccine.[7] Such requests typically include information on vaccine structure, antigens, adjuvants, delivery systems and development processes. In this case, the DCGI sought

---

* A smaller clinical trial carried out in a country than where the original trial was conducted to confirm that a drug or vaccine works similarly in its population.

specific details about the SARS-CoV-2 mRNA and the development of BNT162b2 vaccine.[8]

Some commentators speculated that Pfizer might have had concerns about proprietary data submitted to the DCGI being potentially leaked to Indian vaccine manufacturers, which they could use to quickly re-engineer mRNA vaccine models. Credible reports said the DCGI – through SEC – had specifically sought local safety and immunogenicity data, essentially asking Pfizer to conduct bridging trials to determine how the vaccine performed among Indian populations. In any case, Pfizer withdrew its application on 5 February 2021 after keeping it pending for over a month.[9]

The decision to deny emergency authorization by asking more details to Pfizer-BioNTech appeared to be more geopolitically motivated than purely technical. Primarily, the Indian authorities sought to prioritize the rollout of its domestic vaccines – the locally developed and produced COVAXIN and COVISHIELD, manufactured in India through a collaboration. This strategy helped India showcase its prowess in vaccine production and safeguard the reputation and interests of local vaccine manufacturers.

Despite this, Indian authorities recognized the value of the Pfizer-BioNTech vaccine for two key reasons: first being its mRNA technology, which Indian industries and research institutes had yet to explore and possess, and second, to keep an additional vaccine as a contingency option in case of widespread vaccine shortages. Authorities had not anticipated Pfizer's withdrawal of application, which it had filed on 6 December 2020. They had assumed that given the size of the Indian market and Pfizer's interest therein, the company would keep the application pending and eventually provide the requested details, at least in part.[10]

Pfizer had other considerations to reckon with. The global demand for Covid-19 vaccines was surging by the time the second wave peaked. Vaccines of Pfizer-BioNTech and Moderna were leading the race as the earliest contenders to emerge from the labs. Consequently, wealthy national governments engaged in fierce competition to place orders with these two manufacturers, making even substantial advance payments.[11] This made Pfizer reassess its strategy, taking into account its manufacturing capabilities and the mounting volume of orders.[12] Additionally, Pfizer had no existing obligations or responsibilities to India or the Indian government.

By April, the landscape had shifted with the emergence of new virus variants. The Alpha variant surfaced in the UK in September 2020, followed by the Beta variant in South Africa by November, and the Gamma variant in Brazil shortly after. India encountered Delta and Kappa variants by October, while the Lambda variant emerged in Peru in December 2020.[13] These new variants led to a surge in cases and fatalities, prompting nations to run for vaccine cover from wherever available.

Within weeks of the launch of two vaccines in India, demand skyrocketed. The rich and influential began leveraging their influence to get ahead of everybody else in the vaccination queue, vying for priority access from the first lot of 30 million vaccines allocated for healthcare professionals. The rollout of COVAXIN was constrained by Bharat Biotech's limited production capacity, resulting in COVISHIELD becoming the primary vaccine used in the initial vaccination drive. This stark supply-demand disparity compelled the government to resume discussions with Pfizer and Johnson & Johnson, another US company that had launched its single-dose vaccine in some markets by March.[14]

Pfizer initially indicated it would sympathetically consider offering its vaccine to India. However, weeks passed without action, prompting the Indian government to escalate discussions from the DCGI to the Health Secretary and Pharmaceuticals Secretary and eventually to the Member (Healthcare) in Niti Aayog, Principal Scientific Advisor and a Joint Secretary in the Prime Minister's Office.

Meanwhile, concerns began to surface over adverse events associated with the COVISHIELD vaccine. One notable case involved a volunteer from Chennai who had participated in the clinical trial of COVISHIELD and who later filed a lawsuit, drawing national headlines when the matter reached the Madras High Court. The participant alleged severe side effects following participation in the Phase III clinical trial conducted by the Serum Institute and ICMR. The individual claimed significant neurological damage post-vaccination and sought a compensation of ₹50 million (approximately $700,000) from the Serum Institute of India, the DCGI and the ICMR.[15] This case was dismissed by the court a few years later.

Side effects, technically referred as adverse events, are an inevitable aspect of drug and vaccine use worldwide. To manage this, regulatory bodies have established robust systems for monitoring and reporting such events. In India, this responsibility falls under the pharmacovigilance* programme, which collects data on Adverse Events Following Immunization (AEFI).† These reports are analyzed by an AEFI Secretariat, which operates under the Immunization Division in the Ministry of Health and Family Welfare. The AEFI Secretariat processes the cases and shares relevant details with manufacturers for review and action. Based on periodic causality assessments‡ at the national level, regulatory actions are initiated by the DCGI against the vaccine manufacturers in question.

During the initial months of Covid-19 vaccination, reports of adverse events flooded in, and many such cases ended up in courts. By the end of March 2022, 617 severe adverse events following Covid-19 vaccination had been reported through the AEFI portal, including 180 deaths. However, authorities did not officially attribute any of these fatalities to the vaccine.[16] In this context, the Madras High Court case stood out, as it involved a participant in the COVISHIELD clinical trial, bringing the issue of vaccine-related adverse events into sharper public and judicial focus.

---

* The practice of monitoring the effects and safety of drugs and vaccines after they have been approved and are in use.

† Any negative health effect that happens after a person gets vaccinated. It doesn't necessarily mean the vaccine caused it, but it needs to be investigated.

‡ A scientific process used to determine whether a particular drug or vaccine actually caused a reported health problem.

Using this pretext, Pfizer changed its approach. During subsequent meetings with the government, Pfizer proposed that it could offer its vaccine for immunization if the Government of India indemnified the company against any litigation risks arising from adverse events due to its use. This would mean that any court-awarded compensation for vaccine failures would be the responsibility of the Indian government, not Pfizer.[17]

There are instances in the West where courts have awarded billions of dollars as compensation to victims, leading to companies turning insolvent following such action. In the United States, Purdue Pharma, the maker of OxyContin, filed for bankruptcy in 2019 and later reached a settlement agreement of over $6 billion to resolve thousands of lawsuits related to its role in the opioid crisis. Similarly, Endo International agreed to a $465 million settlement before filing for bankruptcy protection in 2022 due to mounting litigation over its opioid painkillers.

There are no specific provisions under Indian drug law for granting indemnity related to new drug or vaccine approvals; however, indemnity in general has been recognized as a contractual obligation. Indemnity can only take the form of an indemnity bond executed on behalf of the Government of India or by provisioning by a clause within a contract signed with the supplier. There has been no precedent in India of any company receiving such preferential treatment from the government for any drug or vaccine.[18]

While this was happening, the quadrilateral security dialogue between the US, Japan, Australia and India was strengthening through meetings. In one such meeting of heads of the four nations, the group decided to use Covid-19 vaccine as a soft power tool of the alliance to check China in the Asia Pacific. This progressed to action and Johnson & Johnson (J&J) and Biological E. were identified as the American and Indian firms to execute the vaccine diplomacy respectively.[19] However, J&J, which was set to provide its vaccine technology to Biological E. for local production under the initiative, began echoing Pfizer's demand for indemnity as a precondition.[20]

In April 2021, the government offered to expedite emergency approvals for any Covid-19 vaccine already authorized for emergency use in the US, EU, UK and Japan.[21] Two months later, the requirement for post-approval bridging trials for vaccines was entirely waived. These were moves to woo Pfizer and J&J towards ensuring vaccine availability.

Despite efforts like the Quad's announcement to manufacture 1 billion doses of J&J vaccine at Biological E.'s Hyderabad facility,[22] and a special meeting in October 2021 to mark a $50 million US grant for the purpose,[23] the deadlock between Pfizer and the government persisted. J&J continued to align with Pfizer on the issue of indemnity, exerting pressure on the Indian government through multinational drug lobbies and lobbies of transnational drug companies operating in India.[24]

The government eventually realized that Pfizer, preoccupied with piled up global demand and lacking genuine intent to supply vaccines to India, posed the main obstacle. Frustration mounted over Pfizer's stance and the conduct of its officials.

The Quad Vaccine Partnership, conceived as a strategic response to China's assertive vaccine diplomacy, had pledged to deliver 1 billion doses to Indo-Pacific nations by the end of 2022. Despite continuous funding and political backing since 2021, the initiative fell short, achieving only 60 per cent of its target.[25] In contrast, China has distributed a significantly higher volume of doses worldwide, strengthening its global influence.

India's refusal to sign a liability waiver was just one of the factors contributing to delays in vaccine delivery by the Quad. Another issue was the Quad's decision to prioritize J&J and the experimental Corbevax vaccines over that of Pfizer or Moderna, leading to production challenges. Compounding the situation, the US FDA imposed restrictions on J&J's single-dose vaccine following an updated analysis revealing serious risk of blood clots and low platelet counts, further complicating matters. Consequently, Biological E.'s facility in Hyderabad focused primarily on producing Corbevax, which lacked WHO approval, limiting its international distribution.

These obstacles undermined the Quad's ability to effectively compete with China's vaccine initiatives, casting doubt on its potential to manage robust diplomatic and economic initiatives. Such challenges reinforced criticisms that the Quad, often perceived as an opportunistic, military-focused collective, may struggle to address critical economic, diplomatic and humanitarian issues in the Indo-Pacific region.[26]

In fact, within a few months of Covid-19 sweeping across the globe, it became evident to every country that they were on their own in this battle for survival. No nation, particularly the wealthy ones, would extend a helping hand to others until their last citizen was secured. The technological disparity between the West and the rest became glaringly evident. While the US and Europe rapidly developed vaccines using advanced mRNA technology, they were unwilling to share the technology with other countries. This Western attitude was on ugly display when Pfizer withdrew its application for emergency use authorization in India, reluctant to share full clinical-trial data, citing concerns over intellectual property and safety monitoring. Transparency advocates highlighted that the lack of access to raw data could facilitate unauthorized decoding or re-engineering of proprietary mRNA sequences.[27]

Once it was clear that Western nations would hold on to their technologies under the guise of intellectual property (IP) rights, India and South Africa made a strategic move. They initiated a proposal for a waiver of IP rights for Covid-19 vaccines and other medical technologies at the World Trade Organization (WTO) in October 2020. Known as the TRIPS waiver, this proposal meant to address global disparities in vaccine distribution. The goal was to ensure that LMICs could access the necessary technologies to effectively combat the pandemic.[28]

The concept of a waiver from certain obligations, such as in the case of public health emergencies, did exist in the TRIPS Agreement. It emerged in 2001 during WTO discussions on access to medicines.

This discussion led to the adoption of the Doha Declaration on the TRIPS Agreement and Public Health in November 2001. The Doha Declaration affirmed the flexibilities inherent in the TRIPS Agreement which permitted countries to take measures to protect their public health such as invoking compulsory licenses.

A compulsory license allows for the use of a patented invention without the patent holder's consent. India has issued a compulsory license only once, in March 2012, for the drug molecule sorafenib tosylate, marketed as Nexavar by German company Bayer, used in treating kidney and liver cancers. The license was granted to the Indian generic drug manufacturer Natco Pharma, enabling them to produce a more affordable generic version. This decision was made under Section 84 of the Indian Patents Act, 1970, due to the drug's high market price and limited availability.[29]

The India–South Africa TRIPS waiver proposal was unique for seeking a temporary suspension of IP rights obligations for vaccines, treatments, and technologies related to Covid-19. Such a waiver would allow WTO members to suspend patents and IP rights associated with Covid-19 medical products. The proposal received backing from numerous developing countries and public health advocates who asserted that the waiver could expedite global vaccine production and distribution, hastening an end to the pandemic. However, it encountered opposition from wealthy nations and transnational pharmaceutical giants who argued that IP rights were crucial for driving innovation and investment in medical research.[30]

Persistent negotiations have continued at the WTO in search of consensus. Various European and American pharmaceutical lobbies, the US Chamber of Commerce and the Business Roundtable (an association of CEOs from major American companies), staunchly opposed the proposal.[31] These groups emphasized the significance of IP rights in stimulating innovation and cautioned that a waiver could deter future research and development investments. They argued that logistical and manufacturing challenges were the real obstacles to vaccine equity, not access to technology. Despite support from over 100 WTO member countries, negotiations dragged into 2022, eventually resulting in a waiver only for vaccines in June that year. Therapeutics and diagnostics were excluded.[32]

Persistent resistance to such concessions during a pandemic revealed the insecurities of affluent countries, which prioritize pharmaceutical profits over global public health. They argued that waiving IP rights, albeit temporarily, could undermine innovation; however, this stance was widely seen as a move to prioritize corporate interest over equitable access to life-saving treatments. It also exposed the might of transnational corporations in influencing the necessity of a broad spectrum of nations.

Ultimately, the TRIPS waiver had little impact. No country utilized the waiver to produce vaccines using patented technology without consent. By the time it was granted, global vaccine supply had already outpaced the demand. Wealthier nations had succeeded in their mission – of delaying the waiver until it was redundant.

Nevertheless, the TRIPS waiver symbolized an ideological victory for the Global South over the wealthy West. It underscored the widening divide between the resource-rich, protectionist West and an increasingly assertive Global South. The latter recognized its right to access technology and intellectual property for the benefit of humanity, irrespective of who developed it first and at what cost.

This shift reflected a broader realization: the rights of the global citizens cannot be held hostage by a select few who monopolize the development of certain technologies through concentrated wealth and influence. Vaccines serve as a powerful example – a tool that has enabled human civilization to grow exponentially from millions to billions over two centuries. Yet, if equitable access to them is not guaranteed to all, the very survival of humanity on Earth could be jeopardized.

In hindsight, the Covid-19 vaccine episode became a litmus test for the world's commitment to collective action in times of crisis – and it failed spectacularly. The myth of global solidarity gave way to a brutal scramble for survival, with nations fortifying their borders, stockpiling vaccine and drug doses, and turning inward. The TRIPS waiver debate, though ultimately rendered moot by timing, exposed the fragility of the global health architecture and the entrenched power of profit-driven pharmaceutical giants. It revealed the urgent need to rethink the governance of critical technologies – not merely as commodities protected by patents, but as public goods necessary for global security and resilience.

As the world prepares for future pandemics, the lessons of vaccine nationalism, technology hoarding, and corporate lobbying must not be forgotten. The Global South, especially countries like India and South Africa, demonstrated that moral leadership can challenge entrenched power structures and push the boundaries of global policy. Going forward, building truly equitable systems for research, development and distribution of life-saving technologies will require structural changes to global trade rules, stronger South-South cooperation and a renewed understanding that in a deeply interconnected world, the health of one is inseparable from the health of all.

In a world driven by patents and fractured by technological inequality, the right to life must remain sacrosanct.

EPILOGUE

As you have seen in the preceding pages, India's vaccine journey has been anything but linear. It has unfolded with the unpredictability of a thriller – marked by soaring triumphs, moments of paralysis, long stretches of obscurity and sudden breakthroughs that reshaped the nation's public health landscape. Periods of stagnation were often followed by flashes of ingenuity, as the country repeatedly found ways to rebound from setbacks and move forward. It is a story not just of scientific progress, but of resilience, reinvention and collective ambition.

From the colonial era, when nearly half of all children died before reaching their fifth birthday and almost a third of infants failed to survive their first year, India has achieved one of the most remarkable public health transformations of the modern era. By 2024, infant mortality had declined to 2.6 deaths per 100 live births. At the heart of this progress lies one of modern medicine's most powerful and elegant tools: vaccines.

The transformation from colonial laboratories to globally respected Indian manufacturers and research hubs has not been accidental. It is the result of persistent, multi-generational efforts by scientists, policymakers, healthcare workers and institutions that believed in the power of prevention. Today, India stands as one of the largest vaccine producers in the world, supplying essential immunizations to over 170 countries, and helping protect millions of lives each year. In a world where some nations continue to invest heavily in technologies of mass destruction – fuelling death and devastation – India's commitment to disease prevention and public health stands as a compelling counterpoint. The lives saved, the diseases prevented and the trust built through these efforts are proof of what sustained scientific and humanitarian commitment can achieve. It is a promise kept to both global health and the values of human dignity.

Yet past achievements alone cannot guarantee future leadership.

Today, Indian science finds itself at an inflection point. On the one hand, the country possesses an extraordinary ecosystem: a talented scientific workforce, robust institutional capacity, entrepreneurial energy and a growing domestic market that makes it uniquely positioned to shape the next era of vaccinology. India has already demonstrated its prowess in conventional and recombinant platforms, and its potential to be at the forefront of cutting-edge domains – such as mRNA and DNA-based vaccines, thermostable formulations and even cancer immunotherapies – is real and rising.

At the same time, global vaccine science is rapidly moving into more advanced territory. While mRNA vaccines have opened new frontiers, the race is now accelerating toward platforms that can address their shortcomings. Self-amplifying RNA (saRNA), for instance, shows promise in generating stronger immune responses with smaller doses, reducing costs and expanding reach. Circular RNA (circRNA) platforms, with greater stability and longer protein expression, could lead to more durable vaccines that don't require complex cold chains. In a country like India, where logistics and affordability matter as much as innovation, such breakthroughs could be transformative.

India is well-positioned to play a leadership role in these domains; not just as a manufacturing hub but as a pioneer in original vaccine science. However, doing so will require more than technical expertise. It will demand a policy environment that values science for its own sake, supports open inquiry and protects the institutional independence of its research bodies.

That brings us to a sobering challenge. In recent years, there has been a growing trend to bend science to fit political or ideological narratives. Claims not grounded in empirical evidence have gained visibility and even legitimacy when wrapped in the language of nationalism or cultural pride. Pseudoscience has found a platform in places where rigorous science ought to lead. This is not a new risk in the history of nations, but in India today, it threatens to erode the very foundations that have made its scientific achievements possible.

The truth is simple: science flourishes in environments that nurture the four 'D's: disclosure, doubt, debate and diversity of thought. Vaccine development is particularly complex and slow burning. It demands not only high-end laboratories and skilled personnel but also regulatory integrity, long-term investments, public trust and global collaboration. When scientists are expected to conform to political messaging or tailor their findings to fit ideology, the integrity of research suffers – and with it, the safety and effectiveness of public health solutions.

To protect what we have built – and to realize what we are capable of – we must decisively resist the politicization of science. India's vaccine revolution was not fuelled by slogans or spectacle; it was built on sustained rigour, patient experimentation and the courage to challenge assumptions. The path forward must deepen that tradition. We must recommit to nurturing young scientists, expanding research funding, modernizing regulatory frameworks and allowing space for dissent and experimentation within our institutions. The role of public trust and community engagement cannot be overstated either; vaccine acceptance and success depend on transparent communication and inclusive decision-making that respects the concerns of diverse populations.

Moreover, India's position as a leader in global health – especially for the Global South – comes with responsibility. Our innovations must speak to the challenges of other LMICs, not just the affluent world. That means investing in scalable, affordable and context-sensitive solutions. It means not just exporting vaccines, but exporting solidarity, knowledge and collaborative frameworks that empower other nations to build their own capacities.

And yet, this remarkable journey must not be taken for granted. India's vaccine success was never inevitable. It was built brick by brick by generations of scientists, doctors, public health experts, institutions and entrepreneurs who were allowed space to think freely, take risks, and innovate. Along the way, they faced stiff resistance – not only from within a resource-constrained system but also from powerful multinational corporations that saw India's rise as a threat. These companies often denied Indian firms access to critical technologies, used patents as weapons to intimidate local manufacturers and at times even vilified those who dared to develop affordable vaccines for diseases that had long been priced out of reach for most people. Indian patients were denied timely access to essential vaccines because of monopolistic practices and legal barriers, in effect killing millions of newborns.

What enabled India to push through was a commitment to self-reliance, scientific integrity and public health purpose – backed, at least in part, by policies that put national interest and equity above short-term political optics and global corporate pressure.

In the final analysis, the story of India's vaccines is not just a chronicle of scientific advancement. It is a mirror to our values as a society. Do we prize truth over convenience? Do we trust evidence over belief? Are we willing to support institutions that may at times contradict dominant narratives, but do so in pursuit of a deeper, longer-lasting good?

The next chapter of India's vaccine journey will not be written in laboratories alone. It will be shaped in classrooms, on policy tables, in communities and in the public imagination. The choices we make today – about funding, freedom, fairness and fact – will determine whether we continue to lead the world in saving lives or fall back into cycles of missed opportunity. These four 'F's will either become pillars of strength or weakness, depending on how we mobilize them.

Let us move forward, not with chest-thumping, but with clear eyes, steady hands and bold minds. Let India not just remain the vaccine capital of the world but also become its conscience – advancing science not merely for prestige, but for purpose. That, in the truest sense, would make ours a nation built by vaccines.

ACKNOWLEDGEMENTS

Vaccine Nation is not mine alone.

It belongs to the millions of Indians whose stories, sacrifices and everyday acts of courage have shaped our country's immunization journey – to the health workers who have walked through floods and forests to deliver vaccines; the scientists who have toiled for decades with quiet persistence; the policymakers who have dared to make bold decisions, and the parents who roll up their children's sleeves with trust and hope in their eyes. This book is theirs.

When I first shared news of this project, I had not anticipated the tidal wave of support that would follow. From aspiring civil servants and young doctors to senior health administrators, public health workers, scientists and curious citizens, messages began arriving from across the country – and beyond. Some offered facts or figures, others shared forgotten tales or pointed me to new leads. Many simply wrote to say they were waiting, that this story mattered. That support became my compass. It reminded me that this was not just a book about science, but a story about people – and that I was only its narrator.

I am deeply grateful to every single person who contributed, whether with intent or serendipity, to the making of this book. To the librarians and archivists who unearthed brittle documents, the researchers who gently challenged my blind spots, the doctors who walked me through the complexities of immunology and the vaccine pioneers who welcomed me into their lives and laboratories – I thank you for your generosity.

I owe much to public health administrators who offered insight into the inner workings of India's vaccine ecosystem – often unvarnished, always thoughtful. I also extend my gratitude to the dozens of corporate executives who, despite the constraints of their positions, offered their reflections on the condition of anonymity. They spoke not just as industry leaders, but as engaged citizens with a personal stake in India's scientific and public health future.

A few individuals deserve special mention.

Dr T. P. Talwar, now a centenarian, was instrumental in steering India's vaccine research into uncharted territories – from leprosy to reproductive health. His pioneering work will forever remain foundational. Dr K. I. Varaprasad Reddy, whose story reads like a crime thriller, took on the challenge of developing India's first recombinant hepatitis B vaccine through sheer grit and vision. Dr Jacob John, the visionary behind India's pulse polio campaign, brought both scientific clarity and moral urgency to the fight against polio. Dr G. V. G. A. Harshavardhan, who currently heads the Indian Vaccine Manufacturers Association despite his progressing age, is another legend who told me tales from his association with Albert Sabin for India's first polio vaccine at the Pasteur Institute in Coonoor during the 1960s.

Ranjit Shahani, an industry veteran and former managing director of Novartis India, took a deep interest in the journey this book traces. He continued to share valuable insights throughout its development and was eagerly awaiting its release, but sadly passed away in March 2024 before its completion.

Dr V. K. Paul, who guided India's Covid-19 vaccine response from his position at NITI Aayog and Dr Balram Bhargava, who led ICMR's efforts in developing COVAXIN – both played pivotal roles in shaping India's contemporary vaccine landscape. I thank all of them for their participation in the book.

My deepest thanks go to Dr K. S. Jayaraman, former India editor of *Nature* and science editor at the Press Trust of India, who is also my longtime mentor. He was one of the first people I discussed this project with, back in 2021. He not only encouraged me to pursue it but also introduced me to key figures like Dr Talwar and Dr Varaprasad Reddy.

There were others who served as my sounding boards and critical readers, offering insights on structure, flow and substance. Dr Arun Varma, a respected geriatric healthcare expert; P. N. Ranjit Kumar, former Joint Secretary at the Ministry of AYUSH; Sheeba John from the St Vincent's University Hospital, Dublin and Bharat Kumar from the Manipal Academy of Higher Education were all generous with their time and wisdom.

I am equally grateful to veteran science journalists Somashekhar Mulugu, T. V. Padma, Dinesh Sharma and T. V. Jayan, whose informed view helped sharpen the narrative. I also thank senior journalists Shaukat Hussain Mohammed (*Deccan Chronicle/Economic Times*), Ullekh NP (*Open /Economic Times*), Subramani Mancombu (the *Hindu BusinessLine*) and Rajesh Abraham (the *New Indian Express*), for their ongoing encouragement and editorial suggestions over the last four years.

My agent at Labyrinth Literary Agency deserves heartfelt thanks for believing in this book and guiding it into the right hands. I also want to acknowledge the team at Pan Macmillan India – editors, the cover designer, production staff – who brought skill and care to every aspect of this publishing journey. Thank you for your faith in the vision.

Finally, I must thank my family. To my mother, Khadeeja, whose quiet strength has always sustained me; to my wife, Geetha Pillai, who stood by me during relentless deadlines; to my son, Tejus, whose curiosity reminds me why such stories matter. And to Snowy, our husky, who has been my silent companion through it all – thank you for the daily doses of joy.

Vaccine Nation is a product of many voices, but above all, it is a testament to the enduring spirit of Indian science – driven by curiosity, compassion and courage.

NOTES

PART-I: THE EARLY DAYS (1875–1930)

1. SNAKEBITE TURNS SAVIOUR

1. Naazneen Karmali, 'Horse Sense', *Forbes*, 26 November 2007. Available at: https://www.forbes.com/2007/11/14/cyrus-poonawalla-vaccine-biz-07india-cz_nk_1114poonawalla.html.
2. Lauren Frayer, 'The World's Largest Vaccine Maker Took a Multimillion Dollar Pandemic Gamble', WJCT Public Media, 18 March 2021. Available at: https://news.wjct.org/post/worlds-largest-vaccine-maker-took-million-dollar-pandemic-gamble.

2. HAFFKINE'S INDIAN EXPERIMENT

1. P. Chakrabarti, 'Curing Cholera: Pathogens, Places and Poverty in South Asia', *International Journal of South Asian Studies*, 2010, Vol. 3, pp. 153–168. Available at: https://pmc.ncbi.nlm.nih.gov/articles/PMC3160492/.
2. C. C. Manifold, 'Report of a Case of Inoculation with Carbolized Anti-Choleraic Vaccine (Haffkine)', *Indian Medical Gazette*, April 1893, Vol. 28, No. 4, pp. 101–103.
3. W. M. Haffkine, 'Anti-cholera Inoculation: Report to the Government of India', Calcutta: Thacker, Spink & Co., 1895.
4. W. M. Haffkine, 'Anti-Choleraic inoculations in India', *Indian Medical Gazette*, 1895, Vol. 30, pp. 35–41 (Paper read at the First Indian Medical Congress held in Calcutta in December 1894).

3. THE BIRTH OF INDIAN VACCINES

1. M. Ben-Ami, 'The Odessa Pogrom (1881) and the first self-defense (reminiscences)', *Harofé Haivri*, 1964, pp. 1–2, 273–287.
2. H. Friedenwald, 'Notes on Moritz Schiff (1823-1896)', *Bulletin of the History of Medicine*, June 1937, Vol. 5, pp. 589–602.

3. B. J. Hawgood, 'Waldemar Mordecai Haffkine, CIE (1860-1930): Prophylactic Vaccination Against Cholera and Bubonic Plague in British India', *Journal of Medical Biography*, February 2007, Vol. 15, No. 1, pp. 9–19. Available at: https://doi.org/10.1258/j.jmb.2007.05-59.
4. Ilana Lowy, 'From Guinea Pigs to Man, The Development of Haffkine's Anticholera Vaccine', *Journal of the History of Medicine and Allied Sciences*, Vol. 47, No. 3, pp. 270–309. Available at: https://academic.oup.com/jhmas/article-abstract/47/3/270/756916.
5. E. Roux, 'L'oeuvre medicale de Pasteur', A. Comben, R. Girard & G. Griruer (eds), *Agenda du Chimiste* (Paris: Hachette, 1896), pp. 527–548.
6. Haffkine Papers (hereafter HP), Ms. Var 325 file 338, The Manuscripts Department, National Library, The Hebrew University, Jerusalem.
7. Roux, 'L'oeuvre medicale de Pasteur'.
8. W. M. Haffkine, E. H. Hankin, and C. H. Owen, 'Technique of Haffkine's Anti-Cholera Inoculations', *Indian medical Gazette*, 1894, Vol. 29, pp. 201–206.
9. W. M. Haffkine, 'Injections Against Cholera: A Lecture', *Lancet*, February 1893, Vol. 141, pp. 316–318.
10. W. M. Haffkine, 'Inoculation de vaccins anticholériques à l'homme', *Comptes Rendus de la Société de Biologie*, 1892, Vol. 44, pp. 740–741. (Author's translation).
11. Ibid.
12. E. H. Hankin, 'Remarks on Haffkine's Method of Protective Inoculation Against Cholera', *British Medical Journal*, 1892, Vol. 2, pp. 569–571.
13. N. Longmate, 'King Cholera: The biography of a disease', London, 1966, p. 2.
14. J. Ferran, 'A propos de la communication de M. Haffkine sur le cholera asiatique', *Comptes Rendus des Séances de la Société de Biologie*, 1892, Vol. 44, pp. 771–773.
15. G. H. Borns, 'Waldemar Haffkine's Cholera Vaccines and the Ferran-Haffkine Priority Dispute', *Journal of the History of Medicine*, 1982, p. 400, 416.
16. W. M. Haffkine, 'A Lecture on Vaccination against Cholera', (lecture, Examination Hall of the Conjoint Board of the Royal Colleges of Physicians of London and Surgeons of England, 18 December 1895), *Indian Medical Gazette*, March 1896, Vol. 31, No. 3, pp. 81–86.
17. Hankin, 'Remarks on Haffkine's Method of Protective Inoculation Against Cholera'.
18. H. I. Jhala, 'W. M. W. Haffkine, Bacteriologist–A Great Saviour of Mankind', *Indian Journal of Medical History*, October 1967, Vol. 2, No. 2. Available at: https://hps.wisc.edu/wp-content/uploads/sites/366/2018/05/haffkine_jhala-1.pdf.
19. Hawgood, 'Waldemar Mordecai Haffkine, CIE (1860-1930): Prophylactic Vaccination Against Cholera and Bubonic Plague in British India'.

4. FROM CHOLERA TO PLAGUE

1. W. M. Haffkine, 'CIE Record of Services', *India Office List*, compiled from official records by direction of the Secretary of State for India in Council, London: Harrison and Sons, 1916, p. 539.
2. W. B. Bannerman, 'The Plague Research Laboratory of the Government of India', Parel, Bombay, *Proceedings of the Royal Society of Edinburgh*, 1902, Vol. 24, pp. 113–44.
3. W. M. Haffkine, 'A discourse on preventive inoculation', (the Royal Society, London, 8 June 1899), *Lancet*, 1899, Vol. 153, pp. 1694–1699.
4. Ibid.
5. Richard Friedrich Johannes Pfeiffer, 'Biographical Memoirs', The Royal Society, 1858–1945. Available at: https://royalsocietypublishing.org/doi/pdf/10.1098/rsbm.1956.0016.

5. THE BOMBAY PLAGUE

1. 'Administrative Report of the Municipal Commissioner for the City of Bombay 1896-1897', *The Bombay Gazette*, 13th April 1887, p. 633.
2. Robert A. Kyle, 'Colón-Otero, Gerardo; Shampo, Marc A. (1988). *Jaime Ferrán y Clúa: Bacteriologist. Mayo Clinic Proceedings, 63(4), 418–.* doi:10.1016/S0025-6196(12)64867-8; N. Gamaleya, 'Sur la vaccination preventive du cholera asiatique,' C. R. Acad. Sciences, 1888, 106, 432-34, and Louis Pasteur's comments, pp. 434–435.
3. Lowy, 'From Guinea Pigs to Man'.
4. HP, file 438, 'Haffkine's letter to the Secretary of the Department of Education', India Government, Simla, 10 December 1911.
5. Peter Keating, 'Vaccine therapy and the problem of opsonins', *History of Medicine and Allied Sciences*, July 1988, Vol. 43, pp. 275–296.
6. Indian Plague Commission, 'Minutes of evidence taken by the Indian Plague Commission with appendices', printed for H.M.S.O. by Eyre and Spottiswoode, 1900. Available at: https://curiosity.lib.harvard.edu/contagion/catalog/36-990051162450203941.
7. E. Klein, 'Report of the Indian Plague Commission', *Nature*, 1902, Vol. 65, No. 1684, pp. 320–321.
8. Almroth Wright, 'Report of the Indian Plague Commission', *British Medical Journal*, 1902, Vol. 1, No. 2158, pp. 1155–1161. Available at: https://doi.org/10.1136/bmj.1.2158.1155. *See also* 'Report of the Indian Plague Commission', *Lancet*, 1900, pp. 713–714; 'Statistical methods and the Indian Plague Commission', *Lancet*, March 1900, Vol. 155, pp. 724–725.

6. THE MULKOWAL TRAGEDY

1. R. H. Jocelyn Swan, 'THE MULKOWAL DISASTER.1', *Lancet*, 1907, Vol. 169, No. 4353, pp. 299–302. Available at: https://doi.org/10.1016/S0140-6736(01)51920-0.
2. Peter Hobbins, "Immunisation Is as Popular as a Death Adder': The Bundaberg Tragedy and the Politics of Medical Science in Interwar Australia', *Social History of Medicine*, Vol. 24, No. 2, pp. 426–444. Available at: https://doi.org/10.1093/shm/hkq047.
3. Tim Dyson, 'A Population History of India: From the First Modern People to the Present Day', Oxford University Press, 2018, p. 144. Available at: https://doi.org/10.1093/oso/9780198829058.001.0001.

7. ROSS AND THE RESCUE MISSION

1. G. H. F. N., 'Sir Ronald Ross, 1857–1933', *Obituary Notices of Fellows of the Royal Society*, December 1933, pp. 108–115. Available at: https://doi.org/10.1098/rsbm.1933.0006.
2. Ronald Ross, 'Haffkine's anti-plague prophylactic' (Letter to the Editor), *British Medical Journal*, 1900, p. 595.
3. Ronald Ross, 'India and Mr. Haffkine' (Letter to the Editor), *London Times*, March 1907.
4. Ronald Ross, 'India and Mr. Haffkine' (Letter to the Editor), *London Times*, June 1907.
5. Ross et al., 'Mr. Haffkine and the Mulkowal accident', *London Times*, July 1907.

8. HAFFKINE'S HUMILIATION

1. HP, file 397(7), Haffkine to the Secretary of the Government of India, 1 April 1909.
2. HP, file 397(7), Home Department Letter No. 1017 of June 1909; Letter of H. C. Woodman, Adjunct Deputy Secretary to the Government of India, 23 October 1909.
3. Eli Chernin, 'Richard Pearson Strong and the iatrogenic plague disaster in Bilibid Prison, Manila, 1906', *Reviews of Infectious Diseases*, 1989, Vol. 11, pp. 996–1003.
4. HP, file 397(7), Sir Harold Stuart, Secretary of the Government of India, to Haffkine, 6 June 1909.
5. HP, file397(7), Haffkine to the Indian Government, 16 February 1912.
6. HP, file 397(7), L.C. Porter, Secretary of the Government of India, to Haffkine, 27 March 1912.
7. N. K. Dutta, ed., 'Haffkine Institute Diamond Jubilee', Times of India Press, 1959.

8. Walter Laqueur, *The Changing Face of Antisemitism: From Ancient Times to the Present Day*, Oxford University Press, 2006.
9. B. Cvjetanovic, 'Contribution of Haffkine to the concept and practice of controlled field trials of vaccines', *Fortschritte der Arzneimittelforschung* (Progress in Drug Research), 1975, Vol. 10, pp. 481–484.

PART-II: BUILDING BLOCKS (1931–1960)

9. SAHIB SINGH SOKHEY

1. B. B. Dixit, 'Haffkine Institute platinum jubilee commemoration volume: 1899-1974', Haffkine Institute.
2. *The London Gazette*, 9 September 1913, No. 28754, p. 6419. Available at: https://www.thegazette.co.uk/London/issue/28754/page/6419.
3. H. Singh, 'Sahib Singh Sokhey (1887-1971): An Eminent Medico-Pharmaceutical Professional', *Indian Journal of History of Science*, 2015, Vol. 51.2.1, pp. 238–247. Available at: http://dx.doi.org/10.16943/ijhs/2016/v51i2/48435.
4. *The London Gazette*, 1 May 1925, No. 33043, p. 2925. Available at: https://www.thegazette.co.uk/London/issue/33043/page/2925.
5. 'Sahib Singh Sokhey 1887-1971', Biographical Memoirs of INSA Fellows, Indian National Science Academy. Available at: https://www.insaindia.res.in/BM/BM4_7614.pdf.
6. Ibid.
7. Singh, 'Sahib Singh Sokhey'.
8. S. S. Sokhey and M. K. Habbu, 'Casein Hydrolysate Cholera Vaccine', *Bulletin of the World Health Organisation*, 1950, Vol. 3, p. 33.
9. K. Ganapathi, 'Sahib Singh Sokhey', Biographical Memoirs of Fellows, Indian National Science Academy, 1976, Vol. 4, pp. 134–153.
10. Singh, 'Sahib Singh Sokhey'.
11. Ibid
12. S. S. Sokhey and M. K. Habbu, 'Biological Assay of Cholera Vaccine', *Bulletin of the World Health Organisation*, 1950, Vol. 3, p. 43–53.
13. Sub-Committee on National Health (Chairman: Col. S. S. Sokhey) and National Planning Committee, 'Report of the Sub-Committee on National Health', Bombay: Vora & Co. Publishers Ltd., 1947.
14. Ganapathi, 'Sahib Singh Sokhey'.
15. Ibid.
16. 'Report of the Panel on Fine Chemicals, Drugs and Pharmaceuticals', Department of Industries and Supplies, Government of India Press, Simla, 1947, p. 94.
17. Singh, 'Sahib Singh Sokhey'.
18. S. S. Sokhey, 'Pharmaceutical Problems of India', *Indian Journal of Pharmacy*, 1942, Vol. 4, pp. 15–25.

19. S. S. Sokhey, 'The Production of Pharmaceuticals in the Country', *Indian Journal of Pharmacy*, 1959, Vol. 21, pp. 231–234.
20. 'Sahib Singh Sokhey 1887–1971', Biographical Memoirs of INSA Fellows, Indian National Science Academy. Available at: https://www.insaindia.res.in/BM/BM4_7614.pdf Retrieved 16 December 2023.

10. SMALLPOX: A BIG CHALLENGE

1. Ishrat Alam, 'Smallpox and its Treatment in Pre-Modern India', *Disease and Medicine in India*: A Historical Overview, edited by Deepak Kumar, Tulika Books, 2012, p. 85.
2. Kabiraj Nagendra Nath Sengupta, *The Ayurvedic System of Medicine*, Calcutta, 1901, p. 301. *See also* Ian and Jenifer Glynn, *The Life and Death of Smallpox*, Cambridge University Press, 2004, p. 7.
3. A. L. Basham, *The Wonder That Was India*, Rupa Publications, 1992, p. 319, First published 1954.
4. David Arnold, 'Cholera and Colonialism in British India', Oxford University Press, *Past & Present*, November 1986, No. 113, pp. 118–151. Available at: http://www.jstor.org/stable/650982.
5. Stefan Riedel, 'Edward Jenner and the History of Smallpox and Vaccination', *Baylor University Medical Center Proceedings*, 2005, Vol. 18, No. 1, p. 21.
6. 'History of Smallpox', Centers for Disease Control and Prevention, U.S. Government. Available at: https://www.cdc.gov/smallpox/history/history.html.
7. Stanley Plotkin, 'Forward', *Vaccination: A History from Lady Montagu to Genetic Engineering*, by H. Bazin, Montrouge, France / Esher, UK: John Libbey Eurotext, 2011.
8. Haffkine, 'A Lecture on Vaccination Against Cholera'.
9. Ibid.
10. Sanjoy Bhattacharya, Mark Harrison and Michael Worboys, 'Fractured states: smallpox, public health and vaccination policy in British India 1800-1947', Orient BlackSwan, 2005, Vol. 11.
11. Michael Bennett, *War against smallpox: Edward Jenner and the global spread of vaccination*, Cambridge University Press, 2020.
12. John Shoolbred, 'Report on the progress of vaccine inoculation in Bengal', submitted to the Medical Board at Fort William, London, 1805.
13. Ibid.
14. Aparna Alluri, 'The Indian queens who modelled for the world's first vaccine', *BBC News*, 20 September 2020. Available at: https://www.bbc.com/news/world-asia-india-53944723
15. David Arnold, *Colonizing the body: state medicine and epidemic disease in nineteenth-century India*, University of California Press, 1993, p. 138.

16. D. Stewart, 'Report on Smallpox in Calcutta, 1833-4, 1837-8, 1843-4, and Vaccination in Bengal, from 1827 to 1844', Calcutta Government Press, 1845, pp. 50–52.
17. Henry Gelfand, 'A critical examination of the Indian smallpox eradication program', *American Journal of Public Health*, 1966, Vol. 56, No. 10, pp. 1634–1651. Available at: https://ajph.aphapublications.org/doi/pdf/10.2105/AJPH.56.10.1634.
18. WHO, 'Smallpox Eradication Programme - SEP (1966-1980)', 1 May 2010, Available at: https://www.who.int/news-room/feature-stories/detail/the-smallpox-eradication-programme---sep-(1966-1980).
19. Lawrence B. Brilliant, *The management of smallpox eradication in India*, University of Michigan Press, 1985.
20. Lawrence K. Altman, 'India Declared Free of Smallpox', *New York Times*, 3 July 1975. Available at: https://www.nytimes.com/1975/07/03/archives/india-declared-free-of-smallpox-2-countries-left.html.
21. Rohit Sharma, 'WHO dissenter warns against plans to retain smallpox virus', *British Medical Journal*, January 2002, Vol. 324, p. 69. Available at: https://doi.org/10.1136/bmj.324.7329.69/c.

11. TYPHOID MARY

1. Nina Strochlic, 'Typhoid Mary's tragic tale exposed the health impacts of 'super-spreaders'', National Geographic, 18 March 2020. Available at: https://www.nationalgeographic.com/history/article/typhoid-mary-tragic-tale-exposed-health-impacts-super-spreaders.
2. "TYPHOID MARY' DIES OF A STROKE AT 68; Carrier of Disease, Blamed for 51 Cases and 3 Deaths, but She Was Held Immune Services This Morning Epidemic Is Traced', New York Times, 12 November 1938. Available at: https://www.nytimes.com/1938/11/12/archives/typhoid-mary-dies-of-a-stroke-at-68-carrier-of-disease-blamed-for.html.
3. Ibid.
4. Leonard Colebrook, 'Almroth Edward Wright, 1861–1947', *Obituary Notices of Fellows of the Royal Society*, 1948, pp. 297–314.
5. Dieter H. M. Gröschel and Richard B. Hornick, 'Who Introduced Typhoid Vaccination: Almroth Wright or Richard Pfeiffer?', *Reviews of Infectious Diseases*, 1981, Vol. 3, No.6, pp. 1251–1254. Available at: https://doi.org/10.1093/clinids/3.6.1251.
6. D. Semple, 'A Preliminary Note on the Vaccine Therapy of Enteric Fever', *Lancet*, June 1909, Vol. 173, p. 1669. Available at: https://doi.org/10.1016/S0140-6736(01)71819-3.
7. A. E. Wright, 'On the Association of Serous Haemorrhages with Conditions of Defective Blood-Coagulability', *Lancet*, 1896, Vol. 2, pp. 807–809.

8. Ibid.
9. Gröschel and Hornick, 'Who Introduced Typhoid Vaccination', p. 1252.
10. A. E. Wright and D. Semple, 'Remarks on Vaccination Against Typhoid Fever', *British Medical Journal*, 1897, Vol. 1, pp. 256–259.
11. John D. Williamson, Keith G. Gould and Kevin Brown, 'Richard Pfeiffer's typhoid vaccine and Almroth Wright's claim to priority', 2021. Available at: https://doi.org/10.1016/j.vaccine.2021.03.017.
12. Ibid.
13. 'Sir Almroth Wright', *British Medical Journal*, 10 May 1947, Vol. 1, No. 4505, pp. 646–647.
14. Colebrook, 'Almroth Edward Wright, 1861–1947'.
15. J. C. B. Statham, 'The Complex Nature of Typhoid Etiology', *Journal of the Royal Army Medical Corps*, 1908, Vol. 11, pp. 351–367.
16. Aldo Castellani, 'Typhoid-Paratyphoid Vaccination with Mixed Vaccines', *Journal of Tropical Medicine and Hygiene*, 1914, Vol. 1, No. 7, pp. 36–39.
17. 'An Inquiry on Enteric Fever in India, Carried Out at the Central Research Institute, Kasauli, Under the Direction of Lieutenant-Colonel D. Semple, M.D., Director of the Institute, and Captain E. D. W. Greig, M.D. No. 32 of Scientific Memoirs by Officers of the Medical and Sanitary Departments of the Government of India', JAMA, 30 January 1909, Vol. LII, No. 5, pp. 405. Available at: doi:10.1001/jama.1909.02540310065031.
18. 'Enteric Fever in India', *Nature*, 1908, Vol. 79, No. 21. Available at: https://doi.org/10.1038/079021b0.
19. Semple, 'A Preliminary Note on the Vaccine Therapy of Enteric Fever', pp. 1668–1669.
20. A. Hardy, '"Straight Back to Barbarism": Antityphoid Inoculation and the Great War, 1914', *Bulletin of History of Medicine*, February 2000, Vol. 74, pp. 265–290. Available at: https://discovery.ucl.ac.uk.
21. W. D. Tigertt, 'The Initial Effort to Immunize American Soldier Volunteers with Typhoid Vaccine', *Military Medicine*, May 1959, Vol. 124, pp. 342–349.
22. J. Bockemühl, 'Typhoid Vaccination Yesterday and Today', *Immun Infekt*, 1983, Vol. 11, No. 1, pp. 16–22. (Article in German)
23. Ibid.

12. SEMPLE VACCINE: DEAD OR LIVE?

1. 'Pasteur's Method', *Pioneer Mail and Indian Weekly News*, 1896, pp. 26–27.
2. A. R. Kammer and H. C. J. Ertl, 'Rabies Vaccines: From the Past to the 21st Century', *Hybridoma and Hybridomics*, 2002, Vol. 21, No. 2, p. 123.
3. David Semple, 'The Preparation of a Safe and Efficient Antirabic Vaccine', *Scientific Memoirs by the Officers of the Medical and Sanitary Departments of the Government of India*, 1911, pp. 27–28.

4. Ibid.
5. Ibid.
6. William J. Webster, 'Rabies and Antirabic Treatment in India', Delhi: Manager of Publications, 1946, pp. 6.
7. Morrison to director, Bombay Bacteriological Laboratory, 'Anti-rabic Treatment: Opening of Additional Centres', *General Department Maharashtra State Archive*, 1923, G.D. file no. 4761 (I), pp. 5–7.
8. 'India', *British Medical Journal*, October 1925, Vol. 2, pp. 765–766.
9. Ibid.
10. 'Opportunities for Original Research in Medicine in India', Journal of Royal Society of Arts, 1917, Vol. 65, pp. 391–395; quotation on 392.
11. Toby Gelfand, '11 January 1887, the Day Medicine Changed: Joseph Grancher's Defense of Pasteur's Treatment for Rabies', Bulletin of the History of Medicine, 2002, Vol. 76, pp. 698–718.
12. P. Chakrabarti, '"Living versus Dead": The Pasteurian Paradigm and Imperial Vaccine Research', Bulletin of History Medicine, 2010, Vol. 84, No. 3, pp. 387–423. Available at: https://doi.org/10.1353/bhm.2010.0019.
13. Benjamin Bryan, 'A Pasteur Institute for India', *Home-Medical*, August 1894, pp. 373–374. P/4554, Asia Pacific and Africa Collections, British Library, London
14. A. C. Marie, Paul Remlinger, H. Vallée, 'International Rabies Conference Held at the Pasteur Institute, Paris, from April 25th to 29th', League of Nations, Geneva, 1927, p. 48.
15. George M. Baer, ed., 'The Natural History of Rabies', New York: CRC Press, 1991, pp. 15–16.
16. 'Anti-rabies Vaccination and the Public Authorities', Marie, Remlinger and Vallée International Rabies Conference, pp. 154–157.
17. Edward J. Turner, 'Letter to the Secretary, Government of India', *Economic and Overseas Department Papers*, L/E/7/1465, Asia Pacific and Africa Collections, 15 July 1927, p. 6.
18. 'From Private Letters between Col. Graham and Mr. Donaldson', 22 September and 16 November 1927.
19. Arthur Hirtzel, 'Letter to the Medical Adviser', 17 January 1928.
20. William F. Harvey and H. W. Acton, 'An Examination into the Degree of Efficacy of Antirabic Treatment', *Indian Journal of Medical Research*, 1923, Vol. 9, p. 853. *See also* R. Knowles, 'Some Problems in Rabies', *Indian Medical Gazette*, 1927, Vol. 67, pp. 389–391.
21. 'Inadvisability of Extending Anti-rabic Treatment by Present Carbolized Vaccine to District Areas in India until Results of Investigations Are Known', *Department of Education Health and Land, Medical Branch*, 1926, pp. 95–96. (Minutes of a Meeting of a Medical Committee held in the office of the Director-General, Indian Medical Service, on September 28 at 11 am, National Archive of India, New Delhi)

22. Chakrabarti, '"Living versus Dead"'.
23. David Arnold, *Science, Technology and Medicine in Colonial India*, Cambridge University Press, 2000, p. 199.
24. Chakrabarti, '"Living versus Dead"'.
25. 'McKendrick to Cunningham', *Papers and correspondence of John Cunningham*, 9 February 1927, Vol. E. 15, pp. 3–4. Reference code: GB 0237 Gen. 2004, Special Collections, Edinburgh University Library.
26. Chakrabarti, '"Living versus Dead"'.
27. 'McKendrick to Cunningham', 11 May 1927, Vol. E. 16, p. 5.
28. *Thirty Eighth Annual Report of the Pasteur Institute of Southern India, Coonoor*, Pasteur Institute of Southern India, 1940, p. 15.
29. William J. Webster, 'Rabies and Antirabic Treatment in India', Delhi: Manager of Publications, 1946, p. 6.
30. N. Veeraraghavan, 'Phenolized Vaccine Treatment of People Exposed to Rabies in Southern India', *Bulletin of the World Health Organization*, 1954, Vol. 10, pp. 789–796.
31. H, Koprowski and H. R. Cox, 'Studies on chick embryo adapted rabies virus', *Journal of Immunology*, 1948, Vol. 60, pp. 533–554.

13. THE KISS OF DEATH

1. G. Noel, *Princess Alice: Queen Victoria's Forgotten Daughter*, 1985, Constable and Company Limited, London.
2. T. L. Hadfield, P. McEvoy, Y. Polotsky, V. A. Tzinserling and A. A. Yakovlev, 'The Pathology of Diphtheria', *The Journal of Infectious Diseases*, 2000, Vol. 181, No. Supplement_1, pp. S116–S120. Available at: https://doi.org/10.1086/315551.
3. D. B. Benthell and T. T. Hien, 'Diphtheria', in D. A. Warrell et al., eds., *Oxford Textbook of Medicine*, 5th ed., Oxford University Press, 2012. Available at: https://doi.org/10.1093/med/9780199204854.003.070601_update_001.
4. 'Diphtheria: A Popular Health Article', *The Public Health Journal*, 1927, Vol. 18, p. 574.
5. C. Nezelof, 'Pierre Fidèle Bretonneau 1778–1862: A Pioneer in Understanding Infectious Diseases', *Annals of Diagnostic Pathology*, 2002, Vol. 6, No. 1, pp. 74–82.
6. L. Ott, J. Möller and A. Burkovski, 'Interactions between the Re-Emerging Pathogen Corynebacterium diphtheriae and Host Cells', *International Journal of Molecular Sciences*, 2022, Vol. 23, No. 6, p. 3298. Available at: https://doi.org/10.3390/ijms23063298.
7. E. Malito and R. Rappuoli, 'History of Diphtheria Vaccine Development', in Andreas Burkovski, ed., *Corynebacterium diphtheriae and Related Toxigenic Species*, Springer Science, Business Media Dordrecht, 2014, pp. 225–238. Available at: https://doi.org/10.1007/978-94-007-7624-1_11.

8. T. Lampidis and L. Barksdale, 'Park-Williams Number 8 Strain of Corynebacterium diphtheriae', *Journal of Bacteriology*, 1971, Vol. 105, No. 1, pp. 77–85.
9. J. D. Grabenstein, 'Toxoid Vaccines', in Arnold Artenstein, ed., *Vaccines: A Biography*, Springer, 2010, pp. 105–124.
10. P. Ehrlich, 'The Nobel Prize in Physiology or Medicine 1908', *Nobelprize.org*, Nobel Media AB, 1908. Available at: http://www.nobelprize.org/nobel_prizes/medicine/laureates/1908/.
11. D. K. Yadav, N. Yadav and S. M. P. Khurana, 'Vaccines: Present Status and Applications', *Animal Biotechnology: Models in Discovery and Translation*, 2014, pp. 491–508.
12. J. Bland and J. Clements, 'Protecting the World's Children: The Story of WHO's Immunization Programme', *World Health Forum*, World Health Organization, 1998, Vol. 19, No. 2, pp. 162–173.
13. J. Sokhey, R. J. Kim-Farley and I. Bhargava, 'The Expanded Programme on Immunization: A Decade of Progress in India', *Annals of Tropical Paediatrics*, Maney Publishing, 1989, Vol. 9, No. 1, pp. 24–29. Available at: https://doi.org/10.1080/02724936.1989.11748590.
14. Ibid.
15. V. Dietz, J. B. Milstien, F. van Loon, S. Cochi and J. Bennett, 'Performance and Potency of Tetanus Toxoid: Implications for Eliminating Neonatal Tetanus', *Bulletin of the World Health Organization*, World Health Organization, 1996, Vol. 74, No. 6, pp. 619–628.
16. A. Galazka, 'Immunization of pregnant women against tetanus', WHO Geneva, EPI/GEN/83/5.

14. VACCINE RESEARCH AND EARLY INSTITUTIONS

1. David Arnold, ed., *Imperial medicine and indigenous societies*, Manchester University Press, 1988, p. 153.
2. Mridula Ramanna, *Health Care in Bombay Presidency, 1896–1930*, Primus Books, 2012, pp. 19–21.
3. David Arnold, *Science, Technology and Medicine in Colonial India*, Cambridge University Press, 2002, Repr. ed., pp. 142–146.
4. Mark Harrison, *Public Health in British India: Anglo-Indian Preventive Medicine 1859–1914*, Cambridge University Press, 1994, pp. 148.
5. Kalpish Ratna, *The Quarantine Papers*, HarperCollins, New Delhi, 2010.
6. 'Supplement. Imperial Veterinary Research Institute 1890-1940. Golden Jubilee', *Indian Farming*, 1940, Vol. 1, No. 11.
7. Ibid.
8. D. G. Crawford, *A History of the Indian Medical Service 1600–1913, Volume II*, W. Thacker & Co., London, 1914.

9. Ibid.
10. *National Science Policy and Organisation of Scientific Research in India*, UNESCO, 1972, *Science Policy Studies and Documents*, No. 27, Document Code: NS/SPS/27, SC.71/XIII.27/A, pp. 15.
11. Government of India, *The Imperial Gazetteer of India, Vol. IV: Administrative*, Clarendon Press, 1909, New ed. Published under the authority of His Majesty's Secretary of State for India in Council, pp. 457–480.
12. Harrison, *Public Health in British India*.
13. 'ICMR Bulletin', Division of Publication & Information, ICMR, November-December 2011, Vol. 41, No. 11–12, p. 73. Available at: https://main.icmr.nic.in/sites/default/files/icmr_bulletins/ICMR_Bulletin_Nov-Dec_2011.pdf
14. Ibid.
15. John Mathew, 'Ronald Ross to U. N. Brahmachari: Medical Research in Colonial India', *Indian Journal of History of Science*, Indian National Science Academy, 2018, Vol. 53, No. 4, pp. T115–T122. Available at: https://doi.org/10.16943/ijhs/2018/v53i4/49534.
16. K. Park, 'Park's Textbook of Preventive and Social Medicine', M/s Banarsidas Bhanot Publishers, 2005, 18th ed., pp. 679–680.
17. Mathew, 'Ronald Ross to U. N. Brahmachari'.
18. M. U. Mushtaq, 'Public Health in British India: A Brief Account of the History of Medical Services and Disease Prevention in Colonial India', *Indian Journal of Community Medicine*, 2009, Vol. 34, No. 1, pp. 6–14. Available at: https://doi.org/10.4103/0970-0218.45369.
19. Y. Madhavi, 'Transnational Factors and National Linkages: Indian Experience in Human Vaccines', *Asian Biotechnology and Development Review*, RIS: Research and Information System for Developing Countries, 2007, Vol. 9, No. 2, pp. 1–43.

15. SOKHEY, HILL AND BHORE

1. A. M. Das, 'A.V. Hill and Shaping of Modern Science in India', *Journal of Scientometric Research, Wolters Kluwer*, Medknow Publications, 2018, Vol. 7, No. 2, pp. 125–126.
2. A. V. Hill, 'A Report to the Government of India on Scientific Research in India', The Royal Society, 1944.
3. D. Kumar, 'Science and Society in Colonial India: Exploring an Agenda', *Science Technology & Society*, 2001, Vol. 6, No. 2, pp. 375–395.
4. Hill, 'A Report to the Government of India on Scientific Research in India'.
5. 'Training of Doctors: Report by the Goodenough Committee', *British Medical Journal*, 1944, Vol. 2, p. 121. Available at: https://doi.org/10.1136/bmj.2.4359.121.
6. D. Kumar, 'Colonialism and Science in India', *Encyclopaedia of the History of*

Science, Technology, and Medicine in Non-Western Cultures, Springer, Netherlands, 2008.
7. Hill, 'A Report to the Government of India on Scientific Research in India'.
8. UNESCO, 'National Science Policy and Organization of Scientific Research in India', Science Policy Studies and Documents Series, UNESCO, 1972.
9. J. Bhore and Bhore Committee, 'Report of the Health Survey and Development Committee (Bhore Committee Report)', Government of India Press, New Delhi, 1946.
10. Sub-Committee on National Health (Chairman: Col. S. S. Sokhey) and National Planning Committee, 'Report of the Sub-Committee on National Health'.
11. D. Kumar, *Science and the Raj, 1857-1905*, Oxford University Press, 1995.
12. D. Kumar, *Science and Empire: Essays in Indian Context, 1700-1947*, Anamika Publishers & Distributors, New Delhi, 1991.
13. Bhore, 'Report of the Health Survey and Development Committee (Bhore Committee Report)'.
14. Plague Commission, 'Report on the Bombay Plague of 1896–97', Government Central Press, 1904.
15. Bhore, 'Report of the Health Survey and Development Committee (Bhore Committee Report).
16. Ibid
17. Ibid.
18. Sunil Amrith, 'Political Culture of Health in India: A Historical Perspective', *Economic and Political Weekly*, 2007, Vol. 42, No. 2, pp. 114–121.

16. SUPREME SCIENCE COMMANDER

1. Norah Richards, *Sir Shanti Swarup Bhatnagar F. R. S.: A Biographical Study of India's Eminent Scientist*, New Book Society of India, New Delhi, 1948.
2. 'Leadership in a Dynamic Society', *Nature*, Nature Publishing Group, 1943, Vol. 152, pp. 85–87. Available at: https://doi.org/10.1038/152085a0.
3. Roy M. MacLeod, 'Scientific Advice for British India: Imperial Perceptions and Administrative Goals, 1898–1923', *Modern Asian Studies*, Cambridge University Press, 1975, Vol. 9, pp. 343–384. Available at: https://doi.org/10.1017/S0026749X00005813.
4. R. MacLeod and D. Kumar, eds., 'Organisation of Industrial Research: The Early History of CSIR 1934–47', in *Technology and the Raj: Western Technology and Technical Transfers to India 1700–1947*, Sage Publications, 1995, pp. 159–184.
5. U. Das Gupta, ed., *Science and Modern India: An Institutional History, c. 1784–1947*, Longman Pearson Education, 2010, p. 160.
6. T. R. Seshadri, 'Obituary: Shanti Swarup Bhatnagar, 1894–1955', *Biographical Memoirs of Fellows of the Royal Society*, The Royal Society, 1962, Vol. 8. Available at: https://doi.org/10.1098/rsbm.1962.0001.

7. MacLeod and Kumar, eds., 'Organisation of Industrial Research: The Early History of CSIR 1934–47'.
8. 'ICMR Bulletin', Division of Publication & Information.
9. Devinder Sharma, 'When death becomes cheap', *Deccan Herald*, 16 April 2005.
10. 'Shanti Swarup Bhatnagar Prize: An Inspiration for International Recognitions', *Current Science*, 2014, Vol. 107, No. 2, p. 163. Available at: https://www.currentscience.ac.in/Volumes/107/02/0163.pdf.

17. A VACCINE IN FOUR MONTHS

1. 'Manufacture of Antidote to Influenza at Pasteur Institute & Low-Cost Influenza Vaccine', The Parliament Archives, Oral Answers to Questions, Rajya Sabha, 27 August 1957.
2. I. G. K. Menon, 'The 1957 Pandemic of Influenza in India', *Bulletin of the World Health Organization*, 1959, Vol. 20, Nos. 2–3, pp. 199–224.
3. Ibid.
4. N. Veeraraghavan, 'Influenza Virus Isolations at the Government of India Influenza Centre, Coonoor, During 1950–60', *Bulletin of the World Health Organization*, 1961, Vol. 24, pp. 679–686.
5. N. G. Gadekar, 'Lung Lesions in Influenza', *Indian Journal of Medical Sciences*, Indian Council of Medical Research, 1958, Vol. 12, No. 4, pp. 247–256. Available at: doi:10.1159/000464020.
6. Menon, 'The 1957 Pandemic of Influenza in India'.
7. Melissa Cox Norris, 'Vaccination Efforts from Around the Globe: The Story of Dr. Sabin and Dr. Harshavardhan', *LiBlog: The Blog of the University of Cincinnati Libraries*, University of Cincinnati Libraries, 17 June 2015. Available at: https://libapps.libraries.uc.edu/liblog/2015/06/vaccination-efforts-from-around-the-globe-the-story-of-dr-sabin-and-dr-harshavardhan/.
8. Author's interaction with Dr. G. V. J. A. Harshavardhan at the Indian Vaccine Manufacturers Association office in Hyderabad on 4 March 2025.
9. Deepa Alexander, 'How the Pasteur Institute of India Became One of the Pioneers in Vaccine Production', *The Hindu*, 26 May 2021. Available at: https://www.thehindu.com/society/history-and-culture/how-the-pasteur-institute-of-india-became-one-of-the-pioneers-in-vaccine-production/article34649481.ece.
10. 'ICMR Bulletin', Division of Publication & Information, p. 73.

PART-III: SAVING LIVES (1961–1990)

18. TUBERCULOSIS AND THE BCG REVOLUTION

1. Katherine Frank, *Indira: The Life of Indira Nehru Gandhi*, London: HarperCollins, 2001.

2. Ibid, p. 143.
3. Ibid, p. 144.
4. R. A. Hobday, 'Sunlight therapy and solar architecture', *Medical History*, 1997, Vol. 41, No. 4, pp. 455–472. Available at: doi:10.1017/S0025727300063043.
5. Prakash S. Bisen and Ruchika Raghuvanshi, *Emerging Epidemics: Chapter: Tuberculosis*, New York: Wiley Blackwell, 2013, pp. 76–148.
6. Thomas M. Daniel, 'The history of tuberculosis', *Respiratory Medicine*, Vol. 100, No. 11, pp. 1862–1870.
7. I. Barberis, N. L. Bragazzi, L. Galluzzo and M. Martini, 'The history of tuberculosis: from the first historical records to the isolation of Koch's bacillus', *Journal of Preventive Medicine and Hygiene*, 2017, Vol. 58, No. 1, E9–E12.
8. J. Hayman. 'Mycobacterium ulcerans: an infection from Jurassic time', *Lancet*, 1984, Vol. 2, No. 8410, pp. 1015–1016.
9. Aaron E. Hirsh, Anthony G. Tsolaki, Kathryn DeRiemer, Markus W. Feldman and Peter M. Small, 'Stable association between strains of *Mycobacterium tuberculosis* and their human host populations', *Proceedings of the National Academy of Sciences of the United States of America*, 2004, Vol. 101, pp. 4871–4876.
10. Israel Hershkovitz, Helen D. Donoghue, David E. Minnikin, Gurdyal S. Besra, Oona Y-C Lee, Angela M. Gernaey, et al. 'Detection and molecular characterization of 9000-year-old *Mycobacterium tuberculosis* from a neolithic settlement in the Eastern Mediterranean', *PLoS ONE*, 2008, Vol. 3, p. 3426.
11. D. Morse, D. R. Brothwell and P. J. Ucko. 'Tuberculosis in ancient Egypt', *The American Review of Respiratory Disease*, 1964, Vol. 90, pp. 524–541.
12. Lawrason Brown, *The Story of Clinical Pulmonary Tuberculosis*, Baltimore: Williams & Wilkinson Company, 1941.
13. V. S. Daniel and T. M. Daniel, 'Old Testament biblical references to tuberculosis', *Clinical infectious diseases : an official publication of the Infectious Diseases Society of America*, 1999, Vol. 29, No. 6, 1557–1558.
14. Francis Adams, editor. *The genuine works of Hippocrates*. London: The Sydenham Society, 1849.
15. Ralph H. Major, *Classic Descriptions of Disease* (3rd ed), Springfield, IL: Charles C. Thomas, 1945.
16. C. Gradmann. 'Robert Koch and the pressures of scientific research: tuberculosis and tuberculin', *Medical History*, 2001, Vol. 45, No. 1, pp. 1–32.
17. Sol Roy Rosenthal, *BCG Vaccine, Tuberculosis—cancer*, PSG Publishing Company, 1980.
18. Simona Luca and Traian Mihaescu, 'History of BCG Vaccine', *Maedica (Bucur)*, 2013, Vol. 8, No. 1, pp. 53–58.
19. Ibid.
20. Ibid.
21. P. D. Hart and I. Sutherland, 'BCG and Vole Bacillus Vaccines in the Prevention

of Tuberculosis in Adolescence and Early Adult Life', *BMJ*, 1977, Vol. 2, pp. 293–295.

22. G. W. Comstock and C. E. Palmer, 'Long-term Results of BCG Vaccination in the Southern United States', *The American Review of Respiratory Disease*, 1966, Vol. 93, pp. 171–183.
23. World Health Organisation, 'Information Sheet: Observed rate of vaccine reactions. Bacille Calmette-Guerin (BCG) vaccine', 2012. Available at: https://www.who.int/vaccine_safety/initiative/tools/BCG_Vaccine_rates_information_sheet.pdf
24. Ibid.
25. J. Frimodt-Møller, J. Thomas and R. Parthasarathy, 'Observations on the Protective Effect of BCG Vaccination in a South Indian Rural Population', *Bulletin of the World Health Organisation*, 1964, Vol. 30, pp. 545–574.
26. Indian Council of Medical Research, 'Tuberculosis in India. A sample survey 1955-1958', 1959, New Delhi: Special Research Series, No. 34.
27. WHO Tuberculosis Research Office, 1955a, 1955b, 1957, *Bulletin of the World Health Organisation*, 12 & 17.
28. Tuberculosis Prevention Trial, Madras, 'Trial of BCG Vaccines in South India for Tuberculosis Prevention', *Indian Journal of Medical Research*, 1980, Vol. 72, pp. 1–74.
29. Ibid.
30. Tuberculosis Research Centre (ICMR), Chennai, 'Fifteen year follow up of trial of BCG vaccines in south India for tuberculosis prevention', *Indian Journal of Medical Research*, 1999, Vol. 110, pp. 56–69.
31. S. Mayurnath, R. S. Vallishayee, M. P. Radhamani and R. Prabhakar. 'Prevalence study of tuberculous infection over fifteen years, in a rural population in Chingleput district (south India)', *The Indian Journal of Medical Research*, 1991, Vol. 93, pp. 74–80.
32. A. K. Chakraborty, H. Singh, K. Srikantan, K. K. Rangaswamy, M. S. Krishnamurthy and J. A. Stephen, 'Tuberculosis in a rural population of south India: Report on five surveys', Indian Journal of Tuberculosis, 1982, Vol. 29, p. 153.
33. S. S. Goyal, G. P. Mathur and S. P. Pamra, 'Tuberculosistrends in an urban community', *Indian Journal of Tuberculosis*, 1978, Vol. 25, p. 77.
34. C. K. Indumathi, 'Bacillus Calmette–Guérin Vaccination: A Brief Overview', *Pediatric Infectious Disease*, 2012, Vol. 4, No. 2, pp. 71–74.
35. Michael Peel, 'How tackling TB could help win the war on superbugs', *Financial Times*, 24 September 2024. Available at: https://www.ft.com/content/00d5e030-894b-443b-b3ac-375dd530273d
36. World Health Organisation, 'WHO announces plans to establish a TB Vaccine Accelerator council', 17 January 2023. Available at: https://www.who.int/news/

item/17-01-2023-who-announces-plans-to-establish-a-tb-vaccine-accelerator-council.

37. Sergio Lacámara and Carlos Martin, 'MTBVAC: A Tuberculosis Vaccine Candidate Advancing Towards Clinical Efficacy Trials in TB Prevention', *Archivos de Bronconeumología*, 2023, Vol. 59, No. 12, pp. 821–828. Available at: https://doi.org/10.1016/j.arbres.2023.09.009.
38. World Health Organisation, 'Vaccines and immunization: Investigational vaccine candidate M72/AS01E', 19 March 2024. Available at: https://www.who.int/news-room/questions-and-answers/item/vaccines-and-immunization-investigational-vaccine-candidate-m72-as01e.

19. 'COULD YOU PATENT THE SUN?'

1. Linda Rodriquez McRobbie, 'The man in the iron lung', *Guardian*, 26 May 2020. Available at: https://www.theguardian.com/society/2020/may/26/last-iron-lung-Alexander-alexander-polio-coronavirus.
2. Guinness World Records Limited, 'Longest iron lung patient'. Available at: https://www.guinnessworldrecords.com/world-records/longest-iron-lung-patient.
3. Marguerite Yin-Murphy and Jeffrey W. Almond, 'Picornaviruses' in S. Baron, et al. (eds.), *Baron's Medical Microbiology* (4th ed.), Galveston, TX: Univ of Texas Medical Branch, 1996.
4. Amy Berish, 'FDR and Polio', Franklin D. Roosevelt Library & Museum, 2016. Available at: https://www.fdrlibrary.org/polio.
5. David M. Oshinsky, *Polio: An American Story*, New York: Oxford University Press, 2005, pp. 196–198.
6. Carl Kurlander and Randy P. Juhl. 'Lessons from how the polio vaccine went from the lab to the public that Americans can learn from today', *ASBMB Today*, 26 September 2020. Available at: https://www.asbmb.org/asbmb-today/science/092620/lessons-from-how-the-polio-vaccine-went-from-the-1 .
7. William L. Laurences, 'Salk Polio Vaccine Proves Success; Millions Will Be Immunized Soon', *The New York Times*, 13 April 1955.
8. Ibid.
9. J. E. Salk, B. L. Bennett, L. J. Lewis, E. N. Ward and J. S. Youngner, 'Studies in human subjects on active immunization against poliomyelitis: I. A preliminary report of experiments in progress', *Journal of the American Medical Association*, 1955, Vol. 151, No. 13, pp. 1081–1098.
10. J. E. Salk, P. L. Bazeley, B. L. Bennett, U. Krech, L. J. Lewis, E. N. Ward and J. S. Youngner, 'II. A Practical Means for Inducing and Maintaining Antibody Formation', *American Journal of Public Health and the Nation's Health*, 1954, Vol. 44, No. 8, pp. 994–1009. Available at: doi:10.2105/ajph.44.8.994.

11. Jonas Salk, 'Could You Patent the Sun?', video clip from Edward R. Morrow's interview with Dr Jonas Salk, Awesome Stories, 8 December 2013. Courtesy: Global Poverty Project. Last revised 16 December 2019. Available at: https://www.awesomestories.com/asset/view/Jonas-Salk-Could-You-Patent-the-Sun-1.
12. Erling Norrby and Stanley B. Prusiner, 'Polio and Nobel Prizes: Looking Back 50 Years', *Annals of Neurology*, 27 April 2007. Available at: https://doi.org/10.1002/ana.21153.
13. A. B. Sabin and L. R. Boulger, 'History of Sabin attenuated poliovirus oral live vaccine strains', Journal of Biological Standardization, 1973, Vol. 1, pp. 115–118.
14. A. Sabin, M. Ramos-Alvarez, J. Alvarez-Amezquita, et al., 'Live, orally given poliovirus vaccine. Effects of rapid mass immunization on population under conditions of massive enteric infection with other viruses', *JAMA*, 1960, Vol. 173, pp. 1521–1526.
15. William L. Atkinson, J. Hamborsky, L. McIntyre and S. Wolfe, *Epidemiology and Prevention of Vaccine-Preventable Diseases* (11th edition), Washington DC: Public Health Foundation, 2009.
16. Sanofi Pasteur, 'Competition to develop an oral vaccine', 2006. Available at: https://web.archive.org/web/20051214090013/http://www.polio.info/polio-eradication/front/templates/index.jsp.
17. Davide Orsini and Mariano Martini, 'Albert Bruce Sabin: The Man Who Made the Oral Polio Vaccine', *Emerging Infectious Diseases*, 2022, Vol. 28, No. 3, pp. 743–746.
18. Stuart Blume, 'ESSAY ON SCIENCE AND SOCIETY: A Brief History of Polio Vaccines', *Science*, 2000, Vol. 288, No. 5471, p. 1593.
19. M. R. Smallman, *Poliomyelitis: A World Geography: Emergence to Eradication*, New York: Oxford University Press, 2000.
20. Orsini and Martini, 'Albert Bruce Sabin'.
21. Blume, 'Essay on Science and Society', p. 1594.
22. Ibid, pp. 1593–1594.
23. T. Jacob John and Vipin M. Vashishtha, 'Eradicating poliomyelitis: India's journey from hyperendemic to polio-free status', *Indian Journal of Medical Research*, 2013, Vol. 137, 881-894.
24. P. V. Gharpure and P. R. Bhatt, 'Unusual manifestations of human polio', *Indian Journal of Medical Science*, 1952, Vol. 6, pp. 576–578.

20. THE POLIO END GAME

1. R. A. Feldman, S. Christopher, S. George, K. R. Kamath and T. J. John, 'Infection and disease in a group of South Indian Families. IX. Poliovirus infection among pre-school children', *Indian Journal of Medical Research*, 1970, Vol. 58, pp. 551–555.

2. T. J. John, 'Immunization against polioviruses in developing countries', *Reviews in Medical Virology*, 1993, Vol. 3, pp. 149–160.
3. Ibid.
4. John and Vashishtha, 'Eradicating poliomyelitis'.
5. T. J. John, 'Understanding the scientific basis of preventing polio by immunization. Pioneering contributions from India', *Proceedings of the Indian National Science Academy*, 2003, Vol. B69, pp. 393–422.
6. R. N. Basu, 'Expanded Programme on Immunisation in India', *Indian Journal of Pediatrics*, 1980, Vol. 47, pp. 362–368.
7. R. N. Basu and J. Sokhey, 'The Expanded Programme on Immunisation. A Review', New Delhi: EPI Section, Directorate General of Health Services, 1982.
8. H. V. Wyatt, 'Provocation paralysis', *Lancet*, 1993, Vol. 341, pp. 61–62.
9. T. J. John, 'Did India have the world's largest outbreak of poliomyelitis associated with injections of adjuvanted DPT?', *Indian Pediatrics*, 1998, Vol. 35, pp. 73–75.
10. T. J. John, 'The costs and benefits of [polio] immunization in India', *Indian Pediatrics*, 1981, Vol. 18, pp. 513–516.
11. John, 'Understanding the scientific basis of preventing polio by immunization'.
12. World Health Organisation, 'Global eradication of poliomyelitis by the year 2000', Forty-First World Health Assembly, 13 May 1988. Available at: https://polioeradication.org/wp-content/uploads/2016/07/19880513_resolution-2.pdf.
13. T. J. John, R. Pandian, A. Gadomski, M. C. Steinhoff, M. John and M. Ray, 'Control of poliomyelitis by pulse immunisation in Vellore, India', *British Medical Journal*, 1983, Vol. 286, pp. 31–32.
14. Author interaction with Thekkekkara Jacob John in Vellore on 28 March 2025.
15. T. J. John, R. Samuel, V. Balraj and R. John. 'Disease surveillance at district level: a model for developing countries', *Lancet*, 1998, Vol. 352, pp. 58–61.
16. Author interaction with Thekkekkara Jacob John in Vellore on 28 March 2025.
17. Subhadra Menon, 'India's battle to finish off polio', *BBC News*, 25 January 2012. Available at: https://www.bbc.com/news/world-asia-india-16715392.
18. Centre for Disease Control, Department of Health and Human Services, 'Progress Toward Global Eradication of Poliomyelitis', *MMWR Weekly*, 1997, Vol. 46, No. 25, pp. 579–584. Available at: https://www.cdc.gov/mmwr/preview/mmwrhtml/00048061.htm.
19. R. N. Basu, 'Magnitude of problem of poliomyelitis in India', *Indian Pediatrics*, 1981, Vol. 18, pp. 507–511.
20. John and Vashishtha, 'Eradicating poliomyelitis'.
21. Global Polio Eradication Initiative, World Health Organisation, 'Polio Eradication & Endgame Strategic Plan 2013-2018', 2013. Available at: https://polioeradication.org/wp-content/uploads/2016/07/2.8_8IMB.pdf.
22. T. Jacob John. 'Two good reasons to drop type 2 virus from oral polio vaccine', *Lancet*, 2004, Vol. 364, p. 1666.

23. World Health Organisation, 'Meeting of the Strategic Advisory Group of Experts on Immunization, November 2012: conclusions and recommendations', *Weekly Epidemiological Record*, 2013, Vol. 88, pp. 1–16. Available at: https://www.who.int/publications/i/item/WER8901.
24. S. Priya, 'In conversation: T. Jacob John', *Current Science*, 2018, Vol. 114, No. 3, p. 436. Available at: https://www.currentscience.ac.in/Volumes/114/03/0436.pdf.

21. BATTLING MEASLES – THE INDIAN DEBATE

1. T. Jacob John and Valsan P. Verghese, 'Time to re-think the measles vaccination schedule in India', *Indian Journal of Medical Research*, 2011, Vol. 134, pp. 256–259.
2. T. J. John, A. Joseph, T. I. George, J. Radhakrishnan, R. P. D. Singh and K. George, 'Epidemiology and prevention of measles in rural south India', *Indian Journal of Medical Research*, 1980, Vol. 72, pp. 153–158.
3. T. Jacob John, 'Measles in India, a neglected problem', *Indian Journal of Pediatrics*, 1983, Vol. 50, pp. 399–403.
4. John and Verghese, 'Time to re-think the measles vaccination schedule in India'.
5. J. Sokhey, R. J. Kim-Farley and I. Bhargava, 'The expanded programme on immunization: a decade of progress in India', *Annals of Tropical Pediatrics*, 1989, Vol. 9, No. 1, pp. 24–29.
6. Thomas H. Maugh II, 'Maurice R. Hilleman, 85; Scientist Developed Many Vaccines That Saved Millions of Lives', *Los Angeles Times*, 13 April 2005. Available at: https://www.latimes.com/archives/la-xpm-2005-apr-13-me-hilleman13-story.html.
7. Theadore H. Tulchinsky, 'Maurice Hilleman: Creator of Vaccines That Changed the World', *Case Studies in Public Health*, 2018, pp. 443–470.
8. Christopher Reed, 'Medical scientist whose vaccines saved millions of lives: Maurice Hilleman', *Guardian*, 15 April 2005. Available at: https://www.theguardian.com/news/2005/apr/15/guardianobituaries.obituaries.
9. M. R. Hilleman, et al, 'Live Attenuated Mumps Virus Vaccine: 4. Protective Efficacy as Measured in Field Evaluation', *The New England Journal of Medicine*, 1967, Vol. 276, pp. 252–258.
10. Eugene B. Buynak, 'Jeryl Lynn Strain Live Attenuated Mumps Virus Vaccine', *JAMA*, 1968, Vol. 203, No. 1, p. 9. DOI: 10.1001/jama.1968.03140010011002.
11. S. L. Katz, 'John F. Enders and Measles Virus Vaccine – a reminiscence', *Measles*, pp. 3–11. Doi:10.1007/978-3-540-70523-9_1.
12. World Health Organisation, 'History of Measles Vaccination'. Available at: https://www.who.int/news-room/spotlight/history-of-vaccination/history-of-measles-vaccination.
13. Stanley A. Plotkin, John D. Farquhar, Michael Katz and Fritz Buser, 'Attenuation

of RA 27/3 Rubella Virus in WI-38 Human Diploid Cells', *American Journal of Diseases in Children*, 1969, Vol. 118, pp. 178–85.

14. Christian H. Ross, 'Stanley Alan Plotkin's Development of a Rubella Vaccine (1969)', *Embryo Project Encyclopedia*, 28 June 2017. Available at: https://hdl.handle.net/10776/11880.
15. Leonard Hayflick and Paul S. Moorhead, 'The Serial Cultivation of Human Diploid Strains', *Experimental Cell Research*, 1961, Vol. 25, pp. 585–621.
16. Ross, 'Stanley Alan Plotkin's Development of a Rubella Vaccine (1969)'.
17. Maya van den Ent, Satish K. Gupta and Edward Hoekstra. 'Two doses of measles vaccine reduce measles deaths', *Indian Pediatrics*, 2009, Vol. 46, pp. 933–938.
18. World Health Organisation, 'Meeting of the Strategic Advisory Group of Experts on Immunization, November 2008: conclusions and recommendations', *Weekly Epidemiological Record*, 2009, Vol. 84, pp. 1–16.
19. Y. Madhavi, 'Measles-Rubella Vaccine', *Economic and Political Weekly*, 2020, Vol. 55, pp. 26–27. Available at: https://www.epw.in/journal/2020/26-27/notes/measles-rubella-vaccine.html.

22. MISSION INDRADHANUSH

1. Charles Swynnerton, contributor, *Indian Nights' Entertainment, or, Folk-Tales from the Upper Indus*, London: Elliot Stock, 1892.
2. Mohan Rao, ed., *The Lineaments of Population Policy in India: Women and Family Planning (Illustrated Edition)*. London: Taylor & Francis, 2017.
3. Vinod Mehta, *The Sanjay Story*, New Delhi, HarperCollins, 2015.
4. Lewis M. Simons, 'Compulsory Sterilization Provokes Fear, Contempt', *Washington Post*, 3 July 1977. Available at: https://www.washingtonpost.com/archive/politics/1977/07/04/compulsory-sterilization-provokes-fear-contempt/c2e28747-b5f1-4551-9bfe-98b552d8603f.
5. Ibid.
6. Nitin Nadkarni, 'Towards a New Immunization Strategy', *Medico Friend Circle Bulletin*, May 1961, no. 65. Available at: http://www.mfcindia.org/mfcpdfs/MFC065.pdf.
7. Sokhey, Kim-Farley and Bhargava, 'The Expanded Programme on Immunization'.
8. Jawaharlal Nehru, *Glimpses of World History*, New Delhi: Penguin India, 2004.
9. Susan Cohen, *The NHS: Britain's National Health Service, 1948–2020*, Bloomsbury USA, 2021.
10. Stanley A. Plotkin, Walter A. Orenstein and Paul A. Offit (Eds.), *Vaccines: Expert Consult*, Elsevier Saunders, 2017.
11. Ibid.
12. Sokhey, Kim-Farley and Bhargava, 'The Expanded Programme on Immunization'.
13. V. M. Vashishtha and P. Kumar, '50 years of Immunization in India: Progress and

Future', *Indian Paediatrics*, 2013, Vol. 50, pp. 111–118. Available at: https://www.indianpediatrics.net/jan2013/jan-111-118.htm
14. S. Gopalakrishnan and P. Sujitha, 'Vaccination programme in India- the present status: a review', *International Journal of Community Medicine and Public Health*, 2020, Vol. 7, No. 9, pp. 3746–3753.
15. UNICEF, 'Health workers in rural Assam are braving the odds to inoculate children', 11 January 2024. Available at: https://www.unicef.org/india/stories/health-workers-rural-assam-are-braving-odds-inoculate-children.
16. Gopalakrishnan and Sujitha, 'Vaccination programme in India- the present status'.
17. UNICEF, 'Immunization Regional Snapshot 2022', 2023. Available at: https://www.unicef.org/rosa/media/26171/file/Immunization%20Regional%20Snapshot%202022.pdf.
18. World Health Organisation, 'DTP3 immunization coverage among one-year-olds (%)', The Global Health Observatory. Available at: https://www.who.int/data/gho/data/themes/topics/immunization-coverage#:~:text=DTP3%20(third%20dose%20of%20DTP,recovered%20to%2084%25%20in%202023.
19. Vashishtha and Kumar, '50 years of Immunization in India'.
20. E. E. Zhang, *Educate Act Thrive – Eat for the Immune System*, Hong Kong: Red Corporation Limited, 2023.
21. Stanley Plotkin, 'History of vaccination', *Proceedings of the National Academy of Sciences of the United States of America*, 2014, Vol. 111, No. 34, pp. 12283–12287.
22. UN IGME, 'Child mortality, stillbirth, and causes of death estimates'. Available at https://childmortality.org/?indicator=MRM0.
23. Vashishtha and Kumar, '50 years of Immunization in India'.

23. THE EARLY PLAYERS

1. 'Founder's wife given control of Biological E. Limited', *Deccan Chronicle*, 19 November 2017. Available at: https://www.deccanchronicle.com/nation/current-affairs/191117/founders-wife-given-control-of-biological-e-limited.html.
2. Manu Balachandran and Divya J. Shekhar, 'Hyderabad's Biological E: The dark horse in India's vaccine race', *Forbes India*, 7 December 2020. Available at: https://www.forbesindia.com/article/innovation/hyderabads-biological-e-the-dark-horse-in-indias-vaccine-race/64733/1.
3. Ibid.
4. Press release issued by Intercell, 'Intercell AG / other / Intercell AG and Biological E. Ltd Enter into a Strategic Alliance for the Development, Manufacture and Sales of its Japanese Encephalitis Vaccine (E)', 17 March 2005.
5. Mahima Datla, Purnima Mantena, Indira Pusapati vs Renuka Datla and Others,

in Civil Appeal No. 2776, 2777, 2778 (Order of the Supreme Court of India on 6 April 2022).

6. ICRA Reports, 'Biological E. Limited: Ratings Reaffirmed', 20 February 2024. Available at: icra.in.
7. *Pharmaceutical Technology*, 'Biological E's Covid-19 vaccine Corbevax gets DCGI approval as booster dose', 6 June 2022. Available at: https://www.pharmaceutical-technology.com/news/biological-e-corbevax-dcgi-approval/.
8. Vishal Dutta, 'Zydus partners with US-based IDRI for Kala-Azar vaccine', *Economic Times*, 25 July 2013. Available at: https://economictimes.indiatimes.com/industry/healthcare/biotech/pharmaceuticals/zydus-partners-with-us-based-idri-for-kala-azar-vaccine/articleshow/21328455.cms.
9. *Business Standard*, 'Cadila develops India's first virus like particle vaccine for treating flu', 17 November 2016. Available at: https://www.business-standard.com/article/companies/cadila-develops-india-s-first-virus-like-particle-vaccine-for-treating-flu-116111700953_1.html.
10. Panacea Biotec, 'Success Story'. Available at: https://www.panaceabiotec.com/en/content/success-story.

24. A STABLE FOR VACCINES

1. Karmali, 'Horse Sense'.
2. Manu Balachandran, 'Serum Institute: How an Indian horse breeder built Asia's largest vaccine company', *Quartz*, 22 September 2015. Available at: https://qz.com/india/506247/how-an-indian-horse-breeder-built-asias-largest-vaccine-company.
3. Villoo Poonawalla Foundation, 'Cyrus Poonawalla, Chairman and Managing Director of Serum Institute of India'. Available at: https://www.vpcf.org/dr-cyrus-poonawalla.html.
4. Karmali, 'Horse Sense'.
5. T. V. Mahalingam, 'Meet India's biotech giant', *Business Today*, 24 August 2008. Available at: https://www.businesstoday.in/magazine/features/story/meet-indias-biotech-giant-128561-2008-08-06.
6. World Health Organisation, 'Hepatitis B, Key Facts', 18 July 2023. Available at: https://www.who.int/news-room/fact-sheets/detail/hepatitis-b.
7. Shivananda, Virbhadra Somani, B. S. Srikanth, M. Mohan and P. S. Kulkarni, 'Comparison of Two Hepatitis B Vaccines (GeneVac-B and Engerix-B) in Healthy Infants in India', *Clinical and Vaccine Immunology*, 2006, Vol. 13, No. 6, pp. 661–664.
8. Balachandran, 'Serum Institute: How an Indian horse breeder built Asia's largest vaccine company'.
9. Press release issued by the Ministry of Science & Technology, 'Department

of Biotechnology supported efficacy trial with recombinant BCG vaccine, VPM1002 completes enrolment of about 6000 health-workers and high-risk individuals', 27 July 2020. Available at: https://pib.gov.in/PressReleasePage.aspx?PRID=1641519.

25. FROM VAP TO ROTAVAC

1. The National Institute of Allergy and Infectious Diseases, 'Indo-U.S. Vaccine Action Program Overview'. Available at: https://www.niaid.nih.gov/research/indo-us-vaccine-action-program-overview.
2. Nandita Haksar, 'Stranger than fiction: Did the CIA conduct secret mosquito experiments in India in the 1970s?', *Scroll.in*, 17 July 2020. Available at: https://scroll.in/article/967560/stranger-than-fiction-did-the-cia-conduct-secret-mosquito-experiments-in-india-in-the-1970s.
3. Claude Alvares, 'The Great Gene Robbery', *The Illustrated Weekly of India*, 23 March 1986.
4. Praful Bidwai, 'The Indo-US Vaccine Action Programme: A Recipe For Disaster', *Medico Friend Circle Bulletin*, February 1989, No. 148. Available at: http://www.mfcindia.org/mfcpdfs/MFC148.pdf.
5. Praful Bidwai, 'The Indo-US Vaccine Action Programme: A Recipe For Disaster', *The National Medical Journal of India*, February 1989, Vol. 1, No. 1.
6. Jacqueline E. Tate, Anthony H. Burton, Cynthia Boschi-Pinto, Umesh D. Parashar and WHO-coordinated Global Rotavirus Surveillance Network, 'Global, Regional, and National Estimates of Rotavirus Mortality in Children <5 Years of Age, 2000–2013', *Clinical Infectious Diseases*, 2016, 62(Suppl_2), pp. S96–S105. Available at: https://doi.org/10.1093/cid/civ1013.
7. Umesh D. Parashar, Erik G. Hummelman, Joseph S. Bresee, Mark A. Miller and Roger I. Glass (2003). 'Global Illness and Deaths Caused by Rotavirus Disease in Children', *Emerging Infectious Diseases*, 2003, Vol. 9, No. 5, pp. 565–572. Available at: https://doi.org/10.3201/eid0905.020562.
8. Ibid.
9. Roger I. Glass, 'New Indian rotavirus vaccine provides hope', *Global Health Matters*, May/June 2013, Vol. 12, No. 3, p. 10.
10. Immunization Division, Ministry of Health & Family Welfare, Government of India. 'Rotavirus Vaccine: The India Story'.
11. Roger I. Glass, et al. 'Development of candidate rotavirus vaccines derived from neonatal strains in India', *Journal of Infectious Diseases*, 2005, Vol. 192 (September Suppl. 1), pp. S30–S35.
12. K. Vijay Raghavan, 'New paradigms for indigenous vaccines', *Vaccine*, 2014, Vol. 32, pp. A3–A4.
13. A. S. Fauci, 'Results of the ROTAVAC Rotavirus Vaccine Study in India', news

release issued by the National Institute of Allergy and Infectious Diseases, National Institutes of Health, 14 May 2013.

14. Roger I. Glass, Jacqueline E. Tate, Baoming Jiang and Umesh Parashar, 'The Rotavirus Vaccine Story: From Discovery to the Eventual Control of Rotavirus Disease', *The Journal of Infectious Diseases*, 2021, Vol. 224(Supplement_4), pp. S331–S342. Available at: https://doi.org/10.1093/infdis/jiaa598.
15. Raghavan, 'New paradigms for indigenous vaccines'.
16. Nita Bhandari, et al., 'Efficacy of a Monovalent Human-Bovine (116E) Rotavirus Vaccine in Indian Infants: A Randomised Double-blind Placebo-controlled Trial', *Lancet*, 2014, Vol. 383, No. 9935, pp. 2136–2143.
17. K. Ray, 'Made-in-India Rotavac: triumph of a 3-decade-long effort', *Deccan Herald*, 19 February 2018. Available at: https://www.deccanherald.com/content/660440/made-india-rotavac-triumph-3.html
18. World Health Organisation, 'Rotavirus Vaccines: WHO position paper – July 2021', *Weekly Epidemiological Record*, 2021, Vol. 28, pp. 301–319.
19. Roger I. Glass, 'New Indian rotavirus vaccine provides hope', *Global Health Matters*, 2013, Vol. 12, No. 3. Available at: https://www.fic.nih.gov.
20. Ibid.
21. Fauci, 'Results of the ROTAVAC Rotavirus Vaccine Study in India'.
22. Raghavan, 'New paradigms for indigenous vaccines'.
23. Press Information Bureau, Government of India, 'Shri JP Nadda launches Expansion of Rotavirus vaccine under Universal Immunization Programme', 18 February 2017. Available at: https://archive.pib.gov.in/archive2/erelease.aspx.
24. Annika Skansberg, Molly Sauer, Marissa Tan, Mathuram Santosham and Mary C. Jennings, 'Product review of the rotavirus vaccines ROTASIIL, ROTAVAC, and Rotavin-M1', *Vaccine*, 2020, Vol. 38, No. 48, pp. 1223–1234. Available at: https://doi.org/10.1080/21645515.2020.1804245.
25. Prasad S. Kulkarni, et al, 'A randomized Phase III clinical trial to assess the efficacy of a bovine-human reassortant pentavalent rotavirus vaccine in Indian infants', *Vaccine*, 2017, Vol. 35, No. 45, pp. 6228–6237.
26. Sheila Isanaka, et al, 'Efficacy of a low-cost, heat-stable oral rotavirus vaccine in Niger', *New England Journal of Medicine*, 2017, Vol. 376, pp. 1121–1130.
27. The National Institute of Allergy and Infectious Diseases, 'Indo-U.S. Vaccine Action Program Overview'.
28. Department of Biotechnology, Government of India, 'EU-India launches EUR30 million Joint Call on Research and Innovation to develop Next Generation Influenza Vaccine', 26 July 2018. Available at: https://dbtindia.gov.in/sites/default/files/uploadfiles/Guidelines-for-Submission-of-Joint-Proposal_NG.-Influenza-Vaccines.pdf.
29. The Diplomatic Service of the European Union, 'EU–India joint call "Towards a Next Generation Influenza Vaccine to Protect Citizens Worldwide"', European

Union External Action, 1 August 2018. Available at: https://www.eeas.europa.eu/node/49007_en.

26. THE END OF STATE-RUN VACCINE MAKING

1. John, 'Understanding the scientific basis of preventing polio by immunization. Pioneering contributions from India.'
2. Stuart S. Blume, 'Lock in, the state and vaccine development: Lessons from the history of the polio vaccines', *Research Policy*, 2005, Vol. 34, No. 2, pp. 0–173.
3. Melissa C. Norris, 'Vaccination Efforts from Around the Globe: The Story of Dr. Sabin and Dr. Harshavardhan', *LiBlog*, blog of the University of Cincinnati Libraries, 17 June 2015. Available at: https://libapps.libraries.uc.edu/liblog/2015/06/vaccination-efforts-from-around-the-globe-the-story-of-dr-sabin-and-dr-harshavardhan/.
4. R. N. Basu, 'Expanded Programme on Immunisation in India.'
5. Madhavi Yennapu, 'Transnational Factors and National Linkages: Indian Experience in Human Vaccines', *Asian Biotechnology and Development Review*, 2007, Vol. 9, No. 2, pp. 1–43.
6. M. Somasekhar, 'India Halts Vaccine Purchase from Russia', *The Hindu Business Line*, 17 December 1998.
7. M. Somasekhar, 'Indo-Russian Vaccine Project - Focusing on New Formulae', *The Hindu Business Line*, 27 September 2000.
8. Department of Biotechnology, Ministry of Science and Technology, Government of India, 'Annual Report (1999-2000)'.
9. John F. Burns, 'Agreement Eases Way For Connaught Takeover', *The New York Times*, 13 October 1989. Available at: https://www.nytimes.com/1989/10/13/business/agreement-eases-way-for-connaught-takeover.html.
10. Madhavi Yennapu, 'Vaccine Policy in India', *PLoS Med*, Vol. 2, No. 5:127, pp. 387–391. Available at: https://journals.plos.org/plosmedicine/article?id=10.1371/journal.pmed.0020127.
11. Yennapu, 'Transnational Factors and National Linkages: Indian Experience in Human Vaccines.'
12. Department of Biotechnology, Ministry of Science and Technology, Government of India, 'Annual Report (1987-1988)'.

PART-IV: FROM PUBLIC TO PRIVATE SECTOR (1991–2010)

27. LAHORE TO LABS

1. Dominique Lapierre and Larry Collins, *Freedom at Midnight*, New Delhi: Vikas Publishing House, 1975.
2. Stanley Wolpert, *Jinnah of Pakistan*, New York: Oxford University Press, 1984.

3. Taruni Kumar, 'Jinnah's tuberculosis: Could his secret have stopped partition?', *Quint*, 11 September 2019. Available at: https://www.thequint.com/news/world/could-jinnahs-well-kept-secret-have-stopped-the-partition.
4. Lapierre and Collins, *Freedom at Midnight.*
5. Madhusree Mukerjee, 'PROFILE: GURSARAN PRASAD TALWAR Pushing the Envelope for Vaccines', *Scientific American*, July 1996, pp. 39–40.
6. Author interaction with G. P. Talwar at Talwar Research Foundation, New Delhi in October 2021.
7. Gursaran P. Talwar, 'A destiny to fulfill', *Journal of Biosciences*, 2005, Vol. 30, No. 4, pp. 435–447.
8. A. V. Hill, 'A Report to the Government of India on Scientific Research in India', The Royal Society, London, 1944.
9. J. W. Bhore, et al, 'Report of the Health Survey and Development Committee Survey Vol. III', Manager of Publications, Delhi, 1946.
10. All India Institute of Medical Sciences, New Delhi, 'Introduction'. Available at: https://www.aiims.edu/aiims/ritact/aboutaiimsintro.htm.
11. Talwar, 'A destiny to fulfill'.
12. The Leprosy Mission Trust India, 'Leprosy – Social Aspects'. Available at: https://www.leprosymission.in/.
13. Act No. III of 1898. Available at: https://www.indiacode.nic.in/repealedfileopen?rfilename=A1898-3.pdf.
14. Hannah Mudge, 'India's repeal of 1898 Lepers Act is small step but giant leaps remain', The Leprosy Mission, England and Wales, 7 Jul 2016. Available at: https://www.leprosymission.org.uk/latest-news/indias-repeal-1898-lepers-act-small-step-giant-leaps-remain/.
15. Gursaran P. Talwar, 'An immunotherapeutic vaccine for multibacillary leprosy', *International Reviews of Immunology*, 1999, Vol. 18, No. 3, pp. 229–249.
16. W. M. Meyers and D. S. Walsh, D, 'Infections with specific microorganisms', in *Feigin and Cherry's Textbook of Pediatric Infectious Diseases* (Sixth Edition), Elsevier Saunders, 2009.
17. Gursaran P. Talwar, Niyaz Ahmed and Vikram Saini, 'The use of the name Mycobacterium w for the leprosy immunotherapeutic bacillus creates confusion with M. tuberculosis-W (Beijing strain): A suggestion', *Infection, Genetics and Evolution*, 2009, Vol. 8, No. 1, pp. 100–101.
18. Talwar, 'A destiny to fulfill'.
19. Jitendra K. Meena, Amit K. Malhotra, Deepak K. Mathur and Dinesh C. Mathur. 'Intralesional Immunotherapy With Mycobacterium w Vaccine in Patients With Multiple Cutaneous Warts: Uncontrolled Open Study', *JAMA Dermatology*, 2013, Vol. 149, No. 2, pp. 237–239.
20. S. Gupta, A. K. Malhotra, K. K. Verma and V. K. Sharma, 'Intralesional immunotherapy with killed *Mycobacterium* w vaccine for the treatment of ano-

genital warts: an open label pilot study', *Journal of the European Academy of Dermatology and Venereology*, 2008, Vol. 22, No. 9, pp. 1089–1093.

21. Inderpaul S. Sehgal, Ashish Bhalla, Goverdhan Dutt Puri, et al, 'Safety of an immunomodulator Mycobacterium w in Covid-19', *ASE Letters, Lung India*, 2020, Vol. 37, No. 3, pp. 279–281.
22. Gursaran P. Talwar, et al., various articles, *Contraception*, 1976, Vol. 13, pp. 129–268.
23. G. P. Talwar, Om Singh, R. Pal, N. Chatterjee, P. Sahai, K. Dhall, J. Kaur, S. K. Das, S. Suri, K. Buckshee, L. Saraya and B. N. Saxena, 'A vaccine that prevents pregnancy in women', 1994, *Proceedings of the National Academy of Sciences, U.S.A*, Vol. 91, pp. 8532–8536.
24. G. P. Talwar, Rao, Kanury V.S., Chauhan, V.S., eds., 'Recombinant and Synthetic Vaccines', Springer, 1995, Published by Zubal-Books, Since 1961, Cleveland, OH, U.S.A.
25. Madhusree Mukerjee, 'PROFILE: GURSARAN PRASAD TALWAR Pushing the Envelope for Vaccines', Scientific American, July 1996, pp. 39–40.
26. Gursaran P. Talwar, et al., various articles, *Contraception*, 1976, Vol. 13, pp. 129–268.
27. Gursuran P. Talwar, et al., 'Isoimmunization Against Human Chorionic Gonadotropin with Conjugates of Processed S-Subunit of the Hormone and Tetanus Toxoid', *Proceedings of the National Academy of Sciences, U.S.A.*, 1976, Vol. 73, pp. 218.
28. Gursuran P. Talwar, et al., 'The HSD-hCG vaccine prevents pregnancy in women, feasibility study of a reversible safe vaccine', *American Journal of Reproductive Immunology*, 1997, Vol. 37, pp. 153–160.
29. I. Kharat I, et al., 'Analysis of menstrual records of women immunized with anti-hCG vaccines inducing antibodies partially cross-reactive with hLH', *Contraception*, 1990, Vol. 41, pp. 293–299.
30. Talwar, 'A destiny to fulfill'.
31. Gursuran P. Talwar, et al., 'A unique vaccine for birth control and treatment of advanced stage cancers secreting ectopically human chorionic gonadotropin', *Exploration of Immunology*, 2021, Vol. 1, pp. 398–405. DOI: https://doi.org/10.37349/ei.2021.00026
32. Ibid.
33. A. Kaliyaperumal, V.S Chauhan, G. P. Talwar and R. Raghupathy, 'Carrier-induced epitope-specific regulation and its bypass in a protein-protein conjugate', *European Journal of Immunology*, 1995, Vol. 25, No. 12, pp. 3375–3380.
34. G. P. Talwar and Jagdish C. Gupta, 'Immuno-Interception of Human Chorionic Gonadotropin has Two Applications of Extraordinary Utility', *Perceptions in Reproductive Medicine*, 2019, Vol. 1, No. 3, p. 565.

28. RECOMBINANT BREAKTHROUGHS

1. Stuart Blume, 'Towards a history of "the vaccine innovation system" 1950–2000' in Hannaway (ed.), *Biomedicine in the Twentieth Century: Practices, Policies, and Politics*, Amsterdam: IOS Press, 2008.
2. World Health Organisation, 'Hepatitis B, Key Facts.'
3. 'Barry Blumberg,' *Economist*, 28 April 2011. Available at: https://www.economist.com/obituary/2011/04/28/barry-blumberg.
4. Baruch S. Blumberg, *Hepatitis B: The Hunt for a Killer Virus*, New Jersey: Princeton University Press, 2002.
5. Farah Huzair and Steve Sturdy, 'Biotechnology and the transformation of vaccine innovation: The case of the hepatitis B vaccines 1968–2000', *Studies in History and Philosophy of Science Part C: Studies in History and Philosophy of Biological and Biomedical Sciences*, 2017, Vol. 64, pp. 11–21. Available at: https://doi.org/10.1016/j.shpsc.2017.05.004.
6. B. S. Blumberg and H. J. Alter, 'A 'New' Antigen in Leukemia Sera', *JAMA*, 1965, Vol. 191, No. 7, pp. 541–546.
7. B. S. Blumberg, 'Australia antigen and the biology of hepatitis B', *Science*, 1977, Vol. 197, No. 4298, pp. 17–25.
8. Harvey Alter, 'Baruch Blumberg (1925–2011)', *Nature*, 2011, Vol. 473, p. 155. Available at: https://doi.org/10.1038/473155a.
9. Hepatitis B Foundation, 'History: Hepatitis B Vaccine History'. Available at: https://www.hepb.org/prevention-and-diagnosis/vaccination/history-of-hepatitis-b-vaccine/.
10. Bruce Diamond, 'Profile: Govindarajan Padmanaban', *Nature Medicine*, 2003, Vol. 9, No. 8, p. 985. Available at: https://doi.org/10.1038/nm0803-985
11. GBD 2019 Hepatitis B Collaborators, 'Global, regional, and national burden of hepatitis B, 1990–2019: A systematic analysis for the Global Burden of Disease Study 2019', *Lancet Gastroenterology & Hepatology*, 2022, Vol. 7, No. 9, pp. 796–829. Available at: https://doi.org/10.1016/S2468-1253(22)00124-8
12. P. N. Rangarajan, '100 Years of Biochemistry at the Indian Institute of Science', *Current Science*, 2020, Vol. 118, No. 3, pp. 331–332.
13. Madhura Amdekar, 'How a Hepatitis B Vaccine was Made in India', *Connect*, Office of Communications, Indian Institute of Science, 19 March 2020. Available at: https://connect.iisc.ac.in/2020/03/how-a-hepatitis-b-vaccine-was-made-in-india/.

29. SHANVAC-B – THE SHAANDAAR STORY

1. Justin Chakma, Hassan Masum, Kumar Perampaladas, et al., 'Indian vaccine innovation: the case of Shantha Biotechnics', *Global Health*, 2011 Vol. 7, p. 9. Available at: https://doi.org/10.1186/1744-8603-7-9.

2. S. E. Frew, et al., 'India's health biotech sector at a crossroads', *Nature Biotechnology*, 2007, Vol. 25, No. 4, pp. 403–417.
3. Ibid.
4. Oriol Cos, Ramón Ramón, José Luis Montesinos and Francisco Valero, 'Operational strategies, monitoring and control of heterologous protein production in the methylotrophic yeast *Pichia pastoris* under different promoters: A review', *Microbial Cell Factories*, 2006, Vol. 5, No. 1, p. 17.
5. Research Corporation Technologies, 'Pichia Protein Expression System'. Available at: https://rctech.com/technologies/pichia-protein-expression-system-successes/.
6. Porus Munshi, *Making Breakthrough Innovation Possible*, New Delhi: HarperCollins, 2009.
7. Chakma, et al., 'Indian vaccine innovation: the case of Shantha Biotechnics'.
8. Technology Development Board, Department of Science and Technology, 'Shantha Biotechnics Pvt. Ltd.' Available at: https://tdb.gov.in/ms-shantha-biotechnics-pvt-ltd-hyderabad.
9. Sachin Chaturvedi, 'Status and Development of Biotechnology in India: An Analytical Overview', Research and Information System for the Non-Aligned and Other Developing Countries Discussion Papers, RIS-DP #28, 2002.
10. Author interaction with K. I. Varaprasad Reddy in Hyderabad on 2 March 2025.
11. World Health Organisation, 'Cholera vaccines: WHO position paper – August 2017', *Weekly Epidemiological Record*, 2017, No. 34. Available at: https://iris.who.int/bitstream/handle/10665/258764/WER9234-477-498.pdf.
12. Mohammad Ali, et al., 'Updated Global Burden of Cholera in Endemic Countries', *PLoS Neglected Tropical Diseases*, 2015, Vol. 9, No. 6.
13. World Health Organisation, 'Guidelines for the production and control of inactivated oral cholera vaccines TRS 924, 2004, Annex 3', 19 November 2004. Available at: https://www.who.int/publications/m/item/annex-3-trs924-cholera-vax.
14. World Health Organisation, 'Cholera vaccines: WHO position paper – August 2017.
15. Centers for Disease Control and Prevention, 'Cholera Vaccines'. Available at: https://www.cdc.gov/cholera/prevention/cholera-vaccines.html.
16. *Business Standard*, 'Merieux takes 60% in Shantha Biotechnics', 10 November 2006. Available at: https://www.business-standard.com/article/companies/merieux-takes-60-in-shantha-biotechnics-106111001027_1.html.
17. Press Trust of India, 'Sanofi buys 80pc stake in Shantha Biotechnics for Rs 3,000', *Economic Times*, 27 July 2009. Available at: https://economictimes.indiatimes.com/industry/healthcare/biotech/pharmaceuticals/sanofi-buys-80pc-stake-in-shantha-biotechnics-for-rs-3000-cr/articleshow/4826103.cm.
18. VCCircle.com, 'Sanofi infusing $122 million to complete buy-out of Shantha

Biotech, further expansion', *Reuters*, 6 November 2013. Available at: https://www.reuters.com/article/idUSDEE9A507S/.

30. IMMUNIZED AMBITIONS

1. Amdekar, 'How a Hepatitis B Vaccine was Made in India'.
2. 'Revac-B vaccine launched', *The Hindu BusinessLine*, 24 October 1998. Available at: https://www.bharatbiotech.com/pdf/NewsUpdates/1998/Revac-B-vaccine-launched-The-Hindu-Business-Line-Oct-24-1998.pdf.
3. *Express Pharma Plus*, 'Bharat Biotech launches Hepatitis-B vaccine', 5 November 1998. Available at: https://www.bharatbiotech.com/pdf/NewsUpdates/1998/Bharat-Biotech-launches-Hepatitis-B-vaccine-Express-Pharma-Pulse-Nov-05-1998.pdf.
4. 'A major drug scandal in the making: City firm releases harmful hepatitis vaccine', *New Indian Express*, 6 August 2001. Quoted in P. M. Bhargava, Writ Petition No. 20565 of 2001 against Government of Andhra Pradesh (Order by the Andhra Pradesh High Court on 21 November 2001).
5. Latha Jishnu and Gina Singha, 'Allergic Reaction: Interview with Krishna Ella – Why Do I Need Clearance Again?', *Business World*, 17 September 2001.
6. P. M. Bhargava, Writ Petition No. 20565 of 2001 against Government of Andhra Pradesh (Order by the Andhra Pradesh High Court on 21 November 2001).
7. Ibid.
8. Ibid.
9. M.L. Kumawat & Anr. v. M/s Bharat Biotech International Ltd., Consumer Case No. 172 of 2003, National Consumer Disputes Redressal Commission, New Delhi, order dated 9 October 2019.
10. M.L. Kumawat & Anr. v. M/s Bharat Biotech International Ltd., Civil Appeal No. Diary No. 7537 of 2020, Supreme Court of India, order dated 20 November 2020.
11. Bharat Biotech, 'Recombinant Hepatitis B Vaccine IP Revac-B: Manual for Registered Medical Practitioners, Hospitals and Laboratories', Available at: https://www.bharatbiotech.com/images/revac_bpositive/Revac_B+_pres_inform.pdf.
12. Amdekar, 'How a Hepatitis B Vaccine was Made in India'.
13. Ibid.
14. Author interview with Shaukat Hussain Muhammed, former Business Editor, *Deccan Chronicle*, Hyderabad, 6 April 2025.
15. Author interview with Somasekhar Mulugu in Hyderabad on 7 April 2025.
16. Email interaction with Dr P. N. Rangarajan between 3 April 2025 and 12 April 2025.
17. Amdekar, 'How a Hepatitis B Vaccine was Made in India'.

18. 'WHO suspends procurement of hep-B vaccine from Bharat Biotech', *The Hindu BusinessLine*, 15 December 2011. Available at: https://www.thehindubusinessline.com/companies/who-suspends-procurement-of-hep-b-vaccine-from-bharat-biotech/article23063759.ece.
19. S. Bhaumik, 'Rotavirus vaccine in India faces controversy', *Canadian Medical Association Journal*, 2013, Vol. 185, No. 12, pp. E563–E564. Available at: https://doi.org/10.1503/cmaj.109-4543
20. Ibid.
21. Ministry of Health and Family Welfare, Government of India, 'National Immunization Schedule', 2018. Available at: https://nhm.gov.in/New_Updates_2018/NHM_Components/Immunization/report/National_%20Immunization_Schedule.pdf.

31. THREE RAMS, ONE REVOLUTION

1. History, Indian Institute of Science, Bengaluru. Available at: https://www.iisc.ac.in/history/.
2. E. Subramanian, Obituary: G. N. Ramachandran, *Nature Structural Biology*, 2001, Vol. 8, pp. 489–91. Available at: https://doi.org/10.1038/88525.
3. R. Singh, *India's Nobel Prize Nominators and Nominees - The Praxis of Nomination and Geographical Distribution* (Aachen, Germany: Shaker Verlag GmbH, 2016).
4. Rajinder Singh, 'G. N. Ramachandran: A Nobel Prize Nominee and Nominator', *Indian Journal of History of Science*, 2017, Vol. 52. DOI:10.16943/ijhs/2017/v52i1/41303.
5. *Sixth Five Year Plan 1980–85* (New Delhi: Planning Commission), p. 326.
6. S. Ramachandran, 'Government Funding and Support – the Department of Biotechnology', *Current Science*, 1991, Vol. 60.
7. *12th Annual Report 2023–24*, Biotechnology Industry Research Assistance Council, Ministry of Science and Technology, Government of India, 2024.
8. *Indian Bioeconomy Report 2025*, Biotechnology Industry Research Assistance Council, Department of Biotechnology, Government of India, 2025.

32. THE CONJUGATE VACCINE CLASH

1. Oswald T. Avery, Colin M. MacLeod, Maclyn McCarty, 'Studies on the Chemical Nature of the Substance Inducing Transformation of Pneumococcal Types', *The Journal of Experimental Medicine*, 1944, Vol. 79, No. 2, pp. 137–158. DOI:10.1084 jem.79.2.137.
2. O. T. Avery, 'A Further Study on the Biologic Classification of Pneumococci', *Journal of Experimental Medicine*, 1915, Vol. 22, No. 6, pp. 804–819. Available at: https://doi.org/10.1084/jem.22.6.804.
3. S. Mahadevan, 'Oswald Avery and the identification of DNA as the genetic

material', *Resonance*, 2007, Vol. 12, No. 9, pp. 4–11. DOI:10.1007/s12045-007-0089-z.

4. Horace Judson, 'No Nobel Prize for Whining', *The New York Times*, 20 October 2003.
5. D. Goldblatt, 'Conjugate vaccines', *Clinical and Experimental Immunology*, January 2000, Vol. 119, No. 1, pp. 1–3. DOI:10.1046/j.1365-2249.2000.01109.
6. Hussain Ahmad, Edward K. Chapnick, 'Conjugated Polysaccharide Vaccines', *Infectious Disease Clinics of North America*, March 1999, Vol. 13, No. 1, pp. 113–33. DOI:10.1016/s0891-5520(05)70046-5.
7. Centers for Disease Control and Prevention, 'New and Underused Vaccines, Pneumococcus' (Atlanta: CDC, July 2017).
8. B. Wahl, A. Sharan, M. D. Knoll, et al., 'National, regional, and state-level burden of *Streptococcus pneumoniae* and *Haemophilus influenzae* type b disease in children in India: Modelled estimates for 2000–15', *Lancet Global Health*, 2019, Vol. 7, No. 6, pp. E735–E747. Available at: https://doi.org/10.1016/S2214-109X(19)30081-6.
9. R. Verma, P. Khanna, 'Pneumococcal conjugate vaccine: A newer vaccine available in India', *Human Vaccines & Immunotherapeutics*, 2012, Vol. 8, No. 9, pp. 1317–1320. DOI: 10.4161/hv.20654.
10. Serum Institute of India, Press release: 'New Pneumococcal Vaccine from Serum Institute of India Achieves WHO Prequalification', 19 December 2019. Available at: https://www.seruminstitute.com/news_pneumococcal.php.
11. G. Rodgers, 'Time well spent: The complex journey of a life-saving vaccine', Bill & Melinda Gates Foundation, 22 April 2022. Available at: https://www.gatesfoundation.org/ideas/articles/creating-life-saving-pcv-vaccine-for-pneumonia-india.
12. US Patent No. 11,547,752 B2, 'Multivalent pneumococcal vaccine compositions comprising polysaccharide-protein conjugates', 10 January 2023. Available at: https://patents.google.com/patent/US11547752B2.
13. Pfizer, 'U.S. FDA Accepts for Review the Biologics License Application for Pfizer's Investigational Pentavalent Meningococcal Vaccine Candidate (MenABCWY) in Adolescents', 28 December 2022. Available at: https://www.pfizer.com/news/press-release/press-release-detail/us-fda-accepts-review-biologics-license-application-pfizers.
14. 'Multivalent meningococcal meningitis vaccine from Serum Institute of India achieves WHO prequalification', PATH, 12 July 2023. Available at: https://www.path.org/our-impact/media-center/multivalent-meningococcal-meningitis-vaccine-from-serum-institute-of-india-achieves-who-prequalification/.
15. Bill & Melinda Gates Foundation, Press Release: 'The Bill & Melinda Gates Foundation Announces Grant for the Elimination of Epidemic Meningitis in Sub-Saharan Africa', 30 May 2011.

16. Declan Butler, 'Vaccine offers meningitis hope', *Nature*, 9 November 2010, Vol. 468, No. 7321, p. 143. DOI:10.1038/468143a.
17. World Health Organisation, 'Enhanced surveillance of epidemic meningococcal meningitis in Africa: a three-year experience', *Weekly Epidemiological Record*, 16 September 2005, Vol. 80, No. 37, pp. 313–320.
18. 'GAVI must stop giving millions in subsidies to Pfizer and GSK for pneumonia vaccine', Médecins Sans Frontières (MSF), 3 December 2019. Available at: https://www.doctorswithoutborders.org/latest/gavi-must-stop-giving-millions-subsidies-pfizer-and-gsk-pneumonia-vaccine.
19. Global Health Progress, International Federation of Pharmaceutical Manufacturers & Associations, Gavi, The Vaccine Alliance, 2020. Available at: https://globalhealthprogress.org/collaboration/gavi-the-vaccine-alliance/.
20. 'Pneumococcal Vaccine is Launched in Africa, But Are Donors Getting a Fair Deal from Companies?', MSF, 23 February 2011. Available at: https://www.doctorswithoutborders.org/latest/pneumococcal-vaccine-launched-africa-are-donors-getting-fair-deal-companies.

33. DAUGHTERS OF THE TRIAL

1. R. Akhileshwari, 'Were Tribal Girls Guinea Pigs for Cervical Cancer Research', *Deccan Herald*, 10 April 2010. Available at: https://www.deccanherald.com/features/were-tribal-girls-guinea-pigs-2483519.
2. 'Fatal trials', *Frontline*, 7 May 2010. Available at: https://frontline.thehindu.com/other/article30180131.ece.
3. Ibid.
4. A. Dhar, 'HPV vaccine programme: Brinda seeks impartial enquiry', *The Hindu*, 7 April 2010. Available at: https://www.thehindu.com/news/national/HPV-vaccine-programme-Brinda-seeks-impartial-enquiry/article16364734.ece.
5. Committee appointed by the Government of India, 'Final Report of the Committee appointed by the Govt. of India, (vide notification No. V.25011/160/2010-HR dated 15 April 2010) to enquire into "Alleged irregularities in the conduct of studies using Human Papilloma Virus (HPV) vaccine" by PATH in India', 15 February 2011.
6. K. P. N. Kumar, 'Controversial vaccine studies: Why is Bill & Melinda Gates Foundation under fire from critics in India?', *Economic Times*, 31 August 2014.
7. Department-related Parliamentary Standing Committee on Health and Family Welfare, Department of Health and Family Welfare, '72nd report on alleged irregularities in the conduct of studies using Human Papilloma Virus (HPV) vaccine by PATH in India', 30 August 2013.
8. K. S. Jayaraman, 'Pressure mounting on India to explain 'irregularities' in HPV vaccine trials', *Nature India*, 11 September 2013. Available at: https://doi.org/10.1038/nindia.2013.122.

9. N. Sarojini and V. Deepa, 'Trials and tribulations: an expose of the HPV vaccine trials by the 72nd Parliamentary Standing Committee Report', *Indian Journal of Medical Ethics*, October–December 2013, Vol. 10, No. 4.
10. R. Prasad, 'A second chance for the HPV vaccine', *The Hindu*, 4 October 2017. Available at: https://www.thehindu.com/sci-tech/science/cervical-cancer-vaccination-for-delhi-and-punjab-lessons-from-andhra-and-gujarat/article19796877.ece.
11. Committed Grants, Serum Institute of India, Bill & Melinda Gates Foundation, November 2016. Available at: https://www.gatesfoundation.org/about/committed-grants/2016/11/inv-008954.

34. PHILANTHROPY, POWER AND THE GLOBAL SOUTH

1. W. Muraskin, *Revolution in International Public Health? The Origins and Development of the Bill and Melinda Gates Children's Vaccine Program (CVP) and the Global Alliance for Vaccines and Immunization (GAVI)* (Rochester, NY: University of Rochester, 2004).
2. W. Muraskin, *The Politics of International Health: The Children's Vaccine Initiative and the Struggle to Develop Vaccines for the Developing World* (Albany, NY: State University of New York Press, 1998).
3. Bernhard H. Liese, 'The World Bank's partnership with the GAVI alliance (English)', Global program review (Washington, D.C.: World Bank Group, 2014). Available at: http://documents.worldbank.org/curated/en/928871468197087690/The-World-Bank-s-partnership-with-the-GAVI-alliance.
4. H. Gavaghan, 'UN to End Children's Vaccine Initiative', *Science*, 26 March 1999, Vol. 283, No. 5410, pp. 1992–1993. DOI: 10.1126/science.283.5410.1992b.
5. Kumar, 'Controversial vaccine studies.'
6. Claude Alvares, 'The Great Gene Robbery', *The Illustrated Weekly of India*, 23 March 1986.
7. Kumar, 'Controversial vaccine studies.'
8. Department of Vaccines and Biologicals, World Health Organisation, 'Report of a meeting of international public sector vaccinology institutions', Geneva, 16–17 March 2000. Available at: https://iris.who.int/bitstream/handle/10665/66567/WHO_VB_00.30-eng.pdf.
9. J. Henriks, T. Poeloengan, I. Raw, et al., 'Developing Country Vaccine Manufacturers Network (DCVMN), 26–27 April 2001, Bandung, Indonesia', *Vaccine*, 2001, Vol. 20, No. 3–4, pp. 285–287. DOI:10.1016/s0264-410x(01)00333-4.
10. Ibid.
11. S. A. Plotkin, A. A. Mahmoud, J. Farrar, 'Establishing a Global Vaccine-

Development Fund', *The New England Journal of Medicine*, 2015, Vol. 373, No. 4, pp. 297–300. Available at: http://dx.doi.org/10.1056/NEJMp1506820.

12. C. Cookson, 'Davos launch for coalition to prevent epidemics of emerging viruses', *Financial Times*, 18 January 2017. Available at: https://www.ft.com/content/5699ac84-dd87-11e6-86ac-f253db7791c6.
13. 'IFFIm issues NOK600 million Vaccine Bonds', The International Finance Facility for Immunisation (IFFIm), 18 July 2019. Available at: https://iffim.org/press-releases/iffim-issues-nok600-million-vaccine-bonds.
14. 'CEPI partners, IVI and BBIL, launch global Chikungunya vaccine Phase II/III trial in Costa Rica', Global Chikungunya vaccine Clinical Development Program consortium, 24 August 2021.
15. CEPI, Press Release: 'Serum Institute of India joins CEPI global network to boost production of affordable outbreak vaccines', 23 January 2024. Available at: https://cepi.net/serum-institute-india-joins-cepi-global-network-boost-production-affordable-outbreak-vaccines.

35. FROM VIALS TO VOTES

1. K. A. Shaji, V. S. Kumaran and S. Karthick, 'Inter-caste marriage sparks riot in Tamil Nadu district, 148 Dalit houses torched', *The Times of India*, 9 November 2012. Available at: https://web.archive.org/web/20130127015708/http://articles.timesofindia.indiatimes.com/2012-11-09/india/35015844_1_dalit-houses-dalit-youth-dalit-boy.
2. J. Gopikrishnan, 'Health Minister gifts Rs. 3.25 cr to associate's company for a simple seed', *The Pioneer*, 21 May 2008. Available at: https://jgopikrishnan.blogspot.com/2009/03/vaccine-scam-sabotaging-vaccine.html.
3. Y. Madhavi, 'Vaccine PSUs: Chronicle of an Attenuation Willfully Caused', *Medico Friend Circle Bulletin*, June–July 2008, Vol. 329. Available at: http://www.mfcindia.org/mfcpdfs/MFC329.pdf.
4. G. C. Prasad and K. Singh, 'Govt suspends manufacturing licence of 4 drug firms', *The Economic Times*, 28 January 2008. Available at: https://economictimes.indiatimes.com/industry/healthcare/biotech/pharmaceuticals/govt-suspends-manufacturing-licence-of-4-drug-firms/articleshow/2736110.cms.
5. Justice A.M. Khanwilkar and Justice D.Y. Chandrachud, Supreme Court of India, 'S.P. Shukla & Others v. Union of India & Others', Writ Petition (Civil) No. 64 of 2009, Supreme Court Orders, 2016, Order dated 5 October 2016.
6. R. Ramachandran, 'Vaccine Worries', *Frontline*, 11 April 2008, pp. 4–27.
7. J. C. Mathew, 'Committee suggests reviving 3 vaccine units', Rediff, 12 September 2008. Available at: https://m.rediff.com/money/2008/sep/12drug1.htm.
8. Parliament of India, 'Department-related Parliamentary Standing Committee on Health and Family Welfare, Thirty-Fourth Report on the Revival of Vaccine

Public Sector Undertakings', 2008, Kasauli: Central Research Institute (CRI), Coonoor: Pasteur Institute of India (PII) and Chennai: BCG Vaccine Laboratory (BCG VL), Rajya Sabha Secretariat, New Delhi.

9. Parliament of India, 'Forty-Third Report on Action Taken by the Department of Health and Family Welfare on the Recommendations/Observations of the Committee Contained in Its Thirty-Eighth Report on Major Issues Concerning the Three Vaccine Producing PSUs', 2010, Kasauli: CRI, Coonoor: PII and Chennai: BCGVL, Rajya Sabha Secretariat, New Delhi
10. T. Thakker, 'Vaccine units: Report slams 'flawed' move', *The Indian Express*, 12 October 2010. Available at: https://indianexpress.com/article/news-archive/web/vaccine-units-report-slams-flawed-move/. *See also* Government of India, 'Rajya Sabha Unstarred Question No. 1494 on Revival of Vaccine Manufacturing Units, answered by Minister of Health and Family Welfare, Shri Ghulam Nabi Azad', Ministry of Health and Family Welfare, 23 November 2010. Available at: https://sansad.in/getFile/annex/221/Au1494.pdf?source=pqars.
11. B. Karat, 'Letter to Ghulam Nabi Azad, Minister of Health, Shastri Bhavan, New Delhi [Letter Ref No.: BK/2009/IV/119]', 12 October 2009.
12. *The Javed Chaudhary Committee Report*, 'Report on the suspension and revival of public sector vaccine manufacturing units', Ministry of Health and Family Welfare, Government of India, 2010.
13. 'Vaccine Worries', *Frontline*, 23 January 2015. Available at: https://frontline.thehindu.com/science-and-technology/vaccine-worries/article6811538.ece.
14. All India Drug Action Network (AIDAN) & Co-petitioners, Press release: 'Health groups irked by Supreme Court order on vaccine PSUs; mull fresh petition', 19 February 2018. Available at: https://aidanindia.wordpress.com/2018/02/18/health-groups-irked-by-supreme-court-order-on-vaccine-psus-mull-fresh-petition/.
15. V. Varshney, 'Get your Vaccines', *Down to Earth*, 15 July 2009. Available at: https://www.downtoearth.org.in/coverage/health/get-your-own-vaccine-3557#.
16. J. Gopikrishnan, 'Health Ministry barks, doesn't bite', *The Pioneer*, 17 May 2008. *See also* Y. Madhavi, 'Vaccine PSUs: Chronicle of an attenuation willfully caused', *Medico Friend Circle Bulletin*, June–July 2008, p. 329. Available at: https://www.mfcindia.org/mfcpdfs/MFC329.pdf.
17. Smitha T.K., '"Centre's Silence Criminal": Why TN's Billion-Dose Vaccine Facility is Idle', *The Quint*, 8 July 2021. Available at: https://www.thequint.com/coronavirus/integrated-vaccine-complex-chengalpattu-tamil-nadu-shortage-unpaid-wages-funds-crunch-india-centre-hll-bharat-biotech.
18. 'Amid vaccine shortage, this manufacturing plant in Tamil Nadu is lying idle for 9 years', *Business Today*, 28 May 2021. Available at: https://www.businesstoday.in/industry/pharma/story/amid-vaccine-shortage-this-manufacturing-plant-in-tamil-nadu-is-lying-idle-for-9-years-297223-2021-05-28.

19. Smitha T.K., '"Centre's Silence Criminal"'.
20. Krishn Kaushik, 'Modi's BJP receives millions in campaign funding from small electoral trust', Reuters, 12 April 2024. Available at: https://www.reuters.com/world/india/obscure-trust-links-indias-top-businesses-with-modis-election-war-chest-2024-03-14/.
21. Anjana Meenakshi & Project Electoral Bond, 'Covaxin maker Bharat Biotech gave Rs 25 crore to the TDP through electoral bonds', Newslaundry, 22 March 2024. Available at: https://www.newslaundry.com/2024/03/22/covaxin-maker-bharat-biotech-gave-rs-25-crore-to-the-tdp-through-electoral-bonds.
22. Election Commission of India (2024), Government of India, 'Disclosure of Electoral Bonds'. Available at: https://www.eci.gov.in/disclosure-of-electoral-bonds.

36. MONKEYS, TICKS AND NEW FRONTIERS

1. C. G. Iyer, R. L. Rao, T. H. Work, et al., 'Kyasanur Forest Disease VI. Pathological findings in three fatal human cases of Kyasanur Forest Disease', *Indian Journal of Medical Sciences*, 1959, Vol. 13, pp. 1011–1022.
2. K. Banerjee, and H. R. Bhat, 'Kyasanur Forest Disease' in A. Mishra and H. Polasa (eds.), *Virus Ecology* (New Delhi: South Asian Publishers, 1984), pp. 123–138.
3. E. Norrby, 'Yellow fever and Max Theiler: the only Nobel Prize for a virus vaccine', *Journal of Experimental Medicine*, 2007, Vol. 204, No. 12, pp. 2779–2784. Available at: https://doi.org/10.1084/jem.20072290.
4. Nithyanand Rao, 'The Seven-Decade Transnational Hunt for the Origins of the Kyasanur Forest Disease', *The Wire Science*, 19 November 2016. Available at: https://science.thewire.in/science/kyasanur-kfd-rajagopalan-boshell/.
5. K. Banerjee, C. N. Dandawate, P. N. Bhatt and T. R. Rao, 'Serological response in humans to a formolized Kyasanur Forest disease vaccine', *Indian Journal of Medical Research*, 1969, Vol. 57, No. 6, pp. 969–974.
6. G. S. Kasabi, et al., 'Coverage and effectiveness of Kyasanur forest disease (KFD) vaccine in Karnataka, South India, 2005-10', *PLoS Neglected Tropical Diseases*, 2013, Vol. 7, No. 1, p. e2025. DOI: 10.1371/journal.pntd.0002025.
7. P. D. Yadav, et al., 'Phylogeography of Kyasanur Forest Disease virus in India (1957–2017) reveals evolution and spread in the Western Ghats region', *Scientific Reports*, 2020, Vol. 10, p. 1966. DOI: 10.1038/s41598-020-58242-w.
8. Indian Council of Medical Research, 'Expression of Interest (EOI) No. VU/9/2022/ECD Dated 23.006.2023: Joint collaboration for development of vaccine against Kyasanur Forest Disease (KFD)', Department of Health Research, GoI, 2023.
9. S. B. Halstead, 'Dengue', *Lancet*, 2007, Vol. 370, No. 9599, pp. 1644–1652. DOI: 10.1016/S0140-6736(07)61687-0.

10. Sathyamangalam Swaminathan and Navin Khanna, 'Dengue vaccine development: Global and Indian scenarios', *International Journal of Infectious Diseases*, 2019, Vol. 84S, pp. S580–S586. DOI: 10.1016/j.ijid.2019.01.029.
11. World Medical Association, 'WMA Declaration of Helsinki: Ethical Principles for Medical Research Involving Human Participants', 2025. Available at: https://www.wma.net/policies-post/wma-declaration-of-helsinki/.
12. Kaushik Bharati and Hemant Jain, 'Dengue Vaccines: Current Status and Future Prospects', *Journal of Clinical and Diagnostic Research*, 2019, Vol. 13, No. 6, pp. AB01–AB03.
13. Technology Development Board, Ministry of Science and Technology, Government of India, 'Technology Development Board enters into an agreement with M/s Panacea Biotec Pvt Ltd, New Delhi', 14 November 2017. Available at: https://tdb.gov.in/wp-content/uploads/2017/11/Dengue-Press-Release-14-11-2017.pdf.
14. Takeda Inc., Press Release: 'Takeda and Biological E. Limited Collaborate to Accelerate Access to Dengue Vaccine in Endemic Areas', 26 February 2024. Available at: https://www.takeda.com/newsroom/newsreleases/2024/collaboration-to-accelerate-access-to-dengue-vaccine/.
15. 'Sun Pharma partners ICGEB to develop safer, cheaper dengue vaccine', *Economic Times*, 20 October 2016. Available at: https://economictimes.indiatimes.com/industry/healthcare/biotech/pharmaceuticals/sun-pharma-partners-icgeb-to-develop-safer-cheaper-dengue-vaccine/articleshow/54945211.cms.
16. Bharati and Jain, 'Dengue Vaccines'.
17. 'CEPI partners, IVI and BBIL, launch global Chikungunya vaccine Phase II/III trial in Costa Rica'.
18. N. Cherian, A. Bettis, A. Deol, et al., 'Strategic considerations on developing a CHIKV vaccine and ensuring equitable access for countries in need', *Nature*, 18 August 2023. Available at: https://www.nature.com/articles/s41541-023-00722-x.
19. J. Waldron, 'Merck admits defeat in race with Valneva to get first chikungunya vaccine to market', Fierce Biotech, 2 February 2023. Available at: https://www.fiercebiotech.com/deals/merck-admits-defeat-race-valneva-get-first-chikungunya-vaccine-market.
20. E. S. Pronker, T. C. Weenen, H. R. Commandeur, et al., (2011) 'The gold industry standard for risk and cost of drug and vaccine development revisited', *Vaccine*, 2011, Vol. 29, pp. 5846–5849.
21. E. S. Pronker et al., 'Risk in vaccine research and development quantified', *PLoS One*, 2013, Vol. 8, No. 3, p. e57755.
22. D. Wood, and L. Belgharbi, 'Review – 10 years of strengthening vaccines regulatory capacity', WHO Prequalification of Diagnostics, Medicines and Vaccines – 3rd Consultative Stakeholders Meeting, WHO HQ, Geneva, 4 February 2008.

23. B. Hayman and S. Pagliusi, (2020). 'Emerging vaccine manufacturers are innovating for the next decade', *Vaccine X*, Vol. 5, p. 100066. https://doi.org/10.1016/j.jvacx.2020.100066.
24. Plotkin, Mahmoud, Farrar, 'Establishing a Global Vaccine-Development Fund'.

37. EBOLA, ANTHRAX AND BIOTERRORISM

1. Sylvain Baize, Delphine Pannetier, Lisa Oestereich, et al., 'Emergence of Zaire Ebola Virus Disease in Guinea – Preliminary Report', *New England Journal of Medicine*, 16 April 2014, Vol. 371, No. 15, pp. 1418–1425. DOI:10.1056NEJMoa1404505.
2. H. Zheng, C. Yin, T. Hoang, et al., 'Ebolavirus classification based on natural vectors', *DNA and Cell Biology*, 2015, Vol. 34, No. 6, pp. 418–428. Available at: https://doi.org/10.1089/dna.2014.2678.
3. 'Statement on the Meeting of the International Health Regulations Emergency Committee Regarding the 2014 Ebola Outbreak in West Africa', World Health Organisation, 8 August 2014. Available at: https://web.archive.org/web/20140808155521/http://www.who.int/mediacentre/news/statements/2014/ebola-20140808/en/.
4. Press Release: UN senior leaders outline needs for global Ebola response', World Health Organisation, 3 September 2014. Available at: https://web.archive.org/web/20140907161412/http://www.who.int/mediacentre/news/releases/2014/ebola-response-needs/en/.
5. T. Nierle and B. Jochum, 'The failures of the international outbreak response', Médecins Sans Frontières, 29 August 2014. Available at: https://www.msf.org/ebola-failures-international-outbreak-response.
6. S. Baize, 'A single shot against Ebola and Marburg virus', *Nature Medicine*, July 2005, Vol. 11, No. 7, pp. 720–721. DOI:10.1038/nm0705-720.
7. S. M. Jones, H. Feldmann, U. Ströher, et al., 'Live attenuated recombinant vaccine protects nonhuman primates against Ebola and Marburg viruses', *Nature Medicine*, July 2005, Vol. 11, No. 7, pp. 786–790. Available at: https://doi.org/10.1038/nm1258.
8. 'Rod, Nickel, Exclusive: Canada to donate its own Ebola vaccine to WHO for use in Africa', Reuters, 12 August 2014. Available at: https://www.reuters.com/article/us-health-ebola-vaccine-canada-idUSKBN0GC1YU20140812/.
9. H. Branswell, 'Canada urged to cancel Ebola vaccine licence, transfer rights to bigger company', CTV News, 20 October 2014. Available at: https://www.ctvnews.ca/health/canada-urged-to-cancel-ebola-vaccine-licence-transfer-rights-to-bigger-company-1.2062134.
10. T. W. Geisbert, 'First Ebola virus vaccine to protect human beings?', *Lancet*, February 2017, Vol. 389, No. 10068, pp. 479–480. DOI:10.1016/S0140-6736(16)32618-6.

11. WHO, *Ebola Ring Vaccination Results*, Relief Web, 12 April 2019. Available at: https://reliefweb.int/report/democratic-republic-congo/preliminary-results-efficacy-rvsv-zebov-gp-ebola-vaccine-using-ring.
12. University of Oxford, Press Release: 'Oxford Ebola vaccine manufactured and shipped in record time by SII', 15 December 2022. Available at: https://www.ox.ac.uk/news/2022-12-15-oxford-ebola-vaccine-manufactured-and-shipped-record-time-sii.
13. D. Kumar, S. Gauthami, M. Uma, et al., 'Immunogenicity of a candidate Ebola hemorrhagic fever vaccine in mice based on controlled in vitro expression of Ebolavirus glycoprotein', *Viral Immunology*, 2018, Vol. 31, No. 7. Available at: https://doi.org/10.1089/vim.2017.0122.
14. V. Pavot, 'Ebola virus vaccines: Where do we stand?', *Clinical Immunology*, December 2016, Vol. 173, pp. 44–49. DOI:10.1016/j.clim.2016.10.016.
15. Biological Overview, India Fact Sheet, Nuclear Threat Initiative (NTI), 15 June 2015. Available at: https://www.nti.org/analysis/articles/india-biological/.
16. Federal Bureau of Investigation, 'Amerithrax or Anthrax Investigation', Famous Cases and Criminals. Available at: https://www.fbi.gov/history/famous-cases/amerithrax-or-anthrax-investigation.
17. 'Anthrax scare in Rashtrapati Bhawan', *Times of India*, 30 October 2001. Available at: http://timesofindia.indiatimes.com/articleshow/576509195.cms.
18. 'Emergent BioSolutions Announces That BioThrax (Anthrax Vaccine Adsorbed) Receives Market Authorization in India', Emergent BioSolutions, 12 February 2009. Available at: https://investors.emergentbiosolutions.com/news-releases/news-release-details/emergent-biosolutions-announces-biothrax-anthrax-vaccine.
19. S. Majumder, S. Das, V. K. Somani, et al., 'A bivalent protein r-PAbxpB comprising PA domain IV and exosporium protein BxpB confers protection against *B. anthracis* spores and toxin', *Frontiers in Immunology*, 19 March 2019, Vol. 10. Available at: https://doi.org/10.3389/fimmu.2019.00498.
20. 'New anthrax vaccine will come soon', *Times of India*, 6 November 2001. Available at: http://timesofindia.indiatimes.com/articleshow/773150062.cms.
21. A. Chawla, S. Midha, R. Bhatnagar, 'Efficacy of recombinant anthrax vaccine against *Bacillus anthracis* aerosol spore challenge: Preclinical evaluation in rabbits and Rhesus monkeys', *Biotechnology Journal*, 2009, Vol. 4, No. 3, pp. 391–399. Available at: https://doi.org/10.1002/biot.200800213.
22. 'The complex journey of a vaccine: the steps behind developing a new vaccine', International Federation of Pharmaceutical Manufacturers & Associations, 2019. Available at: https://www.ifpma.org/publications/the-complex-journey-of-a-vaccine-the-steps-behind-developing-a-new-vaccine/.
23. 'Panacea Biotec, Inc., B-400776', U.S. Government Accountability Office (US GAO), 21 January 2009. Available at: https://www.gao.gov/products/b-400776.

24. 'Bioterrorism Agents/Diseases', Emergency Preparedness and Response, Centers for Disease Control and Prevention. Available at: https://emergency.cdc.gov/agent/agentlist-category.asp.

PART-V: GLOBAL LEADERSHIP (2011–2025)

38. THE QUEST FOR CANCER VACCINES

1. 'CAR T cells: Engineering patients' immune cells to treat their cancers', National Cancer Institute, 26 February 2025. Available at: https://www.cancer.gov/about-cancer/treatment/research/car-t-cells.
2. Astha Rajvanshi, 'Alka Dwivedi: Lowering Cancer Costs', *TIME*, 2 May 2024. Available at: https://time.com/6968932/alka-dwivedi/.
3. 'Global cancer burden growing, amidst mounting need for services', World Health Organisation, 2024. Available at: https://www.who.int/news/item/01-02-2024-global-cancer-burden-growing--amidst-mounting-need-for-services.
4. 'Latest global cancer data: Cancer burden rises to 19.3 million new cases and 10.0 million cancer deaths in 2020', International Agency for Research on Cancer (IARC), 15 December 2020. Available at: https://www.iarc.who.int/news-events/latest-global-cancer-data-cancer-burden-rises-to-19-3-million-new-cases-and-10-0-million-cancer-deaths-in-2020/.
5. 'Global cancer burden growing, amidst mounting need for services. Lyon, France; Geneva, Switzerland: World Health Organisation, 2024. Available at: https://www.who.int/news/item/01-02-2024-global-cancer-burden-growing--amidst-mounting-need-for-services.
6. 'Report of National Cancer Registry Programme 2020', ICMR-National Centre for Disease Informatics and Research (NCDIR). Available at: https://ncdirindia.org/All_Reports/PBCR_Annexures/Default.aspx.
7. J. Ferlay, M. Ervik, F. Lam, et al., (2024). 'Global Cancer Observatory: Cancer Today', IACR. Available at: https://gco.iarc.who.int/today.
8. G. Humphreys, 'Alka Dwivedi: developing a cancer therapy for all', *Bulletin of the World Health Organization*, 2024, Vol. 102, No. 9, pp. 628–629. Available at: https://doi.org/10.2471/BLT.24.030924.
9. 'Department of Biotechnology supported First CAR-T cell therapy conducted at ACTREC, Tata Hospital in Mumbai', Department of Biotechnology, Ministry of Science & Technology, Government of India, 8 June 2021. Available at: https://dbtindia.gov.in/dbt-press/department-biotechnology-supported-first-car-t-cell-therapy-conducted-actrec-tata.
10. A. Dwivedi et al., 'Robust antitumor activity and low cytokine production by novel humanized anti-CD19 CAR T cells', *Molecular Cancer Therapeutics*, 2021, Vol. 20, No. 5, pp. 846–858. Available at: https://doi.org/10.1158/1535-7163.MCT-20-0476.

11. Humphreys, 'Alka Dwivedi'.
12. A. Dwivedi et al., 'Engineering off-the-shelf gamma delta CAR T cells for the treatment of acute myeloid leukemia', *Blood*, 2023, Vol. 142, No. 1, p. 4827. Available at: https://doi.org/10.1182/blood.2023000344.
13. Ibid.
14. Artkheliyan, 'First Doctor to Cure Cancer in India | Meet Dr Alka Dwivedi' [video]. YouTube, 16 March 2024. Available at: https://www.youtube.com/watch?v=pxbWqgzhl3s.
15. 'CERVAVAC Quadrivalent Human Papillomavirus (Serotype 6, 11, 16 & 18) Vaccine Recombinant', Central Drugs Standard Control Organization (CDSCO), Directorate General of Health Services, Ministry of Health & Family Welfare, Government of India, 2022. Available at: https://cdsco.gov.in/opencms/resources/UploadCDSCOWeb/2018/UploadSmPC/qHPV%20-%20SmPC%202022.pdf.
16. 'Prize Announcement: The Nobel Prize in Physiology or Medicine 2018', NobelPrize.org. Nobel Prize Outreach 2025. Available at: https://www.nobelprize.org/prizes/medicine/2018/prize-announcement/.
17. T. Carvalho, 'Personalized anti-cancer vaccine combining mRNA and immunotherapy tested in melanoma trial', *Nature Medicine*, 2023, Vol. 29, No. 10, pp. 2379–2380. Available at: https://doi.org/10.1038/d41591-023-00072-0.
18. 'World's first TIL therapy approved', *Nature Biotechnology*, 15 March 2024, Vol. 42, p. 349. Available at: https://doi.org/10.1038/s41587-024-02140-3.
19. D. Qian, J. Li, M. Huang, et al., 'Dendritic cell vaccines in breast cancer: Immune modulation and immunotherapy', *Biomedicine & Pharmacotherapy*, 2023, Vol. 162, p. 114685. Available at: https://doi.org/10.1016/j.biopha.2023.114685.
20. I. Y. Filin, K. V. Kitaeva, C. S. Rutland, et al., 'Recent advances in experimental dendritic cell vaccines for cancer', *Frontiers in Oncology*, 2021, Vol. 11. Available at: https://doi.org/10.3389/fonc.2021.730824.
21. C. Shaha, A. Suri and G. P. Talwar, 'Identification of sperm antigens that regulate fertility', *International Journal of Andrology*, 1988, Vol. 11, No. 6, pp. 479–491. DOI: 10.1111/j.1365-2605.1988.tb01022.x
22. H. Dhandapani, A. Suri, et al., 'Dendritic cells matured with recombinant human sperm associated antigen 9 (rhSPAG9) induce CD4+, CD8+ T cells and activate NK cells: a potential candidate molecule for immunotherapy in cervical cancer', *Cancer Cell International*, 2021, Vol. 21, p. 473. DOI: 10.1186/s12935-021-01951-7.
23. N. Jagadish, R. Rana, R. Selvi, et al., 'Characterization of a novel human sperm-associated antigen 9 (SPAG9) having structural homology with c-Jun N-terminal kinase-interacting protein', *Biochemical Journal*, 21 June 2005, Vol. 389, No. 1, pp. 73–82. Available at: https://doi.org/10.1042/BJ20041577.

24. M. Garg, D. Chaurasiya, R. Rana, et al., 'Sperm-associated antigen 9, a novel cancer testis antigen, is a potential target for immunotherapy in epithelial ovarian cancer', *Clinical Cancer Research*, 1 March 2007, Vol. 13, No. 5, pp. 1421–1428. DOI: 10.1158/1078-0432.CCR-06-2340.
25. Press Information Bureau, Ministry of Science & Technology, Press release: 'DBT-NII Receives Trademark for India's First Indigenous Tumour Antigen SPAG9', 4 June 2021.
26. T. V. Venkateswaran and J. Singh, 'Indian scientists testing dendritic therapy against cervix cancer', *India Science Wire*, 2017. Available at: https://vigyanprasar.gov.in/isw/cervixcancer_story.html.
27. Y. Zhang et al., 'Repurposing live attenuated trivalent MMR vaccine as cost-effective cancer immunotherapy', *Frontiers in Oncology*, 2022, Vol. 12. Available at: https://doi.org/10.3389/fonc.2022.1042250.
28. S. K. Nair et al., 'Induction of cytotoxic T cell responses and tumor immunity against unrelated tumors using telomerase reverse transcriptase RNA transfected dendritic cells', *Nature Medicine*, 2000, Vol. 6, No. 9, pp. 1011–1017. Available at: https://doi.org/10.1038/79588.
29. D. Boczkowski, S. K. Nair, D. Snyder, et al., 'Dendritic cells pulsed with RNA are potent antigen-presenting cells in vitro and in vivo', *Journal of Experimental Medicine*, 1996, Vol. 184, No. 2, pp. 465–472. DOI: 10.1084/jem.184.2.465.
30. 'From Covid-19 to HIV-1, Duke Surgical Sciences blazes the trail in vaccine immunology', Duke Surgery, Duke University School of Medicine, 2021. Available at: https://surgery.duke.edu/stories/Covid-19-hiv-1-duke-surgical-sciences-blazes-trail-vaccine-immunology.
31. Author's interaction with Purusharth I. Rajyaguru, Biochemistry Department, Indian Institute of Science, Bengaluru, 13 June 2024.
32. Author's interaction with Keerthana Thekke Veettial and N. Jayaraman, Organic Chemistry Department, Indian Institute of Science, Bengaluru, 13 June 2024.

39. AIDS VACCINES

1. G. Pandey, 'The woman who discovered India's first HIV cases', BBC, 30 August 2016. Available at: https://www.bbc.com/news/magazine-37183012.
2. D. R. Arora, V. Gautam and B. Arora, 'HIV-1 therapeutic vaccine: A ray of hope', *Indian Journal of Medical Microbiology*, 2003, Vol. 21, No. 4, pp. 225–232.
3. K. S. Jayaraman, 'India fast-tracks vaccine candidates', *Nature Medicine*, 1999, Vol. 5, p. 970.
4. T. V. Padma, 'HIV vaccine race underway in India', SciDev.Net, 22 December 2004. Available at: https://www.scidev.net/global/news/hiv-vaccine-race-underway-in-india/.
5. S. Kumar, 'Trials of AIDS vaccine to start in India', *BMJ*, 2003, Vol. 326, No.

7396, p. 952. Available at: https://doi.org/10.1136/bmj.326.7396.952/c.

6. 'IAVI and Indian government announce results of Phase I AIDS vaccine trial', International AIDS Vaccine Initiative (IAVI), 28 February 2014. Available at: https://www.iavi.org/press-release/iavi-and-indian-government-announce-results-of-phase-i-aids-vaccine-trial/.
7. V. D. Ramanathan, M. Kumar, J. Mahalingam, et al., 'A phase 1 study to evaluate the safety and immunogenicity of a recombinant HIV type 1 subtype C-modified vaccinia Ankara virus vaccine candidate in Indian volunteers', AIDS Research and Human Retroviruses, 2009, Vol. 25, No. 11. Available at: https://www.liebertpub.com/doi/abs/10.1089/aid.2009.0096.
8. Padma, 'HIV vaccine race underway in India'.
9. Ibid.
10. G. Murdur, 'Indian doctor's decision to "self test" AIDS vaccine decried as unethical', *BMJ*, 31 July 2004, Vol. 329, No. 7460, p. 252. DOI:10.1136/bmj.329.7460.252-g.
11. D. G. McNeil Jr., 'Trial vaccine made some more vulnerable to H.I.V., study confirms', *The New York Times*, 18 May 2012. Available at: https://www.nytimes.com/2012/05/18/health/research/trial-vaccine-made-some-more-vulnerable-to-hiv-study-confirms.html.
12. R. P. Sekaly, 'The failed HIV Merck vaccine study: A step back or a launching point for future vaccine development?', *Journal of Experimental Medicine*, 2008, Vol. 205, No. 1, pp. 7–12. Available at: https://doi.org/10.1084/jem.20072681.
13. H. L. Robinson, 'HIV/AIDS vaccines: 2018', *Clinical Pharmacology & Therapeutics*, 12 August 2018. Available at: https://doi.org/10.1002/cpt.1208.
14. E. P. Loret et al., 'Intradermal injection of a Tat Oyi-based therapeutic HIV vaccine reduces by 1.5 log copies/mL the HIV RNA rebound median and no HIV DNA rebound following cART interruption in a phase I/II randomized controlled clinical trial', *Retrovirology*, 2016, Vol. 13, No. 21. Available at: https://doi.org/10.1186/s12977-016-0251-3.
15. R. Desikan, R. Raja, N. M. Dixit, 'Early exposure to broadly neutralizing antibodies may trigger a dynamical switch from progressive disease to lasting control of SHIV infection', *PLOS Computational Biology*, 20 August 2020. Available at: https://doi.org/10.1371/journal.pcbi.1008064.
16. R. Murugan, 'Promising alternative to lifelong HIV treatment regime', Kernel – Indian Institute of Science Bangalore, 1 October 2020. Available at: https://kernel.iisc.ac.in/a-promising-alternative-to-lifelong-hiv-treatment-regime/.
17. 'Scientists reveal encouraging findings in first-in-human clinical trial evaluating HIV vaccine approach', IAVI, 2 December 2022. Available at: https://www.iavi.org/press-release/scientists-reveal-encouraging-findings-in-first-in-human-clinical-trial-evaluating-hiv-vaccine-approach/.
18. 'Last large HIV vaccine trial halted', European AIDS Treatment Group, 7

December 2023. Available at: https://www.eatg.org/hiv-news/last-large-hiv-vaccine-trial-halted/.

40. THE LONG ROAD TO MALARIA VACCINES

1. B. Weinraub, 'India has worst Malaria outbreak since '53, but the toll is low', *The New York Times*, 1 May 1975. Available at: https://www.nytimes.com/1975/05/01/archives/india-has-worst-malaria-outbreak-since-53-but-the-toll-is-low.html.
2. 'A Brief History of Malaria Institute of Medicine' in (US) Committee on the Economics of Antimalarial Drugs, K. J. Arrow, C. Panosian and H. Gelband (eds.), *Saving Lives, Buying Time: Economics of Malaria Drugs in an Age of Resistance*, pp. 511–521 (Washington, DC: National Academies Press, 2004).
3. R. Ross, 'On some Peculiar Pigmented Cells Found in Two Mosquitos Fed on Malarial Blood', *BMJ*, 1929, Vol. 2, No. 18 December 1897, pp. 1786–1788. DOI: 10.1136bmj.2.1929.1786.
4. M. Gardner, N. Hall, E. Fung et al., 'Genome sequence of the human Malaria parasite *Plasmodium falciparum*', *Nature*, 2002, Vol. 419, pp. 498–511. Available at: https://doi.org/10.1038/nature01097.
5. R. S. Nussenzweig, J. Vanderberg, H. Most et al., 'Protective Immunity produced by the Injection of X-irradiated Sporozoites of *Plasmodium berghei*', *Nature*, 1967, Vol. 216, pp. 160–162. Available at: https://doi.org/10.1038/216160a0.
6. S. L. Hoffman, L. M. L. Goh et al., 'Protection of humans against Malaria by immunization with radiation-attenuated *Plasmodium falciparum* sporozoites', *The Journal of Infectious Diseases*, 2002, Vol. 185, No. 8, pp. 1155–1164. Available at: https://doi.org/10.1086/339409.
7. M. B. Laurens, 'RTS,S/AS01 vaccine (Mosquirix™): an overview', *Human Vaccines & Immunotherapeutics*, 2020, Vol. 16, No. 3, pp. 480–489. doi:10.1080/21645515.2019.1669415.
8. V. S. Moorthy and J. M. Okwo-Bele, 'Final results from a pivotal phase 3 Malaria vaccine trial'. *Lancet*, 2015, Vol. 386, No. 9988, pp. 5–7. Available at: https://doi.org/10.1016/S0140-6736(15)60767-X.
9. Laurens, 'RTS,S/AS01 vaccine (Mosquirix™): an overview'.
10. Ari Daniel, 'First Malaria Vaccine Hits 1 Million Dose Milestone – Although It Has Its Shortcomings.' NPR, 13 May 2022. Available at: www.npr.org/sections/goatsandsoda/2022/05/13/1098536246/first-malaria-vaccine-hits-1-million-dose-milestone-although-it-has-its-shortcom.
11. M. S. Datoo, A. Dicko, H. Tinto et al., 'A Phase III randomised controlled trial evaluating the Malaria vaccine candidate R21/Matrix-M™ in African children', *Lancet*, 2024. Available at: https://doi.org/10.2139/ssrn.4584076.
12. N. Aderinto, G. Olatunji, E. Kokori et al., 'A perspective on Oxford's R21/

Matrix-M™ Malaria vaccine and the future of global eradication efforts', *Malaria Journal*, 2024, Vol. 23, No. 16. Available at: https://doi.org/10.1186/s12936-024-04846-w.

13. Press release: 'Serum Institute of India ships its first set of R21/Matrix-M™ Malaria Vaccine doses to Africa', Serum Institute of India, 20 May 2024. Available at: https://www.seruminstitute.com/press_release_sii_200524.ph.
14. M. R. Galinski and J. W. Barnwell, '*Plasmodium vivax*: Who cares?', *Malaria Journal*, 2008, Vol. 7, No. 1, p. S9. Available at: https://doi.org/10.1186/1475-2875-7-S1-S9.
15. F. J. Martinez, M. White, M. Guillotte-Blisnick et al., 'PvDBPII elicits multiple antibody-mediated mechanisms that reduce growth in a *Plasmodium vivax* challenge trial', *npj Vaccines*, 2024, Vol. 9, No. 10. Available at: https://doi.org/10.1038/s41541-023-00796-7.

41. mRNA: A CENTURY OF CHALLENGES

1. G. Kolata, 'Long overlooked, Kati Kariko helped shield the world from the coronavirus', *The New York Times*, 8 April 2021. Available at: https://www.nytimes.com/2021/04/08/health/coronavirus-mrna-kariko.html.
2. Nobel Prize (@nobelprize), 'From waiting for copy machines to becoming Nobel Prize laureates …', Instagram, 8 October 2023. Available at: https://www.instagram.com/nobelprize/p/CyI8_y1Oq3l/.
3. 'Best of (Nobel Prize Edition): Katalin Karikó and Drew Weissman', *What it Takes®*, Apple Podcast, 3 October 2023. Available at: https://podcasts.apple.com/in/podcast/best-of-nobel-prize-edition-katalin-karik%C3%B3-and/id1025864075?i=1000629953188.
4. P. Nair, 'QnAs with Katalin Karikó', *Proceedings of the National Academy of Sciences*, 13 December 2021, Vol. 118, No. 51, p. e2119757118. Available at: https://doi.org/10.1073/pnas.2119757118.
5. Kolata, 'Long overlooked, Kati Kariko helped shield the world from the coronavirus'.
6. K. Karikó, H. Muramatsu, F. A. Welsh et al., 'Incorporation of pseudouridine into mRNA yields superior nonimmunogenic vector with increased translational capacity and biological stability', *Molecular Therapy*, 2008, Vol. 16, pp. 1833–1840. Available at: https://doi.org/10.1038/mt.2008.200.
7. B. R. Anderson, H. Muramatsu, S. R. Nallagatla et al., 'Incorporation of pseudouridine into mRNA enhances translation by diminishing PKR activation', *Nucleic Acids Research*, 2010, Vol. 38, pp. 5884–5892.
8. K. Karikó, M. Buckstein, H. Ni, et al., 'Suppression of RNA recognition by Toll-like receptors: The impact of nucleoside modification and the evolutionary origin of RNA', *Immunity*, 2005, Vol. 23, No. 2, pp. 165–175. Available at: https://doi.org/10.1016/j.immuni.2005.06.008.

9. S. Malik, S. Kishore, S. Nag et al., 'Ebola virus disease vaccines: Development, current perspectives & challenges', *Vaccines* (Basel), 2023, Vol. 11, No. 2, p. 268. Available at: https://doi.org/10.3390/vaccines11020268.
10. E. Dolgin, 'The tangled history of mRNA vaccines', *Nature*, 2021, Vol. 597, No. 7876, pp. 318–324. Available at: https://doi.org/10.1038/d41586-021-02483-w.
11. K. Servick, 'This mysterious $2 billion biotech is revealing the secrets behind its new drugs and vaccines', *Science*, 25 March 2020. Available at: https://www.science.org/content/article/mysterious-2-billion-biotech-revealing-secrets-behind-its-new-drugs-and-vaccines.
12. 'BioNTech announces new collaboration to develop HIV and tuberculosis programs', BioNTech, 4 September 2019. Available at: https://investors.biontech.de/news-releases/news-release-details/biontech-announces-new-collaboration-develop-hiv-and.
13. Rebecca Spalding, Joshua Franklin, 'Germany's BioNTech raises $150 million in smaller-than-planned U.S. IPO amid market volatility', Reuters, 9 October 2019. Available at: https://www.reuters.com/article/world/europe/germanys-biontech-raises-150-million-in-smaller-than-planned-us-ipo-amid-mar-idUSKBN1WO29A/.
14. Dolgin, 'The tangled history of mRNA vaccines'.
15. N. Pardi, M. J. Hogan, F. W. Porter et al., 'mRNA vaccines—a new era in vaccinology', *Nature Reviews Drug Discovery*, 2018, Vol. 17, No. 4, pp. 261–279. Available at: https://doi.org/10.1038/nrd.2017.243.
16. R. Ella, S. Reddy, H. Jogdand et al., 'Safety and immunogenicity of an inactivated SARS-CoV-2 vaccine, BBV152: interim results from a double-blind, randomised, multicentre, phase 2 trial, and 3-month follow-up of a double-blind, randomised phase 1 trial', *Lancet*, 2021, Vol. 21, No. 7, pp. 950–961. Available at: https://doi.org/10.1016/S1473-3099(21)00070-0.
17. M. N. Ramasamy, A. M. Minassian, K. J. Ewer et al, 'Safety and immunogenicity of ChAdOx1 nCoV-19 vaccine administered in a prime-boost regimen in young and old adults (COV002): a single-blind, randomised, controlled, phase 2/3 trial', *Lancet*, 2020, Vol. 396, No. 10267, pp. 1979–1993. Available at: https://doi.org/10.1016/S0140-6736(20)32466-1.
18. I. Jones and P. Roy, 'Sputnik V Covid-19 vaccine candidate appears safe and effective', *Lancet*, 20 February 2021, Vol. 397, No. 10275, pp. 642–643. Available at: https://doi.org/10.1016/S0140-6736(21)00191-4.
19. V. Paradkar, 'Developing a protein subunit vaccine for Covid-19', *Vaccine Insights*, Vol. 1, No. 1, pp. 202267–70. DOI: 10.18609/cgti.2022.011.
20. P. J. Hotez, M. E. Bottazzi, 'Whole Inactivated Virus and Protein-Based Covid-19 Vaccines', *Annual Review of Medicine*, January 2022, Vol. 73, No. 1, pp. 55–64. DOI:10.1146/annurev-med-042420-113212.

21. Press release: 'Novavax and Serum Institute of India Announce First Emergency Use Authorization of Novavax Covid-19 Vaccine in Adolescents ≥12 to <18 in India', Novavax, 22 March 2022. Available at: https://ir.novavax.com/press-releases/2022-03-22-Novavax-and-Serum-Institute-of-India-Announce-First-Emergency-Use-Authorization-of-Novavax-Covid-19-Vaccine-in-Adolescents-12-to-18-in-India.
22. J. Abbasi, 'India's New Covid-19 DNA Vaccine for Adolescents and Adults Is a First', *JAMA*, 2021, Vol. 326, No. 14, p. 1365. DOI:10.1001/jama.2021.16625.
23. R. Roy, G. Das, I. A. Kuttanda et al., 'Low complexity RGG-motif sequence is required for Processing body (P-body) disassembly', *Nature Communications*, 2022, Vol. 13, No. 2077. Available at: https://doi.org/10.1038/s41467-022-29715-5.
24. Press release: 'CCMB & AIC-CCMB Leading mRNA Vaccine Technology in India', CSIR-Centre for Cellular and Molecular Biology (CCMB), 13 May 2022. Available: https://www.ccmb.res.in/presscovrg/pressnote_13_05_2022.pdf.
25. K. Mahadik, 'mRNA Vaccine: India's Next Potion in Healthcare', SciTales – CCMB, 21 February 2023. Available at: https://scitales.ccmb.res.in/mrna-vaccine-next-potion-in-healthcare/.
26. Ibid.
27. Press Trust of India, 'Indian Scientists Working on Developing New Vaccine Technology Get Grant', *The Mint*, 5 July 2021. Available at: https://www.livemint.com/science/health/indian-scientists-working-on-developing-new-vaccine-technology-get-grant-11625470727932.html.
28. Press release: 'DBT-BIRAC supported Nation's first mRNA-based vaccine found to be safe gets a nod from the Drugs Controller General of India DCG(I) to move into Phase II/III trial', Department of Biotechnology, Ministry of Science & Technology, 24 August 2021. Available at: https://dbtindia.gov.in/dbt-press/dbt-birac-supported-nation%E2%80%99s-first-mrna-based-vaccine-found-be-safe-gets-nod-drugs.
29. 'India's Biological E. to make Providence Therapeutics' mRNA Covid-19 vaccine', Reuters, 1 June 2021. Available at: https://www.reuters.com/business/healthcare-pharmaceuticals/indias-biological-e-make-providence-therapeutics-mrna-Covid-19-vaccine-2021-06-01/.
30. 'Indian manufacturer new recipient of mRNA technology through the mRNA technology transfer hub', World Health Organisation, 31 March 2022. Available at: https://www.who.int/news/item/31-03-2022-indian-manufacturer-new-recipient-of-mrna-technology-through-the-mrna-technology-transfer-hub.

42. FROM MONKEYS TO MAITRI

1. B. Bhargava, *Going Viral – Making of Covaxin: The Inside Story* (New Delhi: Rupa Publications, 2021), p. 95.

2. B. Jayakumar, 'Serum Institute claims Covid-19 vaccine to be market ready by 2022', *Business Today*, 9 March 2020. Available at: https://www.businesstoday.in/industry/pharma/story/coronavirus-serum-institute-claims-Covid-19-vaccine-to-be-market-ready-by-2022-251700-2020-03-09.
3. Press release: 'UW–Madison, FluGen, Bharat Biotech to develop CoroFlu, a coronavirus vaccine', Bharat Biotech, 2 April 2020. Available at: https://www.bharatbiotech.com/images/press/UW-Madison-FluGen-Bharat-Biotech-to-develop-CoroFlu-a-coronavirus-vaccine.pdf.
4. 'Orangutans among thousands of animals at risk of starvation in Indonesian zoos under coronavirus lockdown, officials warn', ABC News Australia, 2 May 2020. Available at: https://www.abc.net.au/news/2020-05-03/indonesia-orangutans-animals-at-risk-of-starvation-coronavirus/12209354.
5. Bhargava, *Going Viral*.
6. J. Koshy, 'ICMR to get royalty from Covaxin sale: Intellectual property governing use of vaccine jointly developed by Bharat Biotech and ICMR is "shared"', *The Hindu*, 3 May 2021. Available at: https://www.thehindu.com/news/national/icmr-to-get-royalty-from-covaxin-sale/article34474504.ece.
7. S. Mohandas, P. D. Yadav, A. Shete-Aich et al., 'Immunogenicity and protective efficacy of BBV152, whole virion inactivated SARS- CoV-2 vaccine candidates in the Syrian hamster model', *iScience*, 2021, Vol. 24, No. 2, p. 102054. DOI:10.1016/j.isci.2021.102054.
8. P. D. Yadav, R. Ella, S. Kumar, et al., 'Immunogenicity and protective efficacy of inactivated SARS-CoV-2 vaccine candidate, BBV152 in rhesus macaques', *Nature Communications*, 2021, Vol. 12, No. 1386.
9. Press release: 'India's 1st Covid-19 Vaccine – COVAXIN™, Developed by Bharat Biotech gets DCGI approval for Phase I & II Human Clinical Trials', Bharat Biotech, 29 June 2020.
10. R. Prasad, '"I Would Not Take the Vaccine without Efficacy Data": Gagandeep Kang', *The Hindu*, 8 January 2021. Available at: https://www.thehindu.com/sci-tech/health/i-would-not-take-the-vaccine-without-efficacy-data-gagandeep-kang/article33527186.ece.
11. Gagandeep Kang, 'Interview by Karan Thapar: "Why Authorise a Vaccine Without Phase 3 Efficacy?"', *The Wire*, 6 January 2021. Available at: https://science.thewire.in/health/watch-bharat-biotech-covaxin-astrazenca-covid-vaccine-gagandeep-kang/.
12. Balram Bhargava, 'Letter to Clinical Trial Participating Institutes, O.O.No. ECD/Covid-19/Misc./2020', Indian Council of Medical Research, 2 July 2020.
13. T. K. Rajalakshmi, 'Why is the ICMR in a hurry to launch a COVID-19 vaccine?', *Frontline*, 4 July 2020. Available at: https://frontline.thehindu.com/dispatches/article31986304.ece.
14. E. Roy, 'Aug 15 vaccine timeline unrealistic, says Indian Academy of Sciences', *The*

Indian Express, 6 July 2020. Available at: https://indianexpress.com/article/india/aug-15-vaccine-timeline-unrealistic-says-indian-academy-of-sciences-6491903/.

15. Press release: 'ICMR process to develop vaccine to fight Covid-19 pandemic as per globally accepted norms of fast tracking', ICMR, 4 July 2020. Available at: https://www.icmr.gov.in/pdf/press_realease_files/ICMR_Press_Release_04072020.pdf.
16. R. Ella, K. M. Vadrevu, H. Jogdand et al., 'Safety and immunogenicity of an inactivated SARS-CoV-2 vaccine, BBV152: a double-blind, randomised, phase 1 trial', *The Lancet Infectious Diseases*, 2021, Vol. 21, No. 5, pp. 637–646. Available at: https://doi.org/10.1016/S1473-3099(20)30942-7.
17. Ella, R., Reddy, S., Jogdand, H., Sarangi, V., Ganneru, B., Prasad, S., Vadrevu, K. M. (2021). Safety and immunogenicity of an inactivated SARS-CoV-2 vaccine, BBV152: Interim results from a double-blind, randomised, multicentre, phase 2 trial, and 3-month follow-up of a double-blind, randomised phase 1 trial', *The Lancet Infectious Diseases*, Vol. 21, No. 7, pp. 950–961. Available at: https://doi.org/10.1016/S1473-3099(21)00070-0.
18. Press release: 'COVAXIN™ Emergency Use Authorization Approval by DCGI-CDSCO', Bharat Biotech, 3 January 2021. Available at: https://www.bharatbiotech.com/images/press/bharat-biotech-covaxin-emergency-use-authorization-approval-by-dcgi-cdsco-moh-and-fw.pdf.
19. Jacob Koshy, 'Pfizer Withdraws Emergency Use Authorisation Application for Its Covid-19 Vaccine in India', *The Hindu*, 5 February 2021. Available at: https://www.thehindu.com/news/national/pfizer-withdraws-emergency-use-authorisation-application-for-its-Covid-19-vaccine-in-india/article33757258.ece.
20. Press release: 'COVISHIELD completes enrolment of Phase III clinical trials under partnership of ICMR and Serum Institute of India', ICMR, Department of Health Research, GoI, 12 November 2022. Available at: https://www.icmr.gov.in/pdf/press_realease_files/ICMR_Press_Release_COVISHIELD.pdf.
21. Press release: 'Prime Minister reviews status of Covid-19 and preparedness for Covid-19 vaccination', Press Information Bureau, Ministry of Health and Family Welfare, 9 January 2021. Available at: https://pib.gov.in/PressReleseDetailm.aspx?PRID=1687305.
22. S. Biswas, 'Covaxin: What was the rush to approve India's homegrown vaccine?', *BBC News*, 5 January 2021. Available at: https://www.bbc.com/news/world-asia-india-55534902.
23. Shankhyaneel Sarkar (ed.), 'Vaccines 100% safe, rumours of impotency is "absolute rubbish": Somani', *Hindustan Times*, 5 January 2021. Available at: https://www.hindustantimes.com/health/vaccines-100-safe-rumours-of-impotency-is-absolute-rubbish-somani/story-gxScyjopSoc6ZuRT2c9rWN.html.
24. R. Ella et al., 'Efficacy, safety, and lot to lot immunogenicity of an inactivated SARS-CoV-2 vaccine (BBV152): a double-blind, randomised, controlled phase

3 trial'. *medRxiv* preprint, 2021. Available at: https://doi.org/10.1101/2021.06.30.21259439.

25. B. S. Graham, 'Rapid Covid-19 vaccine development', *Science*, 2020, Vol. 368, pp. 945–946.
26. C. A. Rostad, E. J. Anderson, 'Optimism and caution for an inactivated Covid-19 vaccine', *Lancet Infectious Diseases*, 2021, Vol. 21, No. 5, pp. 581–582. Available at: https://doi.org/10.1016/S1473-3099(20)30988-9.
27. Press release: 'Bharat Biotech Concludes Final Analysis for COVAXIN® Efficacy from Phase 3 Clinical Trials', Bharat Biotech, 3 July 2021. Available at: https://www.bharatbiotech.com/images/press/barat-biotech-bbv152-covaxin-phase3-final-analysis-03July2021.pdf.
28. 'World Health Organisation. India Marks One Year of Covid Vaccination', World Health Organisation, 17 January 2022. Available at: https://www.who.int/india/news/feature-stories/detail/india-marks-one-year-of-covid-vaccination.
29. 'WHO Director-General's opening remarks at 148th session of the Executive Board', World Health Organisation, 18 January 2021. Available at: https://www.who.int/director-general/speeches/detail/who-director-general-s-opening-remarks-at-148th-session-of-the-executive-board.
30. Ibid.
31. 'Covid-19 Updates, Vaccine Supply', Ministry of External Affairs, Government of India, 15 June 2023. Available at: https://www.mea.gov.in/vaccine-supply.htm.

43. PATENTS, POWER AND A DIVIDED WORLD

1. 'CBI arrests Biocon executive, four others in bribery case', *The New Indian Express*, 23 June 2022.
2. Central Bureau of Investigation v. S. Eswara Reddy & Ors., W.P. (Crl) 1409/2022, decided on 4 July 2022 by Justice Anu Malhotra.
3. Ibid.
4. V. Krishnan and A. John, 'The massive failures of India's drug regulatory system', Pulitzer Center, 12 March 2025. Available at: https://pulitzercenter.org/stories/massive-failures-indias-drug-regulatory-system. *See also* V. Krishnan, 'Panel exposes flaws in India's drug approval procedure', Livemint, 8 May 2012. Available at: https://www.livemint.com/Politics/N1ChhXsgrSB4qp8nJXxeAI/Panel-exposes-flaws-in-India8217s-drug-approval-procedure.html.
5. 'Rule 101, CLINICAL TRIALS RULES, 2019, GSR 227(E)', Central Drugs Standard Control Organisation, Ministry of Health and Family Welfare, Government of India, 19 March 2019.
6. Press release: 'FDA approves first Covid-19 vaccine: Approval signifies key achievement for public health', U.S. Food & Drug Administration, 23 August 2021. Available at: https://www.fda.gov/news-events/press-announcements/fda-

approves-first-Covid-19-vaccine.

7. S. Das, 'Pfizer compiling data to answer DCGI queries on coronavirus vaccine', *Business Standard,* 12 January 2021. Available at: https://www.business-standard.com/article/companies/pfizer-compiling-data-to-answer-dcgi-queries-on-coronavirus-vaccine-121011200085_1.html.
8. Ibid.
9. P. Raghavan, 'Expert panel turns down emergency use plea for Pfizer's shot', *The Indian Express,* 6 February 2021. Available at: https://indianexpress.com/article/india/pfizer-withdraws-emergency-use-authorisation-application-in-india-7175600/.
10. 'Pfizer's lack of 'safety data' results in withdrawal of emergency use of its COVID vaccine in India', ABP News Bureau, 5 February 2021. Available at: https://news.abplive.com/news/india/pfizer-s-lack-of-safety-data-results-in-withdrawal-of-emergency-use-of-its-covid-vaccine-in-india-1442724.
11. K. Kelland, 'Report - Rich nations stockpiling a billion more COVID-19 shots than needed', Reuters, 19 February 2021. Available at: https://www.reuters.com/business/healthcare-pharmaceuticals/rich-nations-stockpiling-billion-more-covid-19-shots-than-needed-report-2021-02-19/
12. 'Shot of a lifetime: How two Pfizer manufacturing plants upscaled to produce the COVID-19 vaccine in record time', Pfizer. Available at: https://www.pfizer.com/news/articles/shot_of_a_lifetime_how_two_pfizer_manufacturing_plants_upscaled_to_produce_the_covid_19_vaccine_in_record_time.
13. K. Katella, 'Omicron, Delta, Alpha, and More: What To Know About the Coronavirus Variants', Yale Medicine, 1 September 2023. Available at: https://www.yalemedicine.org/news/Covid-19-variants-of-concern-omicron.
14. Neha Arora and Krishna N. Das, 'Exclusive: Pfizer wants to make vaccine in India if faster clearance, export freedom assured – sources', Reuters, 10 March 2021. Available at: https://www.reuters.com/article/health-coronavirus-india-pfizer/exclusive-pfizer-wants-to-make-vaccine-in-india-if-faster-clearance-export-freedom-assured-sources-idUSKBN2B21AN. *See also* Krishna N. Das, 'J&J in talks to bring COVID-19 vaccine to India with Biological E – source', Reuters, 10 February 2021. Available at: https://www.reuters.com/business/healthcare-pharmaceuticals/jj-talks-bring-covid-19-vaccine-india-with-biological-e-source-2021-02-09.
15. R. Roy, 'Madras High Court issues notice to SII, DCGI, ICMR on plea by volunteer alleging side effects after "COVISHIELD" trial', LiveLaw, 19 February 2021. Available at: https://www.livelaw.in/news-updates/madras-high-court-notice-sii-dcgi-icmr-volunteer-alleging-side-effects-covishield-trial-170095.
16. K. R. Antony, 'The secrecy around deaths after vaccination', *The Hindu,* 15 April 2021. Available at: https://www.thehindu.com/opinion/op-ed/the-secrecy-around-deaths-after-vaccination/article34320223.ece.

17. 'Indemnity demand holding up Pfizer jab's India approval', *The Economic Times*, 17 May 2020. Available at: https://economictimes.indiatimes.com/industry/healthcare/biotech/pharmaceuticals/indemnity-demand-holding-up-pfizer-jabs-india-approval/articleshow/82422985.cms.
18. K. Venkataramanan, 'What is indemnity, and how will it affect Covid-19 vaccine pricing and availability in India?', *The Hindu*, 6 June 2021. Available at: https://www.thehindu.com/sci-tech/health/explained-what-is-indemnity-and-how-will-it-affect-Covid-19-vaccine-pricing-and-availability-in-india/article60678840.ece.
19. Quad, 'Joint Leaders' Statement', The White House, 24 May 2022. Available at: https://www.whitehouse.gov/briefing-room/statements-releases/2022/05/24/quad-joint-leaders-statement/.
20. 'Still discussing indemnity issue with Pfizer, Moderna, Johnson: Health Ministry', Livemint, 23 July 2021. Available at: https://www.livemint.com/news/still-discussing-indemnity-issue-with-pfizer-moderna-johnson-health-ministry-11627055447165.html. *See also* Sahil Pandey, 'Johnson and Johnson still in discussion with Centre over indemnity issue: Sources', ANI, 2 August 2021. Available at: https://www.aninews.in/news/national/general-news/johnson-and-johnson-still-in-discussion-with-centre-over-indemnity-issue-sources20210802192355/.
21. Press Information Bureau, 'Centre fast tracks Emergency Approvals for foreign produced Covid-19 Vaccines', Ministry of Health and Family Welfare, 13 April 2021. Available at: https://pib.gov.in/PressReleasePage.aspx?PRID=1711381.
22. K. Das, 'India's Biological E. to produce J&J Covid-19 vaccine', Reuters, 18 May 2021. Available at: https://www.reuters.com/business/healthcare-pharmaceuticals/indias-biological-e-make-jj-vaccine-alongside-own-shot-managing-director-says-2021-05-18/.
23. 'India's Biological E., U.S. body finalise $50 mln COVID-19 shot financing deal', Reuters, 25 October 2021. Available at: https://www.reuters.com/business/healthcare-pharmaceuticals/indias-biological-e-us-body-finalise-50-mln-covid-19-shot-financing-deal-2021-10-25/.
24. 'Deadlock on Indemnity Clause Keeps US Vaccines From Indian Market', The Wire Science, 11 November 2021. Available at: https://science.thewire.in/health/deadlock-indemnity-clause-preventing-us-vaccines-indian-market/.
25. Suhasini Haidar, 'A year on, Quad initiative for 1 billion India-made vaccines runs into rough weather', *The Hindu*, 15 May 2022. Available at: www.thehindu.com/news/national/a-year-on-quad-vaccine-initiative-for-1-billion-indian-made-vaccines-runs-into-rough-weather/article65414436.ece.
26. S. Nagar and S. Imparato, 'The Disappointment of the Quad Vaccine Partnership', *The Diplomat*, 1 July 2022. Available at: https://thediplomat.com/2022/07/the-disappointment-of-the-quad-vaccine-partnership/.
27. Transparency International Global Health, 'Lack of transparency over vaccine

trials, secretive contracts and "science by press release" risk success of global Covid-19 response', 25 May 2021. Available at: https://www.transparency.org/en/press/covid-19-vaccines-lack-of-transparency-trials-secretive-contracts-science-by-press-release-risk-success-of-global-response.

28. 'Waiver from Certain Provisions of the TRIPS Agreement for the Prevention, Containment and Treatment of Covid-19', Communication from India and South Africa, 2 October 2020, IP/C/W/669, World Trade Organisation.
29. S. Vijayakumar and D. Rajagopal, 'Natco's compulsory licence for selling generic copies of Bayer's cancer drug Nexavar upheld by IPAB', *The Economic Times*, 5 March 2013. Available at: https://economictimes.indiatimes.com/industry/healthcare/biotech/pharmaceuticals/ipab-upholds-compulsory-licence-issued-to-natco-for-cancer-drug-nexavar/articleshow/18784178.cms.
30. L. Ford, 'WTO fails to reach agreement on providing global access to Covid treatments', *The Guardian*, 14 February 2024. Available at: https://www.theguardian.com/global-development/2024/feb/14/wto-fails-to-reach-agreement-on-providing-global-access-to-covid-treatments.
31. 'U.S. Chamber opposes WTO waiver of vaccine intellectual property rights', Reuters, 2 March 2021. Available at: https://www.reuters.com/article/business/us-chamber-opposes-wto-waiver-of-vaccine-intellectual-property-rights-idUSKBN2AU241. *See also* 'Industry lobbyists work to influence U.S. position in critical global health negotiations', Public Citizen, 28 October 2024. Available at: https://www.citizen.org/wp-content/uploads/Lobbyists-Work-to-Influence-U.S.-Position-in-Critical-Global-Health-Negotiations-10.28.24.pdf.
32. 'Ministerial decision on the TRIPS Agreement adopted on 17 June 2022', Ministerial Conference: Twelfth Session, WTO, Geneva, 12–15 June 2022, pp. 1–2.

INDEX